Neuroimaging

Neuroimaging
A Window to the Neurological Foundations of Learning and Behavior in Children

edited by

G. Reid Lyon, Ph.D.
Human Learning and Behavior Branch
National Institute of Child Health
and Human Development

and

Judith M. Rumsey, Ph.D.
Child Psychiatry Branch
National Institute of Mental Health
and
Child Development Center
—— Georgetown University Medical Center ——

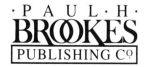

·P·A·U·L·H·
BROOKES
PUBLISHING CO

Baltimore · London · Toronto · Sydney

RJ
492
.N48
1996

Paul H. Brookes Publishing Co.
Post Office Box 10624
Baltimore, Maryland 21285-0624

Copyright © 1996 by Paul H. Brookes Publishing Co., Inc.
All rights reserved.

This work may be reproduced in whole or in part for the official use of the U.S. Government or any authorized agency thereof.

The following chapters were written by government employees within the scope of their official duties and, as such, shall remain in the public domain: Chapters 1, 2, 3, 5, 6, 9, and 11.

Typeset by Wilsted & Taylor Publishing Services, Oakland, California.
Manufactured in the United States of America by
The Maple Press Co., York, Pennsylvania.

Library of Congress Cataloging-in-Publication Data

Neuroimaging : a window to the neurological foundations of learning and behavior in
    children / edited by G. Reid Lyon, Judith M. Rumsey.
        p.   cm.
    Includes bibliographical references and index.
    ISBN 1-55766-256-8
    1. Brain—Imaging.   2. Pediatric neurology—Diagnosis.   3. Pediatric diagnostic
imaging.   I. Lyon, G. Reid, 1949– .   II. Rumsey, Judith M.
        [DNLM: 1. Brain Diseases—in infancy & childhood.   2. Brain Diseases—diagnosis.
    3. Diagnostic Imaging—in infancy & childhood.   4. Developmental Disabilities—
diagnosis.   5. Learning Disorders—diagnosis.   WS 340 N4923 1996]
    RJ492.N48   1996
    618.92'804754—dc20
    DNLM/DLC
    for Library of Congress   96-22543
                                                                                      CIP

British Library Cataloguing-in-Publication data are available from the British Library.

34724605

To Dr. Gary Adamson—the father who I never had—who along the way taught me the need to learn the science to maximum depth but never to lose sight of the bigger picture. I only hope I can emulate his courage, character, and strength in making that long journey back.

—G. Reid Lyon

To my daughter, Cynthia Rumsey

—Judith M. Rumsey

Contents

List of
___ Tables and Figures ___

About the Editors

G. Reid Lyon, Ph.D., Psychologist, Human Learning and Behavior Branch, National Institute of Child Health and Human Development, National Institutes of Health, 6100 Executive Building, Room 4B05, 9000 Rockville Pike, Bethesda, Maryland 20892. Dr. Lyon directs and manages the National Institute of Child Health and Human Development research programs in learning disabilities, dyslexia, language disorders, and disorders of attention in children.

Judith M. Rumsey, Ph.D., Psychologist, Child Psychiatry Branch, National Institute of Mental Health, National Institutes of Health, Building 10, Room 6N240, Bethesda, Maryland 20892, and Child Development Center, Georgetown University Medical Center, 3307 M Street, NW, Washington, D.C. 20007. Dr. Rumsey is a research psychologist at the National Institute of Mental Health and a clinical associate professor of pediatrics at Georgetown University Medical Center. Her research interests include the neuropsychology, clinical follow-up, and neuroimaging of developmental disorders, in particular, dyslexia and autism.

_ About the Contributors _

Richard A. Bronen, M.D., Associate Professor, Departments of Diagnostic Radiology and Surgery, Yale University School of Medicine, 333 Cedar Street, New Haven, Connecticut 06510. Dr. Bronen's research interests include relating functional magnetic resonance imaging findings to underlying brain anatomy and investigating cerebral disorders using anatomical magnetic resonance imaging.

Pim Brouwers, Ph.D., Head, Neuropsychology Group, Pediatric Branch, National Cancer Institute, 9000 Rockville Pike, Building 10, Room 13N240, Bethesda, Maryland 20892. Dr. Brouwers' research interests are in the neurobehavioral consequences of chronic medical illness, such as cancer and human immunodeficiency virus type-1 disease, and in treatment thereof in children and adults.

Lucy A. Civitello, M.D., Assistant Professor, Departments of Neurology and Pediatrics, George Washington University; and Attending Pediatric Neurologist, Children's National Medical Center, 111 Michigan Avenue, NW, Washington, D.C. 20010. Dr. Civitello is a consulting neurologist for the Pediatric Branch of the National Cancer Institute, National Institutes of Health. Her research interests include evaluating the neurological sequelae of human immunodeficiency virus infection in children.

R. Todd Constable, Ph.D., Physicist, Department of Diagnostic Radiology, Yale University School of Medicine, 333 Cedar Street, New Haven, Connecticut 06510. Dr. Constable works on developing magnetic resonance imaging and analysis techniques to optimize functional magnetic resonance imaging studies.

Charles DeCarli, M.D., Senior Clinical Investigator, Epilepsy Research Branch, National Institute of Neurological Disorders and Stroke, National Institutes of Health, Building 10, Room 5C205, 9000 Rockville Pike, Bethesda, Maryland, 20892. Dr. DeCarli is a neurologist with special interests in neuroimaging and the study of dementia.

Martha Bridge Denckla, M.D., Kennedy Krieger Institute, Suite 501, 707 North Broadway, Baltimore, Maryland 21205. Dr. Denckla is Professor of Neurology and Pediatrics at the Johns Hopkins University School of Medicine and Director of the Department of Developmental Cognitive Neurology at the Kennedy Krieger Institute. Dr. Denckla is also Principal Investigator and Director of a National Institute of Child Health and Human Development learning disabilities research center, National Institutes of Health.

Monique Ernst, M.D., Ph.D., Senior Staff Fellow at the National Institute on Drug Abuse, National Institutes of Health, Brain Imaging Section, Post Office Box 5180, Baltimore, Maryland 21224. Dr. Ernst's research interests lie in the identification of neural substrates underlying neuropsychiatric disorders and vulnerabilities to substance abuse by using positron emission tomography.

Jack M. Fletcher, Ph.D., Psychologist and Professor, Department of Pediatrics, MSB 3.136, The University of Texas Medical School at Houston, 6431 Fannin, Houston, Texas 77030. Dr. Fletcher's research has focused on the classification of reading disabilities and on the development of children with different types of brain injuries.

Robert K. Fulbright, M.D., Assistant Professor of Neuroradiology, Yale University School of Medicine, 333 Cedar Street, New Haven, Connecticut 06510. Dr. Fulbright is Co-Director of Clinical Neuro-MR Imaging. His research includes functional magnetic resonance imaging of language, memory, motor-sensory, auditory processing, and chemical senses and magnetic resonance imaging of epilepsy.

William D. Gaillard, M.D., Assistant Professor of Pediatrics and Neurology, Department of Neurology, The Children's National Medical Center of George Washington University, 111 Michigan Avenue, NW, Washington, D.C. 20010. Dr. Gaillard's research interests are in the functional neuroimaging of children with epilepsy, and a major portion of this research is conducted as a guest researcher at the Epilepsy Research Branch, National Institute of Neurological Disorders and Stroke, National Institutes of Health.

John C. Gore, Ph.D., Professor of Diagnostic Radiology and Applied Physics and Director of NMR Research, Department of Diagnostic Radiology, Yale University School of Medicine, Post Office Box 208042, New Haven, Connecticut 06510. Dr. Gore's research is concerned with the development of magnetic resonance imaging techniques and applications with special emphasis on functional brain imaging. Recent studies have involved the use of functional magnetic resonance imaging to study language, memory, auditory and visual processing, and sensory motor processes.

Barry Horwitz, Ph.D., Laboratory of Neurosciences, National Institute on Aging, National Institutes of Health, Building 10, Room 6C414, Bethesda, Maryland 20892. Dr. Horwitz is Chief of Unit on Brain Imaging and Computers. His research has focused on using computational techniques applied to functional neuroimaging data to determine how different brain regions interact with one another during cognition.

Judy Howard, M.D., Department of Pediatrics, University of California–Los Angeles Medical Center, Room 23-10, 1000 Veterans Avenue, Los Angeles, California 90095. Dr. Howard is Professor of Clinical Pediatrics and is engaged in research investigating the effects of prenatal drug exposure on cognitive and behavioral outcomes.

Leonard Katz, Ph.D., Professor, Department of Psychology, University of Connecticut, Storrs, Connecticut 06269. Dr. Katz is a senior investigator at Haskins Laboratories, New Haven, Connecticut. His research focuses on spoken and printed word recognition in several languages.

Jack Krasuski, M.D., Senior Staff Fellow, Laboratory of Neurosciences, National Institute on Aging, National Institutes of Health, Building 10, Room 6C414, 9000 Rockville Pike, Bethesda, Maryland 20892. Dr. Krasuski's research interests include applications of anatomical and functional neuroimaging modalities in the study of neuropsychiatric disorders.

Cheryl Lacadie, B.S., Research Support Specialist, Department of Diagnostic Radiology, Yale University School of Medicine, Fitkin Basement, New Haven, Connecticut 06510. Mrs. Lacadie's research activities include functional magnetic resonance imaging of neurological disorders, including dyslexia, autism, and Tourette syndrome, and specific tasks, including motor functions, olfactory perception, and attention.

Alvin M. Liberman, Ph.D., Professor Emeritus of Psychology, University of Connecticut, and of Linguistics, Yale University; and Research Associate, Haskins Laboratories, 270 Crown Street, New Haven, Connecticut 06511. Dr. Liberman's research is concerned most broadly with the place of speech in the biological scheme of things and, more narrowly, with the relation between the sounds of speech and the phonological message they convey.

Karen E. Marchione, R.N., M.A., Coordinator, Center for the Study of Learning and Attention, Department of Pediatrics, Yale University School of Medicine, LMP 4093, Post Office Box 208064, New Haven, Connecticut 06510. Ms. Marchione's research interests in educational psychology include attention deficit disorder and reading disability in children.

Kenneth R. Pugh, Ph.D., Research Scientist, Department of Pediatrics (Neurology), Yale University School of Medicine, Post Office Box 208064, New Haven, Connecticut 06510; and Research Scientist, Haskins Laboratories, New Haven, Connecticut. Dr. Pugh's research interests include psycholinguistics/neurolinguistics (with a primary emphasis on reading development and reading disability), attention, and memory. Recent work has focused on using neuroimaging techniques (particularly functional magnetic resonance imaging) to relate cognitive performance with functional brain organization.

Allan L. Reiss, M.D., Behavioral Genetics and Neuroimaging Research Center, Kennedy Krieger Institute, Johns Hopkins University School of Medicine, 707 North Broadway, Baltimore, Maryland, 21205. Dr. Reiss directs the Behavioral Genetics and Neuroimaging Research Center and is Vice President of Psychiatry and Behavioral Neurosciences at the Kennedy Krieger Institute. He is also an associate professor of psychiatry and pediatrics at the Johns Hopkins University School of Medicine. In addition to his interests in the genetic and neurological bases of children's developmental disorders, Dr. Reiss is developing advanced software modules for the quantitative analysis of neuroimaging data.

Donald P. Shankweiler, Ph.D., Haskins Laboratories, 270 Crown Street, New Haven, Connecticut 06511. Dr. Shankweiler is a professor of psychology at the University of Connecticut and a member of the research staff of Haskins Laboratories. His research is concerned with the origin and interpretation of reading difficulties and with the basis of language disorders in aphasia. Much of his recent work concerns the role of working memory in sentence understanding and its disorders.

Bennett A. Shaywitz, M.D., Professor of Pediatrics and Neurology and Chief of Pediatric Neurology, Department of Pediatrics, Yale University School of Medicine, 333 Cedar Street, New Haven, Connecticut 06510. Dr. Shaywitz's primary and long-standing research has focused on the neurobiological influences in learning and attention disorders. His most recent area of investigation involves the nosology and classification of learning and attention disorders. Most recently, Dr. Shaywitz has been named Co-Director of the Yale Center for the Study of Learning and Attention Disorders, one of three federally funded centers for the study of learning and attention disorders. He has served on advisory boards of the National Institute of Child Health and Human Development and the National Institute of Neurological and Communicative Disorders and Stroke, National Institutes of Health, and the National Academy of Sciences and on the editorial board of *Pediatric Neurology*. He currently serves on the professional advisory boards of the National Center for Children with Learning Disabilities and the Reye Syndrome Foundation.

Sally E. Shaywitz, M.D., Director, Learning Disorders Unit, and Professor, Department of Pediatrics, Yale University School of Medicine, 333 Cedar Street, New Haven, Connecticut 06510. Dr. Shaywitz is particularly interested in utilizing epidemiological and biological strategies to elucidate more clearly the nature of learning and attention disorders. She has addressed issues relating to gender; measurement; and conceptual models for, and the emergence of, learning and attention disorders over time. Co-Author of the *Report to Congress on Learning* and Co-Director of the Yale Center for the Study of Learning and Attention Disorders, Dr. Shaywitz currently serves on the professional advisory board of the National Center for Learning Disabilities, on the editorial board of the *Journal of Learning Disabilities*, and as Editorial Consultant to the National Institute of Child Health and Human Development, National Institutes of Health, and the Department of Education.

Pawel Skudlarski, Ph.D., Physicist, Yale University School of Medicine, NMR Research, 333 Cedar Street, New Haven, Connecticut 06510. Dr. Skudlarski is working on the development of methods for the data analysis and experimental design in the functional magnetic resonance imaging of the human brain.

Rachelle Tyler, M.D., Developmental Studies Program, Department of Pediatrics, University of California–Los Angeles Medical Center, Room 23-10, 1000 Veterans Avenue, Los Angeles, California 90024. Dr. Tyler is a clinical instructor in the Department of Pediatrics and is pursuing research on the effects of prenatal exposure on cognitive and developmental outcomes in children.

Preface

Since the mid-1980s, there has been an explosion of activity within the neurosciences. Much of this activity has centered on the development of neuroimaging methods that have provided unprecedented views of the anatomical structures of the human brain and of how specific brain structures and neural networks function as behavior is produced. Although many of the technical advances associated with neuroimaging have been addressed in the basic scientific literature, particularly from 1991 on, little information about the clinical applications of different neuroimaging modalities has been published. This disparity is seen, in particular, in the area of children's developmental disorders.

With this volume, Dr. Judith M. Rumsey and I have sought to bring together some of the most talented neuroscientists working in the area of children's brain disorders and diseases to begin to identify, through the lens of neuroimaging technology, links between variations in behavior and associated variations in the developing brains of youngsters. Within this context, we encountered several challenges. First, which brain-related disorders should we address in the book? Second, how much emphasis should we give to anatomical neuroimaging methods and how much to functional neuroimaging methods? Third, and most important, how should we present the information? With respect to the developmental disorders of interest and to the relative emphasis on the different types of neuroimaging methodologies, we simply let the data show the way. We found that some of the most methodologically and clinically advanced neuroimaging studies were being conducted in the areas of dyslexia, attention-deficit/hyperactivity disorder, autism, epilepsy, pediatric acquired immunodeficiency syndrome, fragile X syndrome, Turner syndrome, and neurofibromatosis-1. The fact that these particular disorders also affect significant numbers of children motivated us to attempt to provide the information in a clear manner that would be accessible and interesting to both basic and clinical scientists.

The chapters in this book, therefore, reflect the substantial thought and effort involved in presenting highly technical information as clinically useful prose without, we hope, detracting from the integrity of the science in which we engage each day. It is our hope that the manner in which the information is presented will interest those professionals who are not directly involved in the neurosciences, but who, as physicians, psychologists, speech-language pathologists, educators, and occupational and physical therapists, are active in helping all children achieve their fullest potentials. It is also our hope that this book provides the neuroscientific community with a useful summary of where we have been and a vision of where we can go.

G. Reid Lyon, Ph.D.
Bethesda, Maryland

_____ Acknowledgments _____

The editors wish to thank Brian Donohue, B.A., and Guinevere Eden, Ph.D., for their helpful reviews of some of the chapters. Duane Alexander, M.D., Director of the National Institute of Child Health and Human Development, deserves a special note of thanks for his courageous leadership in ensuring that neurobehavioral research becomes a priority in the study of children. Finally, the editors are deeply grateful for the guidance and support provided by the professionals at the Paul H. Brookes Publishing Co. Melissa Behm continues to push the envelope, and her decision to provide the readership with a book devoted to neuroimaging is a gutsy one. Theresa Donnelly worked tirelessly on this project, and her perspectives, perseverance, strength, and wisdom are greatly appreciated and admired. Special acknowledgments go to Melissa Furrer, whose deft editing was truly a gift from above.

About the Cover

On the cover are the [^{18}F]fluorodeoxyglucose and ^{15}O-water positron emission tomography images of a 9-year-old girl with Rasmussen syndrome and epilepsia partialis continua of approximately 9 months duration. Shown is a striking reduction in glucose metabolism over the right hemisphere without a concomitant reduction in cerebral blood flow.

Images courtesy of Charles DeCarli, M.D., Senior Clinical Investigator, Epilepsy Research Branch, National Institute of Neurological Diseases and Stroke, National Institutes of Health, Bethesda, Maryland.

Neuroimaging

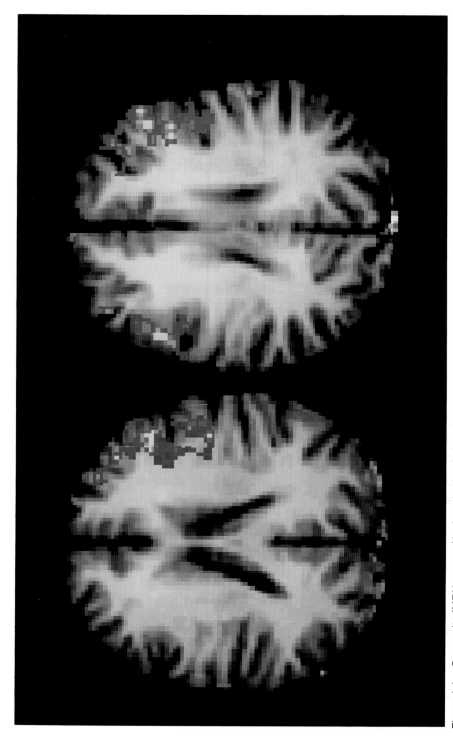

Figure 4.4. Composite fMRI images of brain activation during phonological processing in 19 men (left) and 19 women (right). Activations are shown on an axial section 20 mm above and parallel to the intercommissural line and are oriented as if viewed from below so that the left side of the brain is on the right side of the image. During phonological processing, men activate primarily the left IFG; in contrast women activate both the left and right IFG. However, both men and women perform the phonological task equally well.

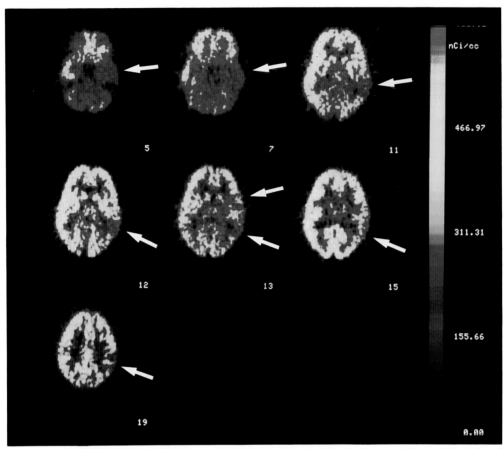

Figure 8.2. FDG PET (right brain is shown on the right) showing extensive right temporal (arrows), frontal, and parietal hypometabolism in a 9-year-old girl with a right temporal lobe seizure focus. Results of MRI studies were normal. Color scale reflects glucose utilization: red, high consumption; blue, low consumption.

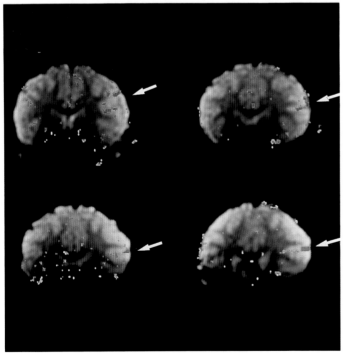

Figure 8.3. fMRI (right brain is shown on the left) study of a 10-year-old right-handed boy with cystic right temporal lobe dysplasia, right temporal lobe ictal focus, and left hemispheric language dominance. Images are serial coronal images of frontal lobe; orange and yellow pixels are areas activated during a word generation task. Broca's area is identified in the inferior frontal gyrus (arrows).

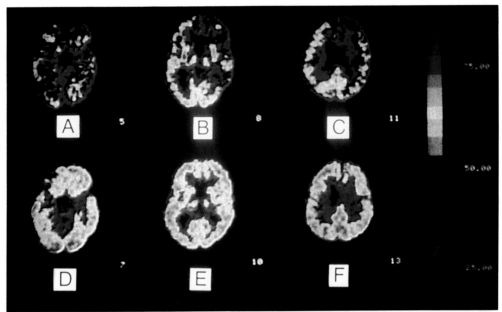

Figure 9.5. PET scan of regional glucose metabolism in the brain before AZT treatment (A–C) and after 2 months of continuous infusion AZT treatment (D–F). All images are scaled from 0% to 100% of the maximal glucose activity in the brain regions. The pretreatment scan shows diffuse cortical hypometabolism and several focal areas of markedly reduced glucose utilization. The posttreatment scan shows an increase in global cerebral metabolic rate with only mild focal abnormalities remaining. (From Pizzo, P.A., Eddy, J., Falloor, J., Balls, F., Murphy, R., Moss, H., Wolters, P., Brouwers, P., Jarosinski, P., Rubin, M., Broder, S., Yarchoan, R., Brunetti, A., Maha, M., Nusinoff-Lehrman, S., & Poplack, D. [1980]. Effect of continuous intravenous infusion of zidovudine [AZT] in children with symptomatic HIV infection. *New England Journal of Medicine, 319,* p. 893; reprinted by permission. All rights reserved.)

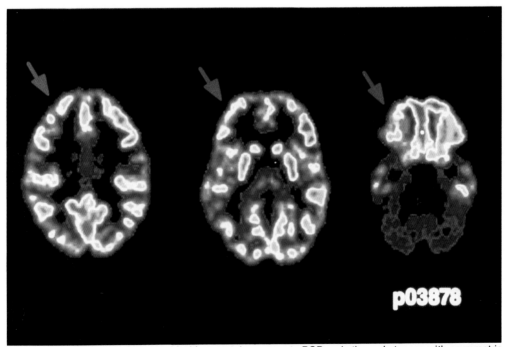

Figure 10.2. PET scan of 5-year-old with prenatal exposure to PCP and other substances with asymmetric frontal glucose uptake. Arrows indicate areas of decreased glucose metabolism. (Note that arrows on left depict right frontal glucose metabolism.)

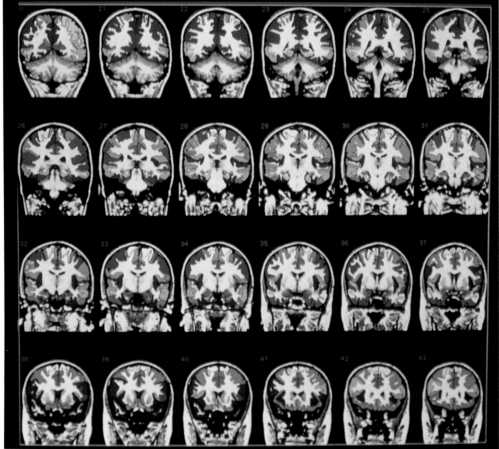

Figure 11.1.　Sequential contiguous 3.0-mm coronal anatomical magnetic resonance images (24 selected from a total of 60 slices) with superimposed neocortical systems units delineated by a new method of cortical parcellation. The different colors represent brain regions and indicate the location of borders between functionally discrete processing areas. This represents a promising new method for the analysis of anatomical MRI data.

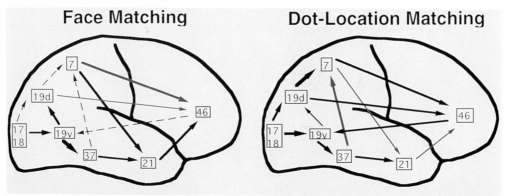

Figure 11.2.　Graphic representation of the functional networks involved in face matching (left) and dot-location matching (right). Numbered boxes correspond to functional areas (Brodmann's areas); arrows indicate anatomical pathways. Solid black and red arrows indicate functional interactions (path coefficients). Black arrows indicate positive coefficients; red arrows indicate negative coefficients. Arrow widths indicate the value of the coefficient, which corresponds to the strength of the interaction. Dotted blue arrows indicate a lack of functional interaction. (ˈ=0.7–1.0 [black], ⁻0.7–⁻1.0 [red]; ·=0.4–0.6 [black], ⁻0.4–⁻0.6 [red]; /=0.1–0.3 [black], ⁻0.1–⁻0.3 [red]; ---·=0 [blue].) Face matching was shown to predominantly involve occipitotemporal pathways; dot location predominantly involved occipitoparietal pathways. The dot-location task involved strong feedback from area 46 in the frontal lobe to occipital cortex (area 19), an effect that was absent in face matching. (From McIntosh, A.R., Grady, C.L., Ungerleider, L.G., Haxby, J.V., Rapoport, S.I., & Horwitz, B. [1994]. Network analysis of cortical visual pathways mapped with PET. *Journal of Neuroscience, 14*, p. 659; adapted by permission.)

I

Basic Biological and Methodological Concepts

Since the mid-1980s, there has been a tremendous growth of knowledge and sophistication concerning the developing brain and both subtle and hard neurological disorders in children. The sources of this information are many, inasmuch as developmental neuropsychologists, developmental psychologists, neurophysiologists, neuroanatomists, and cognitive neuroscientists have begun an era of collaboration and interdisciplinary research to better understand the neurobiology of the developing brain. Unlike decades past, when one could only infer brain development and functions from observable behavior, noninvasive and comprehensive neuroimaging methodologies now provide a window to the neurological bases of sensory, motor, attentional, perceptual, linguistic, and cognitive development. To grasp the impact that these technological advances in developmental neuroimaging have had on our current understanding and conceptualizations of the developing brain, certain terms and models relevant to neuropsychology and neuroanatomy, as well as those relevant to the nomenclature and technical foundation of different types of neuroimaging procedures, should be understood.

Within this context, the two chapters in this section are designed to provide an overview of critical theoretical, conceptual, and methodological issues that are essential to the interpretation of neuropsychological and neuroimaging studies of children. In Chapter 1, Dr. G. Reid Lyon provides a brief introductory review of human brain anatomy and developmental neuropsychology with an emphasis on acquainting the reader with the methods and tools that are used to identify relationships between the developing brain and emerging behavior in the child. In Chapter 2, Drs. Jack Krasuski, Barry Horwitz, and Judith M. Rumsey provide a clear, cogent, and masterful review of the major neuroimaging methods that are used in the study of children's brain development and disorders. Within this chapter, critical information about the design, purpose, and workings of both anatomical and functional neuroimaging methods is presented. Different neuroimaging procedures and methods are used to address different questions about brain development and disorders, and the chapter is organized and written to explicate how these decisions are made and how the different neuroimaging methods do the job.

To provide the audience with clear explanations and examples as to how one goes about viewing the developing brain through the lens of neuroimaging technology, the chapters in this section were written with the understanding that readers will differ with respect to their backgrounds in neuropsychology, neuroanatomy, and neuroimaging. As such, the level of detail provided in sections devoted to brain structures and functions and the technical aspects of different neuroimaging methods is geared toward the nonspecialist and, therefore, is written in more general language. The goal of this section is to communicate background information that will enhance the reader's understanding of how far developmental neuroscience has truly come in mapping the neurological underpinnings of children's cognition and behavior, in general, and of specific developmental disorders, in particular.

1

Foundations of
Neuroanatomy and Neuropsychology
G. Reid Lyon

The human brain is a fascinating and complex organ. Its intricate systems and delicate structures provide the basis for our rational existence. Without the brain, our hearts could not beat; our lungs could not breathe; we could not detect a chill in the air; we could not see a sunset, hear a symphony, read a novel, solve a mathematics problem, remember, or believe in a system of values. Although the adult brain weighs only approximately 3 pounds, it stores more information than all of the libraries in the world. The workings of the human brain are remarkably complicated, and it is not unexpected to find many neuroscientists questioning whether the human brain, as it works inside of us, can ever fully understand the human brain.

However, since the 1970s, in particular, since the mid-1980s, neuroscientists have accrued a sizable and solid body of information about the structure of the brain and its specific functions. This knowledge has been made accessible through a number of elegant neuroanatomical, neurophysiological, and neuropsychological studies. Of importance to this chapter and to this book are those mysteries of the brain that have been unraveled through the application of neuroimaging technologies. These relatively new tools of modern neuroscience have enabled researchers and clinicians to gain important insights into the structure and function of the normally developing brain and to begin to understand the differences in brain structure and function that are associated with dyslexia, attention-deficit/hyperactivity disorder, autism, epilepsy, and genetic disorders, such as neurofibromatosis, Turner syndrome, and fragile X syndrome.

To help readers understand the findings that have been amassed via neuroimaging technology, this chapter focuses on a brief review of human neuroanatomy and neuropsychology, with special attention paid to brain structure–function relationships. For more detailed and in-depth coverage of neuroanatomy, neurophysiology, and neuropsychology, the reader is referred to Barr and Kiernan (1993), Brodal (1992), Carpenter (1978), and Luria (1973).

SELECTED STRUCTURES OF THE BRAIN
AND THEIR DEVELOPMENT

Neuroanatomical Frames of Reference and Direction

Before one can understand the literature on neuroanatomy and neurophysiology, it is necessary to understand a few common terms that are used to describe how various neuroanatomical structures are located in the brain in relation to each other. That is, in writing about neuroanatomy, it is common practice to identify a neuroanatomical structure or region with reference to its position with other areas (i.e., in front of, on top of, behind). Neuroanatomists use a specialized vocabulary that has emerged from brain dissections and physiology studies of humans and animals to describe locations within the brain. To make matters more confusing, for several of these terms, we have synonyms that frequently are used as substitutes (depending on whether an animal or human is being discussed).

As Walsh (1978) noted, in animals, the head-to-tail direction typically is described by the Latin-derived terms *rostral* and *caudal*, and the belly-to-back direction typically is described by the terms *ventral* and *dorsal*. These positions usually are at right angles to one another in animals but not in humans. Specifically, in the human, the belly and the nose point in the same direction so that the terms *anterior* and *posterior* may take the place of rostral and caudal, and the terms *superior* and *inferior* may take the place of dorsal and ventral. Figure 1.1 displays the regions of the head (and the brain) that correspond to these relational and directional terms. Figure 1.1 also shows that the term *medial* is used to indicate toward the middle of the brain, and the term *lateral* is used to indicate toward the side or outer surface of the brain.

An additional set of terms that denote position and direction has evolved from studies of sections of the brain that are cut in different planes to reveal different neuroanatomical structures and regions. These terms are particularly relevant to neuroimaging studies because the neuroimaging scanners collect data and construct images of brain "slices" in the coronal or frontal plane; the sagittal or longitudinal plane; or the horizontal, axial, or transverse plane. Figure 1.2 displays the relationship of these planes to the head and brain.

As illustrated in Figure 1.2, coronal slices lie parallel to a vertical plane through both ears. Sagittal sections are perpendicular to the coronal plane and run longitudinally from the front to the back of the brain. A midsagittal slice lies at or near the midline, whereas parasagittal slices are lateral sagittal slices. A horizontal, transverse, or axial slice is at right angles to the other two planes.

The Developing Brain

The development of the human brain is a complex and dynamic process of sequential and somewhat predictable anatomical, functional, and organizational changes that enable an individual to adapt to his or her environment (Chugani, 1994). According to

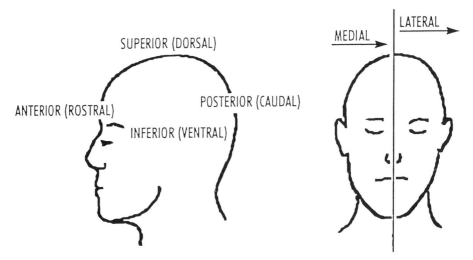

Figure 1.1.   Terms of relationship in neuroanatomy. (Adapted from Walsh [1978].)

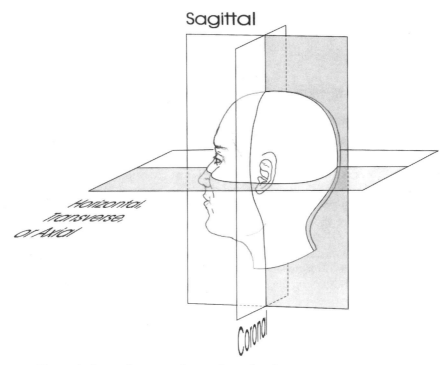

Figure 1.2.   Planes of reference in neuroanatomy and neuroimaging.

Huttenlocher (1994), the general development of the human cerebral cortex can be divided into two major phases. During the first phase, neuronal precursors are born from embryonic tissue situated near the cerebral ventricles (small cavities within the depths of the brain) and begin to travel or migrate to the cortical plate in a systematic and orderly manner. The cortical plate is a thick initial layer of cells from which nerve fibers migrate to form various brain structures. The neurons that migrate first form the lower cortical layers, and those that migrate later form the upper layers of the brain. This differentiation, proliferation, and migration of cells takes place in utero and begins at a gestational age of approximately 10 weeks. By approximately 18 weeks of gestational age, all of the neurons of the human cerebral cortex have been generated and have arrived at their destined location (Sidman & Rakic, 1973).

During the second phase, existing neurons develop and elaborate their connections with other neurons. Neurons establish synaptic circuits with connecting neurons by growing axon nerve fibers (axons) that extend from the neuron and carry electrical impulses that generate the release of neurotransmitters from dendritic structures, which are at the ends of the axons (Huttenlocher, 1994). These events begin during the second trimester of gestation and continue well into the postnatal period. According to Huttenlocher (1994), the size of the infant's brain at birth is only approximately one third that of an adult's brain. Despite the smaller size, the gross anatomy of the neonatal brain is similar to that of the adult brain. Brain weight increases rapidly from approximately 300 grams–370 grams at birth to approximately 40% of its adult weight of 1,250 grams–1,500 grams during the first 4 years of life (Chugani, 1994; Hooper & Willis, 1989). This tremendous increase in the volume of the brain during the first years of life primarily is a result of growth in the number of neuronal and axonal connections (Schade & van Groenigen, 1961). The anatomical development of the brain continues well into childhood (Huttenlocher, 1979; Huttenlocher & de Courten, 1987). For example, the elimination of redundant synapses can be observed in the visual cortices of humans until approximately 10 years of age (Wilson, 1988). In a similar manner, development within the association areas of the brain that are involved with language appear to complete their development by the onset of adolescence (Huttenlocher, 1979). The myelination of axons, a process that increases the speed and efficiency by which electrical impulses travel down the axonal process, continues to develop into the adult years (Yakovlev & Lecours, 1967).

During this period of general brain development, there exists a very interesting nonlinear pattern of production, proliferation, and elimination of neurons of cell processes and synaptic contacts. These phases of neuronal and synaptic exuberance and elimination do not coincide with the above-described general growth and weight gain of brain. For example, neurons in the developing brain actually are overproduced prenatally and then are reduced in the latter stages of prenatal development (Rabinowicz, 1979). In contrast, the overproduction and pruning (elimination) of neuronal processes and their synaptic contacts occurs postnatally over a fairly long period of time (Chugani, in press; Huttenlocher, 1979; Huttenlocher & de Courten, 1987). As Huttenlocher (1979) showed, synaptic density in children up to 11 years of age actually exceeded that observed in the adult. This overproduction of synaptic processes may allow an individual brain to retain and increase the efficiency of connections that are used repeatedly during a critical period and to eliminate those contacts that are used to a lesser degree (Chugani, in press). In addition, Changeux and Danchin (1976), Chugani (in press), and Jacobson (1978) have noted that the overabundance of connections among neurons may reduce the genetic load that otherwise would be required to specifically program the tremendous number of synaptic contacts in the nervous system.

The Tissue Substrate

The tissue mass of the brain comprises nerve cell bodies (neurons), nerve fibers (axons), dendrites, which stream out from the cell body and serve to transmit information via electrical and chemical means, and supporting cells (glia). The cerebral cortex comprises the mantle of gray matter that resides within the cerebral hemispheres. The cerebral cortex is the most recently elaborated structure in the central nervous system, and it has been thought of as the site of higher cognitive functions.

It has been estimated that the cerebral cortex of the human brain contains from 10 billion to 18 billion neurons, and some estimates run as high as 25 billion. Each of these neurons has at least one point of contact with another neuron, and the majority actually communicate with multitudes of others to form neural networks. These neural networks provide the interaction sites that mediate the complexity of human behavior. Unlike all of the other cells in the body, the neuronal cells within the brain do not divide, multiply, or regenerate. When nerve cells die, new nerve cells cannot replace them. Connective tissue may, however, fill the space left by the dead neurons, or surrounding neurons may fill the gaps. The neurons within the cerebral cortex are organized in one of six layers depending on the type and size of the cells, their density, and the arrangement of the cells. One of the most striking features of cortical organization is this cellular layering or lamination. For a brief, yet excellent, discussion of the six layers of the cerebral cortex, the reader is referred to Netter (1972).

Within the cerebral cortex, three types of cells predominate: pyramidal cells, which are the most numerous, have the shape of a pyramid and vary in size from 10 micra to 50 micra, although some may be as large as 100 micra in the motor regions of the brain; stellate or granule cells, which have a polygonal shape and range in size from 4 micra to 8 micra; and fusiform or spindle cells, which typically are located in the deepest layers of the cortical mantle and send their long axons upward toward the surface of the cortex.

Neurons that communicate with the sensory regions of the brain and provide information about the world around us are labeled afferent (sensory) neurons. The ability to see, hear, and feel pressure on our skin are some examples of the functions of afferent neurons. In other words, afferent neurons are responsible for sending information about both the body and the outside world to the brain for analysis. Efferent (motor) neurons enable us to speak, move, and manipulate features within our environment. The efferent system enables parts of the body to carry out the motor plans and programs that are constructed in the brain. Neurons also can be classified as either excitatory, when their actions increase the probability of activity in downstream and surrounding neurons, or inhibitory, when they participate in attenuating or blocking excitatory nerve impulses.

Neurons that populate different cortical regions of the brain have different functional properties (specific regions and lobes of the brain are discussed later in this chapter). For example, the neurons that compose the primary projection areas of the cortex primarily reside in cell layer IV and possess high specificity (Hubel & Wiesel, 1963). As an example of how these primary projection areas work, consider the cortical visual system: The neurons in cell layer IV in the cortical visual system (occipital lobe) primarily respond to discrete features of visual stimuli, such as the angle of a line, the direction of movement, or a shade of color. In a similar manner, primary projection neurons in the auditory (temporal lobe) and somatosensory (parietal lobe) cortices also respond to highly specific stimuli that reflect highly differentiated properties of acoustic input and tactile and kinesthetic input, respectively.

Neurons that reside in the secondary association regions (cell layers II and III) of the visual, auditory, and parietal cortices, however, respond to several properties of modality-specific stimuli. These neurons organize or synthesize the individual elements of information processed by cells in the primary projection areas (cell layer IV) and combine the information into functional patterns (Luria, 1973). Modality specificity, in general, means that neurons within the visual cortex respond primarily to visual stimuli, neurons in the auditory cortex activate primarily in the presence of verbal and nonverbal sound, and neurons within the somatosensory cortex respond primarily to tactile and kinesthetic information (touch). It should be noted, however, that modality-specific neurons are not as tightly contained within the artificial boundaries of lobes or cell layers as this discussion suggests. Brain stimulation studies have shown, for example, that electrical activation within the occipital lobe (typically thought of as responsible for visual functions) can stimulate or inhibit some aspects of verbal function.

General Neuroanatomical Principles and Structures

After an initial differentiation of embryonic tissue during the first 4 weeks after conception, three enlargements or primary brain vesicles (pouches) form at the front or anterior end of the neural tube (Hooper & Willis, 1989; Hynd & Willis, 1988). These primary brain vesicles are shown in Figure 1.3A, as is the isthmus, which connects the vesicles and the neural tube. Figure 1.3A indicates that the three major subdivisions of the embryonic brain, the prosencephalon (forebrain), mesencephalon (midbrain), and

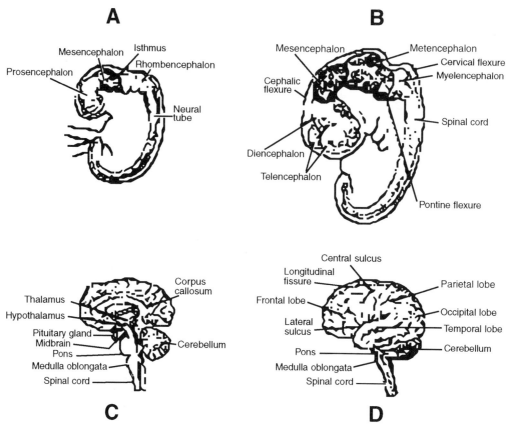

A

Mesencephalon Isthmus

Prosencephalon Rhombencephalon

Neural tube

B

Mesencephalon Metencephalon

Cervical flexure

Cephalic flexure Myelencephalon

Spinal cord

Diencephalon

Telencephalon

Pontine flexure

C

Corpus callosum

Thalamus

Hypothalamus

Pituitary gland

Midbrain Cerebellum

Pons

Medulla oblongata

Spinal cord

D

Central sulcus

Longitudinal fissure

Parietal lobe

Frontal lobe

Occipital lobe

Lateral sulcus Temporal lobe

Pons Cerebellum

Medulla oblongata

Spinal cord

Figure 1.3. Differentiation of the brain at three levels of development. (A, lateral view of primary brain vesicles; B, lateral view of secondary brain vesicles; C, midsagittal section of mature brain; D, lateral view of mature brain.) (From Hynd, G.W., & Willis, W.G. [1988]. *Pediatric neuropsychology*, p. 29. New York: Grune & Stratton; reprinted by permission.)

rhombencephalon (hindbrain), further divide into five secondary brain vesicles during prenatal development. Figure 1.3B shows that the prosencephalon comprises the telencephalon (end brain or forebrain) and the diencephalon (twice, twin, or between brain). The telencephalon, in turn, serves as the substrate for the development of the cerebral cortex (the outer mantle of nerve cells and most evolved neural tissue) and the basal ganglia (masses of neurons situated deep within the cerebral hemispheres), and the diencephalon differentiates into the thalamus and hypothalamus (Figure 1.3C). A detailed presentation of diencephalic structures is provided in the midsagittal view depicted in Figure 1.4.

The mesencephalon, shown in Figure 1.3A and 1.3B, differentiates during development into specific midbrain structures known as the quadrigeminal plate, the tectum, the cerebral peduncles, and the cerebral aqueduct. The midbrain tectum and cerebral aqueduct are shown in Figure 1.4. After this initial formation, the mesencephalon does not subdivide further.

The rhombencephalon, shown in Figure 1.3A, subdivides into the myelencephalon to form the medulla oblongata and the fourth ventricle, which is located between the cerebellum and medulla (see Figures 1.3C and 1.4). The hindbrain also subdivides into the metencephalon, which comprises the pons and cerebellum (Figures 1.3C and

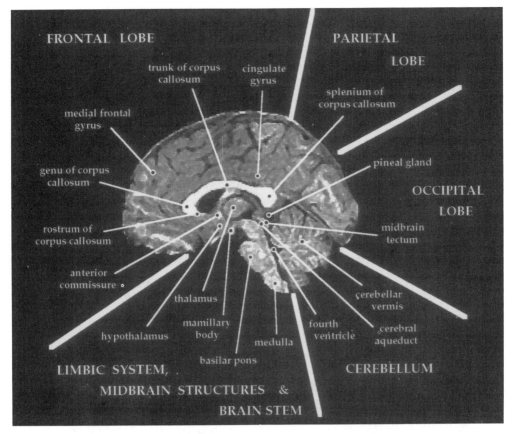

Figure 1.4.   Midsagittal view of the human brain.

1.4). As Lezak (1976) noted, those brain regions that are the farthest back or most posterior on the neural tube axis are the most simply organized. In structures in the front or anterior aspects of the brain, the anatomical organization of the brain becomes much more complex and diverse. As expected, the more simply organized structures in the hindbrain are the first to develop and are responsible for regulating relatively primitive functions that are critical to survival, such as respiration, blood pressure, and beating of the heart, whereas the anterior or frontal systems help to mediate higher cognitive functions, such as language use, planning, intention, and judgment. In contrast, midbrain structures serve as way stations for many different nerve tracts connecting the brain and spinal cord and for a number of cranial nerve nuclei.

Additional, albeit brief, descriptions of some of the brain structures that are referred to in later chapters follow. More detailed descriptions of these structures, as well as complete coverage of additional neuroanatomy, can be found in a number of excellent sources (Carpenter, 1978; Crelin, 1974; Huttenlocher, 1990).

Some Specific Brain Structures

Differences in a number of brain structures and systems are linked to the developmental disorders discussed in later chapters. For this reason, the anatomy and basic functions of some of the most frequently cited brain structures are reviewed in this section.

The cerebrum is the most recently evolved and sophisticated region of the brain. It derives from the telencephalon or forebrain. As mentioned previously, the cerebrum contains an outer layer or mantle of cells (neuronal gray matter), called the cerebral cortex, and underlying white matter that is composed of axons that relay information to different regions within the cortex. The cerebrum is composed of two cerebral hemispheres that appear to be fairly symmetrical to the naked eye, but in fact, are not identical mirror images of each other. A lateral (side) view of the left hemisphere of the cerebrum is shown in Figure 1.3D, and a more detailed view of the right hemisphere is provided in Figure 1.5. Note that the right hemisphere depicted in Figure 1.5 is angled toward the right to show that the longitudinal fissure partially separates the left and right hemispheres from each other. Both Figure 1.3D and Figure 1.5 indicate that each hemisphere contains a number of sulci (grooves or trenches on the surface of the brain), gyri (elevations or convolutions of the surface of the brain), and lobes (frontal, temporal, parietal, and occipital). For example, the longitudinal fissure or sulcus runs from the anterior aspect of the brain to the posterior aspect. As mentioned, it practically separates the right and left hemispheres. The lateral sulcus or sylvian fissure runs along the lateral aspect of each hemisphere in a relatively horizontal plane. The central sulcus or fissure of Rolando runs downward from the superior aspect of each hemisphere, traverses the lateral portion of the hemisphere, and blends into the lateral sulcus.

The lateral and central sulci divide the cerebral hemispheres into general, and somewhat arbitrary, brain regions. These divisions are artificial, because areas of the cerebral hemispheres that are different anatomical areas are, in many instances, in-

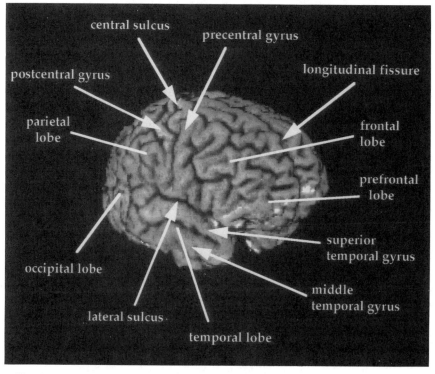

Figure 1.5.   Lateral view of the right cerebral hemisphere.

volved in a single behavioral function. For example, although language-based auditory processes, such as the ability to discriminate speech sounds, typically are associated with the functioning of the temporal lobe within the left hemisphere, cells within the parietal, occipital, and frontal lobes also may contribute to this process.

As shown in Figures 1.3D and 1.5, the frontal lobe, the largest of the lobes, constitutes all of the cerebral tissue in front of, or anterior to, the central sulcus. Directly in front of the central sulcus is the precentral gyrus. The precentral gyrus houses the primary motor area, which enables movement on the opposite or contralateral side of the body (the motor region in the left hemisphere controls the motor output on the right side of the body and vice versa). Lesions in this region typically result in paralysis. In front of the precentral gyrus of each hemisphere is the premotor cortex, which organizes complex motor movements. Such movements are critical for the performance of manual dexterity tasks and to the ability to perform complex, skilled motor movements necessary for activities such as speaking, writing, playing the piano, and the like (see Figure 1.5 for a view of premotor cortex of the right hemisphere).

The area in front of the premotor cortex is the prefrontal lobe (Figure 1.5), which is implicated in a number of functions, including language expression, the formulation of plans and strategies for behavior, and the verification that behavior has taken place. The integrity of the prefrontal lobes is essential to the development of verbal strategies to guide behavior, the ability to direct and sustain attention, the ability to make complex judgments, and the ability to inhibit impulsive responses to extraneous stimuli in the environment. Deficits in frontal lobe functions are implicated in a number of developmental disorders, including attention-deficit/hyperactivity disorder (see Chapter 5), autism (see Chapter 6), fragile X syndrome, Turner syndrome and neurofibromatosis (see Chapter 7), epilepsy (see Chapter 8), and pediatric acquired immunodeficiency syndrome (AIDS) (see Chapter 9). In addition, the cognitive and behavioral effects of maternal drug abuse during pregnancy that are discussed in Chapter 10 seem to reflect the negative effects of the drugs on the development of the frontal lobes.

Figures 1.3D and 1.5 show that the temporal lobe constitutes a good deal of the neural tissue below the lateral sulcus. Toward the posterior regions of the brain, the tissue of the temporal lobe seems to blend imperceptibly with the tissue of the occipital lobe. In general, the cells in the temporal lobe in each hemisphere are involved in hearing and memory. The left temporal lobe usually is reserved for the receipt, analysis, and storage of verbal linguistic information, whereas the right temporal lobe receives and analyzes nonverbal auditory information (tone perception, melody, environmental sounds, etc.). The temporal lobes also contribute to our senses of time and spatial relationships and play a critical role in emotions, such as anger and jealousy, primarily because of their connections with the limbic system. The temporal lobes frequently are discussed in the chapters addressing dyslexia (see Chapters 3 and 4), Turner syndrome (see Chapter 7), and epilepsy (see Chapter 8).

The parietal lobe is shown in Figures 1.3D and 1.5. As shown, the parietal lobe occupies space behind, or posterior to, the central sulcus. As do the temporal lobes, the parietal lobe in each hemisphere merges with the occipital lobe. The parietal lobe in each hemisphere serves as the primary neuronal substrate for receiving input from sensory receptors that provide information about touch, pain, pressure, temperature, and the like. As do the motor systems in the frontal lobes, the sensory systems in the parietal lobes have a contralateral influence on the body; that is, somesthetic and kinesthetic information that impinges on the right side of the body is received, analyzed, and stored in the left parietal lobe, and sensory information from the left side is processed by the right parietal lobe. In addition, the neurons within the parietal lobe are arranged precisely and systematically, such that sensations from the body are perceived in specific corresponding regions in the postcentral gyrus.

The occipital lobe, depicted in Figures 1.3D and 1.5, is located at the back of the brain, behind the temporal lobe and parietal lobes. It has been noted previously that the boundaries between the occipital lobe and the temporal and parietal lobes are poorly defined. The cells within the primary and association areas of the occipital lobe primarily are involved in the receipt, analysis, and synthesis of visual information. The ability to see and perceive visual information, therefore, is the prime responsibility of each occipital lobe within each hemisphere. Because of the occipital lobe's role in vision, occipital lobe lesions have been linked to some types of acquired reading disorders (e.g., alexia) (see Luria, 1973), although developmental dyslexia typically is associated with linguistic impairments (see Chapters 3 and 4).

The corpus callosum (see Figures 1.3C and 1.4) is included in this discussion of the cerebrum because it connects the two hemispheres via commissural fibers (axons) and plays a significant role in the interhemispheric transfer of sensory experiences, learned discriminations, and memory. A number of neuroimaging studies also have reported that differences in the structure of the corpus callosum may be related to dyslexia (see Chapter 3) and attention-deficit/hyperactivity disorder (see Chapter 5).

The diencephalon, which comprises the thalamus and hypothalamus (see Figures 1.3C, 1.4, and 1.6), lies in the midline of the two cerebral hemispheres. The cerebral hemispheres sit on the top of the thalamus (Greek for "couch"). The thalamus can be considered a way station or switchboard for sensory information that arrives at the periphery of the body. All information must pass through the thalamus on its way to the cerebral hemispheres, where it is received, analyzed, and synthesized in great detail. In fact, all of the senses, except smell, relay their impulses through the thalamus. Portions of the thalamus interact with the limbic system and seem to be involved in emotional experience. Insults to the thalamus resulting from injury or disease may produce intellectual impairments associated with limitations in alertness and arousal, difficulties in focusing or shifting attention, or memory impairments.

The hypothalamus, although it weighs less than 4 grams and comprises less than 1% of total brain tissue, plays a remarkable and crucial role in regulating the body's most critical activities. For example, blood pressure, pulse, and body temperature are associated with the functions of the hypothalamus. In addition, the hypothalamus serves as the control center for food intake by letting us know when we are hungry or full. It controls endocrine levels via secretion of gonadotrophin-releasing hormones and is critically influential in the maintenance of water balance and libido and in the operation of the autonomic nervous system. Some of our emotions also seem to be strongly influenced by hypothalamic function. For example, fatigue, fear, and rage can be induced via stimulation of nuclei within the hypothalamic system.

The basal ganglia are nuclei, or collections of gray matter, located deep within the cerebral hemispheres beneath the cerebral cortex (see Figure 1.6). Structures within the basal ganglia include the putamen and the globus pallidus, which together constitute the lenticular nucleus, and the caudate nucleus (see Figure 1.6). The corpus striatum includes the caudate and lenticular nuclei, whereas the striatum includes the caudate and the putamen. The striatum receives major inputs from widespread areas of the cerebral cortex, especially from the motor cortices in the frontal lobes and the somatosen-

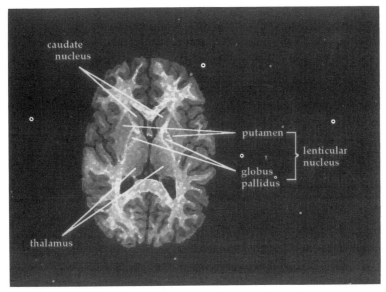

Figure 1.6. Horizontal (axial) section of the brain at two levels showing structures of the basal ganglia.

sory cortices in the parietal lobes. The striatum relays information to the globus pallidus, which, in turn, relays information to the thalamus.

Because the thalamus forwards information to the motor and premotor regions of the frontal lobes, the basal ganglia can influence motor activity via this route. Additional neural loops that involve the basal ganglia are grafted onto this major circuit. Disorders that involve the basal ganglia are typified by involuntary movements. Examples are Parkinson's disease, characterized by rigidity (caused by increased tone), tremor, and difficulty in moving, and Huntington disease, a hereditary disorder characterized by involuntary movements.

Neuroimaging studies have linked abnormalities in basal ganglia structures to attention-deficit/hyperactivity disorder (see Chapter 5), autism (see Chapter 6), and fragile X syndrome, Turner syndrome, and neurofibromatosis (see Chapter 7). In addition, children who were prenatally exposed to teratogens, such as cocaine and phencyclidine, also display anomalous development in some structures of the basal ganglia (see Chapter 10).

The cerebellum (little brain), which is located in the posterior fossa (cavity in the back of the skull), is attached to the brain stem and consists of two large hemispheres and three lobes (flocculonodular, anterior, and posterior) (Figures 1.3D and 1.4). Each hemisphere of the cerebellum contains a vermal region, a paravermal region, and a lateral region. The most clearly established role of the cerebellum is to coordinate postural and locomotor mechanisms involved in muscular activity, movement, and motor control and coordination. It provides guidance with respect to body position and enables us to make delicate, graceful movements without conscious awareness. A high degree of muscular synergism and motor control is achieved by the cerebellum via its ability to integrate afferent information from the skin, muscles, tendons, joints, semicircular canals of the ears, and the auditory and visual systems of the cerebral cortex. In turn, the cerebellum provides efferent input to the cerebral cortex and the spinal cord so that muscle and motor activity and coordination are well coordinated, organized, and smooth. Until the 1980s, the cerebellum's functions were thought to be solely motor. New research, however, has raised the possibility that the cerebellum plays a role in a number of nonmotor functions involved in the perception of temporal sequences, language, and social behavior.

Lesions in the region of the cerebellum typically result in jerky movements and a tremor in the extremities (e.g., the hands) when a deliberate movement is made (intention tremor). Balance also may be affected when the cerebellum is damaged. In the 1980s and 1990s, the cerebellum was found to be implicated in a number of developmental cognitive and social disorders, including autism (see Chapter 6).

The limbic system (Latin for "rim") is composed of a number of anatomical structures that serve to both border (hence the term *rim*) and include the diencephalon. The limbic system contains a number of deep brain structures, including the amygdala, septal nuclei, anterior thalamus, nuclei within the hypothalamus, cingulate gyrus, fornix, mammillary bodies, and hippocampus. Although the anterior thalamus, hypothalamus, and cingulate gyrus can be visualized nicely in Figure 1.4, other structures within the system, including the hippocampus and amygdala, are situated deep within the temporal lobes.

Beginning with the writings of Papez (1937), the limbic system has been thought of as the seat of emotions (Benes, in press; Spreen et al., 1984). The limbic system also plays a major role in memory, in particular, via the neurons within the hippocampus. Structures within the limbic system are discussed in this book in chapters addressing attention-deficit/hyperactivity disorder (see Chapter 5), autism (see Chapter 6), fragile X syndrome, Turner syndrome, and neurofibromatosis (see Chapter 7), and epilepsy (see Chapter 8).

The position of the midbrain is shown in Figure 1.3C, and the midbrain tectum is depicted in Figure 1.4. The midbrain constitutes the smallest division in the brain stem; other divisions of the brain stem are the medulla oblongata and pons, which are discussed below. The midbrain includes four small colliculi, which are small structures that look like little hills and are involved in elementary visual and hearing functions. Nuclei in the midbrain also contribute to the integration of reflexes with the visual and auditory systems and play a major role in the smooth integration of muscle movements.

The medulla oblongata and the pons, shown in Figures 1.3C, 1.3D, and 1.4, are considered components of the hindbrain and also comprise portions of the brain stem, which they share with the midbrain. The medulla is essential to biological functions, such as respiration, blood pressure, and, in part, heart rate. All of the efferent fibers leaving the cerebral cortex to carry motor messages to the limbs cross the midline, or decussate, in the medulla; this results in contralateral control (i.e., the left cerebral hemisphere controls the right side of the body and vice versa). The pons (bridge), also located in the hindbrain (see Figures 1.3C, 1.3D, and 1.4), contains a broad band of fibers that provides a neural link between the cerebral cortex and the cerebellum.

This overview of human neuroanatomy is provided to acquaint the reader with the major brain structures and systems that are discussed throughout this book. In reality, human neuroanatomy is far more complex and elegant than what is described here, and readers are urged to pursue additional study by consulting the above-mentioned resources. In the following section of this chapter, a brief review of neuropsychological principles is provided. This review is intended to acquaint the reader with theories and methods that attempt to explain the way the activity of the brain is expressed in observable behavior.

NEUROPSYCHOLOGY: RELATING BRAIN AND BEHAVIOR

Purposes of Neuropsychological Study

Neuropsychology attempts to relate what is known about the functioning of the brain to what is understood about behavior. More specifically, clinical neuropsychology seeks to define the role of the brain in thought and action by studying empirically the behavioral phenomena associated with the neural changes induced by disease, injury, or dysfunction of the nervous system in children and adults (Lyon et al., 1991). Regardless of the age of an individual, the primary goal of neuropsychology is to investigate the functional status of the brain by analyzing behavioral responses by administering various tests and/or tasks (Rourke et al., 1983; Teeter, 1986). Developmental neuropsychology, a subspecialty of neuropsychology, is a scientific and clinical field that combines the study of the development of the brain with the study of the development of behavior. Developmental neuropsychology, by necessity, capitalizes on research and clinical methodologies that can identify and assess rapidly changing brain–behavior relationships during childhood and adolescence.

Differences Between
Developmental and Adult Neuropsychology

The study of brain–behavior relationships in children differs substantially from the neuropsychological investigation of adults in several ways. First, the nervous systems of children are quite different from those of adults in terms of both physiological characteristics and functional capabilities. By definition, the developing nervous system is in a state of continuing change, whereas, for the most part, the adult brain is relatively static with respect to growth. For example, some neural structures are not fully developed in children, but, as myelination occurs and dendritic connections develop, cognitive, motor, linguistic, and behavioral changes can be observed.

Second, disease or dysfunction affecting the nervous systems of children typically are reflected in deficient development of cognitive, perceptual, linguistic, attentional, and behavioral skills. In contrast, trauma to the adult brain generally results in the loss of previously acquired skills.

Third, before the mid-1980s, little was understood regarding the status of neural development and brain function among children with reading disorders (e.g., dyslexia), attention-deficit/hyperactivity disorder, autism, epilepsy, pediatric AIDS, acquired closed brain injury, and genetic disorders, such as neurofibromatosis and fragile X syndrome. This dearth of information primarily existed because a large number of the neuropsychological assessment tasks that comprise the most widely used neuropsychological batteries for children are downward extensions of batteries initially developed and validated on adult clinical populations. Although such tasks have provided the basis for an extensive and appropriate literature that is relevant to adult brain damage and dysfunction, they are not as relevant to our knowledge base in developmental neuropsychology. It is important to note that these tasks and their content primarily are based on models of adult brain function and dysfunction that occur after a period of *normal* development. In addition, many tasks are designed to assess the effects of focal neuropathology typically seen in adults (e.g., tumors, cerebral vascular accidents, penetrating brain wounds), rather than the more generalized neural disorders usually observed in children (e.g., anoxia, acquired brain injury, epilepsy, postnatal infections). More developmentally appropriate neuropsychological tasks and measures have been developed since the mid-1980s; these tasks assess aspects of various cognitive abilities, such as language, reading, and attention. These tasks are sensitive to developmental changes in these cognitive abilities over time and are more appropriate for mapping brain–behavior relationships in children. In addition, a number of these tasks have been correlated explicitly with the results obtained from neuroimaging studies so that valuable information related to how a given task activates different regions of the brain and how this activation changes during development can be documented. Several of the chapters that follow discuss these neuropsychological tasks and their relationship to brain function in children.

Increased Demand for Neuropsychological Knowledge

Since the mid-1980s, neuropsychological studies of children increasingly have been charged with making relevant and informed contributions to the assessment and treatment of children with known brain damage and disorders (i.e., cerebral trauma, epilepsy) and putative brain dysfunctions (i.e., dyslexia, attention-deficit/hyperactivity disorder). The increase in the application of neuropsychological principles to the understanding and treatment of developmental disorders can be attributed to several factors. First, advances in the basic neurosciences have provided new technologies for investigating the means by which the brain develops and processes information, thereby stimulating a robust scientific and clinical interest in the developing brain. This book addresses the ways in which emerging neuroimaging technology has provided exciting new views of the neurological correlates of individual differences in children's learning and behavior.

Second, the survival rates for children who have experienced acquired brain injuries have increased markedly. In addition, improvements in neonatal intensive care practices have decreased the mortality rate of infants who are born with significantly low birth weight (<1,500 grams) (Obrzut & Hynd, 1986) (see Chapter 10). Children recovering from these types of conditions, however, frequently display persistent learning and behavioral difficulties associated with their neurological history, thereby increasing the need for a more precise understanding of brain–behavior relationships within a developmental context (Lyon et al., 1991). As a result, diagnostic practices that are based on knowledge of brain development *and* cognitive and behavioral development are critical for 1) documenting the nature of developmental disorders; 2) monitoring the recovery and/or development of linguistic, perceptual, motor, and attentional skills; and 3) delineating treatment options.

Finally, there is a growing awareness that some relatively subtle learning and behavioral difficulties frequently seen in school settings (e.g., dyslexia, attention-deficit/hyperactivity disorder) are related to intrinsic neurological differences in brain structures and functions that are responsible for linguistic processing, alertness, motor activity, and arousal levels (Lyon & Krasnegor, 1996). Because increasing numbers of children are identified each year as manifesting neurodevelopmental learning and behavior disorders, there is a substantial need for rapid improvements in neuropsychological instruments and neuropsychological assessment procedures. To that end, the chapters that follow provide a number of examples of how state-of-the-art neuropsychological studies and assessments, conducted in conjunction with neuroimaging studies, can be performed for various disorders.

Neuropsychological Theories and Models

Significant changes have occurred over time with respect to how neuropsychological theories and models represent relationships among the functioning of the brain, development of the brain, and emergence of complex behaviors (see Gaddes, 1983; Lenneberg, 1967; Luria, 1970, 1973, 1980; Moscovitch, 1973). Theories attempting to explicate these relationships have ranged from parochial localization theories to antilocalization mass action theories to synergistic functional systems theories, which incorporate the most valid principles of the theoretical extremes. A brief examination of this theoretical evolution follows.

Consider that, in the Middle Ages, philosophers and naturalists proposed that sensations, perceptions, and complex mental functions, such as speech, language, memory, emotion, and the like, were located in three cerebral ventricles (described by Luria, 1973). Gall, in the early 19th century, reported that human faculties were located in specific and strictly localized regions of the brain. For example, the sense of time was thought to be located in the left anterior region of the frontal lobe, creative skill and wit were assigned to a region also in the anterior aspects or front of the brain (later known as Broca's area), and courage and pugnacity were thought to be located in the left posterior quadrants of the brain in the occipital–temporal regions. This practice of ascribing circumscribed mental, emotional, and physical faculties to specific areas of the brain (loosely based on bumps on the skull) came to be known as Gall's phrenology. (For a historical review of Gall's contributions, see Walsh, 1978.)

As peculiar as these early localization theories of brain structure–function relationships may seem to the modern reader, they were the guiding tools for thinking about linkages between brain function and behavior. Not until the mid-1800s did Broca (1865) begin the first genuine scientific investigations of localized brain lesions and their effects on behavior. Three major advances resulted from this work. First, Broca reported that the inability to speak (expressive aphasia) resulted from damage localized to the third left frontal convolution of the left hemisphere. Second, speech seemed to be lateralized to the left hemisphere, because damage to the homologous frontal region in the right hemisphere did not result in a loss of expressive language. Third, the relationship between anterior left frontal damage and loss of speech was invariant in right-handed individuals.

Localization theory also was reinforced by the findings of Wernicke (1874), who reported that difficulties in understanding speech (receptive aphasia) were caused by damage localized to the posterior third of the left superior temporal gyrus. Despite such examples of how specific areas of the brain seemed critical to specific behaviors, localization theory could not account for other clinical observations that localized damage to a small area of the cortex did not necessarily result in the loss of a single isolated behavioral function. For example, although lesions to the superior temporal gyrus typically did result in impairments in the ability to understand speech, difficulties in reading, writing, and performing mathematical functions also were noted (Hooper & Boyd, 1986).

By the late 1800s, John Hughlings Jackson had reported clinical data that suggested that brain–behavior relationships were not so simply organized within a localization framework and that complex mental processes, such as thinking, language, and reading, required the activity of many brain regions, if not the whole brain (for review, see Taylor, 1958). Jackson's views were echoed by Goldstein (1948), Head (1926), and Monakow (see Luria, 1973), who also suggested that complex forms of mental activity could not be localized in highly focal regions of the cerebral cortex but were subserved by the mass action of undifferentiated brain tissue. Given this conceptualization, Head (1926), Jackson (see Taylor, 1958), and others postulated that any type of brain damage had a generalized negative effect on all thinking and behavior. Unfortunately, this particular view also was problematic, given that many types of specific and localized brain lesions could be identified that did not result in a pervasive lowering of cognitive function.

Not until the mid-20th century were the divergent, and seemingly polar, views espoused by localization theorists and mass action theorists reconciled in a more scientifically and clinically meaningful way. Specifically, Luria (for review, see Luria, 1947, 1965, 1969, 1970, 1973), on the basis of his substantial clinical studies of World War I and World War II veterans who experienced brain injuries and the research of Leontiev (1959), Pavlov (1949), and Vygotsky (1956), proposed a theory of functional systems of higher cortical function that helped to account for the various clinical findings left unexplained by both localization and mass action theories.

Luria (for an excellent review, see Luria, 1973) proposed that mental operations, such as thinking, attention, oral language, reading, writing, mathematics, and so forth, all were affected by means of complex functional systems of cooperating zones of the cerebral cortex and subcortical structures (for examples, see Hooper & Boyd, 1986; Lyon et al., 1991). In turn, the functional systems responsible for different complex behaviors use three functional units within the brain. These functional units are organized hierarchically and integrated functionally and are essential to the execution of any type of mental activity (Hooper & Boyd, 1986; Luria, 1980). A brief review of each of these functional units follows.

The first functional unit is responsible for arousal and for maintaining an optimal level of cortical excitation. Anatomical structures subserving this first functional unit principally are located in the upper and lower parts of the brain stem (pons, medulla) and have substantial reciprocal connections with nuclei within the midbrain, the thalamus and hypothalamus, and the cortex. Damage or dysfunction in the first functional unit is reflected in the impaired ability to maintain wakefulness and attentional states.

The second functional unit is located in the outer cell layers of the posterior regions of the two hemispheres; these regions include the temporal (auditory), parietal (somatosensory), and occipital (visual) lobes. Damage to, or dysfunction of, zones in the second functional unit leads to difficulties in receiving, analyzing, and storing auditory, visual, and tactile and kinesthetic information.

The third functional unit, which consists of structures in the frontal lobes, is responsible for the processes by which goals and plans are developed, the motor programs that carry out such plans, and the monitoring systems that determine whether a goal or plan has been achieved. Impairments in the functions of the third functional unit are, for example, related to difficulties in initiating and/or completing tasks, using verbal strategies to guide performance on a task, inhibiting impulsive responses, and sustaining attention to tasks for required lengths of time.

Developmental Neuropsychological Theory

Luria (1965, 1970, 1973) has provided the field of neuropsychology with a compelling theory of the development of brain–behavior relationships, and Hooper and Boyd (1986) have nicely summarized the stages within the theory. As Hooper and Boyd noted, implicit to Luria's model of hierarchical development of functional units and functional systems is the notion of sequential neurological development. The sequence of development depends on the physiological and functional changes that occur during five stages of neural development.

During stage 1, the development of the first functional unit is a biological priority. Specifically, the reticular activating system (RAS), which is composed of nuclei and fibers that pass through the brain stem, midbrain, diencephalon, and frontal cortex, undergoes extensive differentiation and development in utero and, in general, is functional by approximately 12 months after conception (or 3 months of age). The RAS is essential to arousal from sleep, wakefulness, and focusing attention (Luria, 1973). Although the exact neurochemistry and neurophysiology of attention and the neuropathophysiology of attention-deficit/hyperactivity disorder remain elusive (see Chapter 5; also see Lyon & Krasnegor, 1996), damage to the RAS, particularly during the prenatal period, has been implicated in attentional disorders and hyperkinesis (Douglas, 1983; Zentall, 1975). For example, Rutter (1983) reported a distinction between early (before 12 months postconception) and later onset insults to the RAS, suggesting that a more biologically driven form of hyperkinesis results from early onset damage (see Hooper & Boyd, 1986, for discussion).

In stage 2, the primary sensory zones within temporal, parietal, and occipital lobes (second functional unit) and primary motor cortex (third functional unit) develop rapidly. The cortical cell layers involved in basic motor functions develop before the sensory zones located in the posterior aspects of the hemispheres develop. This differential maturation between motor and sensory brain zones and functions most likely ensures the early adaptability of the newborn to the environment. Spinal reflexes can be detected during the second fetal month (Hooper & Boyd, 1986), and all motor reflexes, except functional respiration and vocalization, are present by the fourth fetal month (Reinis & Goldman, 1980). By birth, the primary motor areas of the brain are operational and are responsible for the reflexive motor repertoires that can be observed in newborns.

The effects of damage or lesions to the brain during this stage of development differ, as in any stage, depending on a host of transient factors, including, but not limited to, the following: 1) amount of destruction of cells at the site of damage; 2) disruption of cellular activity of adjacent cells; 3) changes in the blood vessels at and around the site of damage; 4) possibility of edema (swelling) in the region; 5) buildup of intracranial pressure, which damages healthy cells; 6) changes in cerebrospinal fluid; 7) loss of the innervation of cells that were in contact with the destroyed cells; 8) degree of new growth or proliferation of collateral white matter (i.e., axons, dendrites) into regions once occupied and controlled by damaged cells; and 9) changes in the size and cellular makeup of the brain, particularly when the damage occurs early in life (Isaacson, 1976; Teeter, 1986).

As Hooper and Boyd (1986) have reported, unilateral damage (injury to one side of the brain only) to the primary motor and sensory cortices that occurs shortly after birth may not disrupt the development of motor, visual, and/or language abilities, because the remaining intact hemisphere can deploy neural resources to compensate for the loss. Unilateral injuries that occur after the first year of life and bilateral damage that occurs at any time, however, typically produce long-term negative effects on behavior.

Brain development during stage 3 is characterized by the development of the association areas of the sensory and motor cortices. Each sensory modality (hearing, vision, and somatothesis), its associated brain region (temporal lobe, occipital lobe, and parietal lobe), and the motor regions (frontal lobe) undergo quantitative and qualitative changes during stage 3. In fact, developmental events during stage 3 are initiated concurrent with those of the first two stages but continue through the fifth year of life (Hooper & Boyd, 1986). In regard to behavior, stage 3 is marked by the development of verbal skills (Golden, 1981) and by the initiation of Luria's (1973) concept of progressive lateralization, whereby language capabilities are subserved primarily by the left hemisphere. From a neuropsychological perspective, the earlier a unilateral injury to the left hemisphere occurs before the age of 2 years, the greater the likelihood that verbal functions will be transferred to the right hemisphere (for a discussion of this process, see Kinsbourne, 1981). After 2 years of age, compensation of linguistic function resulting in near-normal capabilities after damage to the left hemisphere is more remote (Hooper & Boyd, 1986).

During stage 4, maturation of the tertiary areas of the posterior second functional unit occurs (Luria, 1973). The tertiary areas are overlapping zones, such that, within these zones, neural cells have the capability to respond to multiple sensory inputs. That is, a given cell in the tertiary areas can respond to visual, auditory, or tactile and kinesthetic input. In general, these overlapping zones are located at the juncture of the temporal, occipital, and parietal lobes of each hemisphere, and their development is critical to the development of complex symbolic abilities, including reading, mathematics, written expression, and spelling. Consider that each of these abilities requires the development of associations among sensory stimuli. For example, to read or spell, one must associate auditory (phonemic) and visual (graphic) information.

Typically, injury or dysfunction within these posterior (second functional unit) tertiary systems results in significant learning impairments (Hooper & Boyd, 1986). For example, limitations in bimodal integration (association between visual and auditory information) can, as mentioned previously, lead to difficulties in decoding and recognizing words, as well as to impairments in higher-order language skills (Golden & Anderson, 1979). More substantial impairments in these regions are associated with more pervasive learning difficulties, such as mental retardation (Golden, 1981).

Stage 5 of brain development is characterized by the development of the tertiary areas of the prefrontal (third functional unit) cortices. Although these cortical zones are the last to achieve maturation, some controversy exists as to when development is complete (Huttenlocher, 1994). Luria (1973) reported that the tertiary zones in the prefrontal regions did not become functional until between 4 and 7 years of age, and then they continued to develop through adulthood. In contrast, Passler et al. (1985) hypothesized that the development of the tertiary prefrontal areas is a multistage process in which the most rapid period of development occurs between 6 and 8 years of age, and the mastery of tasks subserved by these cortical regions is evident by 12 years of age.

The prefrontal tertiary zones of the cortex can be considered the tertiary region for the entire brain. Specifically, these zones possess a highly integrated network of afferent and efferent fibers that place the prefrontal cortices in contact with all other subcortical and cortical systems (Luria, 1973). Given the overarching role that the prefrontal tertiary zones play in ensuring contact and communication with the entire brain, damage to or dysfunction of these zones typically is reflected in limitations in attention, difficulty in formulating language to plan sequences of behavior, difficulties in making appropriate judgments, impairments in monitoring and self-evaluation of performance, and limitations in mental and behavioral flexibility (Denckla, 1994, 1996, in press; Luria, 1973; Pennington, in press; Stuss & Benson, 1984).

SUMMARY

As a child matures, substantial developmental changes occur in the brain; these changes can be identified by the application of neuropsychological theories, assessment tasks, and clinical evaluation procedures that identify predictable relationships between brain development and behavior. Commensurate with ontogenetic development, the child's behavioral repertoire becomes increasingly automatized and fluent in the execution of complex behaviors (Hooper & Boyd, 1986). Of critical importance to clinical study, these changes in brain–behavior relationships are regular and predictable (Luria, 1973). Because of this predictability, it is understood that differential effects of childhood brain injury on the development of cognitive, linguistic, perceptual, attentional, and motor abilities occur at different ages (Boll & Barth, 1981; Luria, 1973; Rourke, 1994; Spreen et al., 1984). The nature, extent, and persistence of a neurodevelopmental learning and/or behavior disorder, therefore, depend on a number of factors, including the developmental stage at which the injury occurred, the significance of the disturbed functional system(s) at that stage of development, and the availability of alternate functional systems to compensate for the impairments incurred (Golden, 1981; Hooper & Boyd, 1986).

In summary, a neuropsychological analysis of developing brain–behavior relationships depends on an understanding of neural development; the development of sensory, motor, cognitive, linguistic, and perceptual systems; and the interaction of developmental trajectories in these domains. An understanding of neuropsychological theory and methodology provides a foundation for the accurate interpretation of behavioral predictions based on structural and functional neuroimaging studies, and this brief overview is provided primarily to aid the reader in gaining such an understanding.

REFERENCES

Barr, M.L., & Kiernan, J.A. (1993). *The human nervous system: An anatomical viewpoint.* Philadelphia: J.B. Lippincott.

Benes, F.M. (in press). Corticolimbic circuitry and the development of psychopathology during childhood and adolescence. In N.A. Krasnegor, G.R. Lyon, & P. Goldman-Rakic (Eds.), *Development of the prefrontal cortex: Evolution, neurobiology, and behavior.* Baltimore: Paul H. Brookes Publishing Co.

Boll, T.J., & Barth, J.T. (1981). Neuropsychology of brain damage in children. In S.B. Filskov & T.J. Boll (Eds.), *Handbook of clinical neuropsychology* (pp. 418–452). New York: John Wiley & Sons.

Broca, P.P. (1865). Sur la siège du faculté de langage articulé. *Bulletin de la Société d'Anthropologie de Paris, 6,* 377–393.

Brodal, P. (1992). *The central nervous system: Structures and function.* New York: Oxford University Press.

Carpenter, M.B. (1978). *Core text of neuroanatomy* (2nd ed.). Baltimore: Williams & Wilkins.

Changeux, J.P., & Danchin, A. (1976). Selective stabilization of developing synapses as a mechanism for the specification of neuronal networks. *Nature, 264,* 705–712.

Chugani, H.T. (1994). Development of regional brain glucose metabolism in relation to behavior and plasticity. In G. Dawson & K.W. Fischer (Eds.), *Human behavior and the developing brain* (pp. 153–175). New York: Guilford Press.

Chugani, H.T. (in press). Neuroimaging of developmental non-linearity and developmental pathologies. In R.W. Thatcher, G.R. Lyon, J. Rumsey, & N.A. Krasnegor (Eds.), *Developmental neuroimaging: Mapping the development of brain and behavior.* New York: Academic Press.

Crelin, E.S. (1974). *Development of the nervous system: Ciba Clinical Symposium No. 26.* Basel, Switzerland: Karger.

Denckla, M.B. (1994). Measurement of executive function. In G.R. Lyon (Ed.), *Frames of reference for the assessment of learning disabilities: New views on measurement issues* (pp. 117–142). Baltimore: Paul H. Brookes Publishing Co.

Denckla, M.B. (1996). A theory and model of executive function: A neuropsychological perspective. In G.R. Lyon & N.A. Krasnegor (Eds.), *Attention, memory, and executive function* (pp. 263–278). Baltimore: Paul H. Brookes Publishing Co.

Denckla, M.B. (in press). Prefrontal-subcortical circuits in developmental disorders. In N.A. Krasnegor, G.R. Lyon, & P. Goldman-Rakic (Eds.), *Development of the prefrontal cortex: Evolution, neurobiology, and behavior.* Baltimore: Paul H. Brookes Publishing Co.

Douglas, V.I. (1983). Attention and cognitive problems. In M. Rutter (Ed.), *Developmental neuropsychiatry* (pp. 280–329). New York: Guilford Press.

Gaddes, W. (1983). Applied educational neuropsychology: Theories and problems. *Journal of Learning Disabilities, 16,* 511–514.

Golden, C.J. (1981). *Diagnosis and rehabilitation in clinical neuropsychology.* Springfield, IL: Charles C Thomas.

Golden, C.J., & Anderson, S. (1979). *Learning disabilities and brain function.* Springfield, IL: Charles C Thomas.

Goldstein, K. (1948). *Language and language disorders.* New York: Grune & Stratton.

Head, H. (1926). *Aphasia and kindred disorders of speech.* London: Cambridge University Press.

Hooper, S.R., & Boyd, T.A. (1986). Neurodevelopmental learning disorders. In J.E. Obrzut & G.W. Hynd (Eds.), *Child neuropsychology: Vol. 2. Clinical practice* (pp. 15–49). New York: Academic Press.

Hooper, S.R., & Willis, W.G. (1989). *Learning disability subtyping: Neuropsychological foundations, conceptual models, and issues in clinical differentiation.* New York: Springer-Verlag.

Hubel, D.H., & Wiesel, T.N. (1963). Visual areas of the lateral suprasylvian cortex of the cat. *Journal of Physiology, 202,* 251–260.

Huttenlocher, P.R. (1979). Synaptic density in human frontal cortex: Developmental changes and effects of aging. *Brain Research, 163,* 195–205.

Huttenlocher, P.R. (1990). Morphometric study of human cerebral cortex development. *Neuropsychologia, 28,* 517–527.

Huttenlocher, P.R. (1994). Synaptogenesis in human cerebral cortex. In G. Dawson & K.W. Fischer (Eds.), *Human behavior and the developing brain* (pp. 137–152). New York: Guilford Press.

Huttenlocher, P.R., & de Courten, C. (1987). The development of synapses in striate cortex of man. *Human Neurobiology, 6,* 1–9.

Hynd, G.W., & Willis, W.G. (1988). *Pediatric neuropathology.* New York: Grune & Stratton.

Isaacson, R.L. (1976). Recovery "?" from early brain damage. In T.D. Tjossem (Ed.), *Intervention strategies for high risk infants and young children* (pp. 21–57). Baltimore: University Park Press.

Jacobson, M. (1978). *Developmental neurobiology* (2nd ed.). New York: Plenum Press.

Kinsbourne, M. (1981). The development of cerebral dominance. In S.B. Filskov & T.J. Boll (Eds.), *Handbook of clinical neuropsychology* (pp. 399–417). New York: John Wiley & Sons.

Lenneberg, E.H. (1967). *The effect of age on the outcome of central nervous system disease in children.* New York: John Wiley & Sons.

Leontiev, A.N. (1959). *Problems in mental development.* Moscow: Nauk Academy of Pedagogy.

Lezak, M.D. (1976). *Neuropsychological assessment.* New York: Oxford University Press.

Luria, A.R. (1947). *Traumatic aphasia.* The Hague, The Netherlands: Mouton.

Luria, A.R. (1965). Neuropsychological analysis of focal brain lesions. In B.B. Wolman (Ed.), *Handbook of child psychology* (pp. 122–174). New York: McGraw-Hill.

Luria, A.R. (1969). The frontal syndrome. In P.J. Vinken & G.W. Bruyn (Eds.), *Handbook of clinical neurology* (pp. 216–292). Amsterdam: North Holland.

Luria, A.R. (1970). The functional organization of the brain. *Scientific American, 222,* 66–78.

Luria, A.R. (1973). *The working brain.* New York: Basic Books.

Luria, A.R. (1980). *Higher cortical functions in man.* New York: Basic Books.

Lyon, G.R., & Krasnegor, N.A. (Eds.). (1996). *Attention, memory, and executive function.* Baltimore: Paul H. Brookes Publishing Co.

Lyon, G.R., Newby, R.E., Recht, D., & Caldwell, J. (1991). Neuropsychology and learning disabilities. In B.Y.L. Wong (Ed.), *Learning about learning disabilities* (pp. 376–407). New York: Academic Press.

Moscovitch, M. (1973). Language and the cerebral hemispheres. In P. Pilner, L. Krames, & T. Alloway (Eds.), *Communication and affect* (pp. 172–211). New York: Academic Press.

Netter, F.H. (1972). *The CIBA collection of medical illustrations: Vol. 1. The nervous system.* Summit, NJ: CIBA.

Obrzut, J.E., & Hynd, G.W. (Eds.). (1986). *Child neuropsychology: Vol. 2. Clinical practice.* New York: Academic Press.

Papez, J.W. (1937). A proposed mechanism of emotion. *Archives of Neurology and Psychiatry, 38,* 725–743.

Passler, M.A., Issac, W., & Hynd, G.W. (1985). Neuropsychological development of behavior attributed to frontal lobe functioning in children. *Developmental Neuropsychology, 1,* 349–370.

Pavlov, I.P. (1949). *Complete collected works.* (6 vols.). Moscow: Nauk Academy of Pedagogy.

Pennington, B.F. (in press). Dimensions of executive functions in normal and abnormal development. In N.A. Krasnegor, G.R. Lyon, & P. Goldman-Rakic (Eds.), *Development of the prefrontal cortex: Evolution, neurobiology, and behavior.* Baltimore: Paul H. Brookes Publishing Co.

Rabinowicz, Y. (1979). The differential maturation of the human cerebral cortex. In F. Falkner & J.M. Tanner (Eds.), *Human growth: Neurobiology and nutrition* (Vol. 3, pp. 97–123). New York: Plenum Press.

Reinis, S., & Goldman, J.M. (1980). *The development of the brain: Biological and functional perspectives.* Springfield, IL: Charles C Thomas.

Rourke, B.P. (1994). Neuropsychological assessment of children with learning disabilities: Measurement issues. In G.R. Lyon (Ed.), *Frames of reference for the assessment of learning disabilities: New views on measurement issues* (pp. 475–509). Baltimore: Paul H. Brookes Publishing Co.

Rourke, B.P., Bakker, D.J., Fisk, J.L., & Strang, J.D. (1983). *Child neuropsychology: An introduction to theory, research, and clinical practice.* New York: Guilford Press.

Rutter, M. (Ed.). (1983). *Developmental neuropsychiatry.* New York: Guilford Press.

Schade, J.P., & van Groenigen, D.B. (1961). Structural organization of the human cerebral cortex. I. Maturation of the middle frontal gyrus. *Acta Anatomica, 47,* 74–111.

Sidman, R.L., & Rakic, P. (1973). Neuronal migration with special reference to developing human brain: A review. *Brain Research, 62,* 1–35.

Spreen, O., Tupper, D., Risser, A., Tuokko, H., & Edgell, D. (1984). *Human developmental neuropsychology.* New York: Oxford University Press.

Stuss, D.T., & Benson, D.F. (1984). Neuropsychological studies of the frontal lobes. *Psychological Bulletin, 95,* 3–28.

Taylor, J. (Ed.). (1958). *Selected writings of John Hughlings Jackson.* New York: Basic Books.

Teeter, P.A. (1986). Standard neuropsychological batteries for children. In J.E. Obrzut & G.W. Hynd (Eds.), *Child neuropsychology: Vol. 2. Clinical practice* (pp. 187–228). New York: Academic Press.

Vygotsky, L.S. (1956). *Selected psychological investigations.* Moscow: Nauk Academy of Pedagogy.

Walsh, K.W. (1978). *Neuropsychology: A clinical approach.* London: Churchill Livingstone.

Wernicke, C. (1874). *Der aphasic Symptomenkomplex.* Berlin: Breslau, Cohn, & Wiegert.

Wilson, H.R. (1988). Development of spatiotemporal mechanisms in infant vision. *Vision Research, 28,* 611–628.

Yakovlev, P.I., & Lecours, A.R. (1967). The telogenetic cycles of regional maturation of the brain. In A. Minkowsky (Ed.), *Regional development of the brain in early life* (pp. 3–70). Oxford, England: Blackwell.

Zentall, S. (1975). Optimal stimulation as theoretical basis of hyperactivity. *American Journal of Orthopsychiatry, 45,* 549–561.

2

A Survey of Functional and Anatomical Neuroimaging Techniques

Jack Krasuski,
Barry Horwitz, and Judith M. Rumsey

Neuroimaging has had a dramatic impact on both clinical medicine and research. New technologies enable clinicians and researchers to acquire high-resolution images of the human brain in a matter of minutes and from a variety of vantage points by using imaging protocols or parameters that maximize chances of seeing the particular sort of pathology in question. These technologies permit us to view both brain structure and brain function, thereby opening endless research possibilities for exploring dysfunctions and disorders in which anatomical correlates are subtle at best, such as developmental disorders and childhood neuropsychiatric disorders.

Although the underlying physics of these techniques may be complex, we hope that clinicians and researchers interested in this important area of neuroimaging of developmental and childhood neuropsychiatric disorders will develop a working knowledge of some technical aspects of these methods. Such an understanding undoubtedly will permit readers of the applied chapters to appreciate more fully the issues that affect interpretations of findings and to evaluate more critically the current and future work in this area. To this end, this chapter describes state-of-the-art neuroimaging techniques, primarily focusing on structural magnetic resonance imaging (MRI), positron emission tomography (PET), single photon emission computed tomography (SPECT), and functional magnetic resonance imaging (fMRI). Computed tomography (CT), because of the radiation exposure it entails, its poorer resolution and contrast, and the likelihood of artifacts caused by bone, has been superseded by MRI as the preferred neuroimaging research tool for studying children and, therefore, is not addressed in this chapter.

In clinical situations, visual inspection of a set of images by a trained physician frequently is sufficient for interpretation and diagnosis, although this is not always the case. Sometimes, images from a single patient taken at different times must be compared. For example, a patient might be scanned before and after treatment for a tumor or at different stages of a degenerative disease. In research settings, images taken from groups of people with different pathologies or taken under different experimental conditions (e.g., at rest, during a memory task) may be compared. In such situations, the differences between images may be too subtle, or the images' signal-to-noise ratios may be too low for subjective readings to suffice. To meet the challenge such situations present, ingenious and elegant statistical image analysis techniques have been developed to localize and quantify differences. Image analysis

The authors thank Monika Krasuski for generating Figures 2.2 and 2.3 and Dr. Cheryl Grady for the use of Figure 2.4. The authors further thank Drs. Wei Huang, Dan Pavel, and Terri Strassberger for providing useful suggestions.

techniques and experimental design considerations, therefore, also are addressed in this chapter.

Each section begins with a brief overview of the method, its significance, and its advantages and disadvantages; this overview is followed by an in-depth discussion of various aspects of image acquisition, experimental design, and data analysis. The principles, promise, and limitations of each of these techniques are presented. Because the functional imaging techniques share many elements of design and methodology that build on PET methods, the section on PET is somewhat extended. For readers who are familiar with these techniques and who may be interested in more technical discussion, a series of footnotes is provided.

PET

PET became available as recently as the 1980s and has improved dramatically in its short life. It remains a research technique primarily for constructing images of brain function by using radioactive isotopes (also known as radionuclides) that are injected into an arm vein. This technique measures a variety of physiological processes, including glucose utilization/metabolism, oxygen utilization, blood flow, and various neurotransmitter concentrations. The isotopes used with PET are positron emitters (e.g., ^{11}C, ^{18}F, ^{15}O, ^{13}N) incorporated into various tracer molecules (e.g., [^{18}F]fluoro-deoxyglucose [FDG], [^{15}O]H_2O). The PET scanner uses a ring of external detectors to measure this radioactivity, and its computers construct images of radioactivity counts emanating from the organ of interest, such as the brain, by using computed tomographic algorithms. Then, a mathematical model is used to transform the information contained in the radioactivity counts collected by the PET scanner into quantitative measures of the physiological process of interest.

Advantages of PET include its ability to yield true quantitative measures of regional cerebral blood flow (rCBF) and glucose metabolism, both of which reflect neuronal activity. Spatial resolution, the ability to discern two objects as separate, is on the order of several millimeters. Temporal resolution, the time period captured in the image, depends on the particular isotope being used. For ^{15}O, used frequently in cognitive studies, temporal resolution is on the order of 15 s to 1 min.

Disadvantages include the fact that PET exposes patients and subjects to low-dose radiation. Although these dosages are considered safe for healthy adult subjects, children are more sensitive to radiation effects, which makes it problematic to study physically healthy children, such as those with learning disabilities and normal control subjects. Furthermore, PET requires a local cyclotron to manufacture radioisotopes, which restricts its availability to a limited number of biomedical research facilities and makes it a relatively expensive technique.

Image Acquisition

Radionuclides

Radionuclides are radioactive isotopes of either elements that are ubiquitous in the body, such as ^{15}O, ^{11}C, or ^{13}N, or replacements for common elements, such as an ^{18}F atom that replaces an H atom in deoxyglucose. Some radionuclides decay by emitting gamma rays directly, and others decay by emitting positrons. PET uses these positron emitters, whereas SPECT uses gamma-ray emitters (see Table 2.1).

Radionuclides are incorporated into tracer molecules to permit the assessment of a physiological parameter. For instance, the radionuclide ^{18}F is incorporated into de-

Table 2.1. Characteristics of functional neuroimaging methods

Method	Radionuclide and tracer	Physiological parameter	Time resolution (min)	Spatial resolution (mm)	Maximum scans per session
Two-dimensional surface imaging	^{133}Xe	rCBF	5–7	25	3
SPECT	^{99}Tc-HMPAO	rCBF	1–2	7	2
	^{99m}Tc-ECD	rCBF	1–2	7	2
	^{133}I-IMP	rCBF	1–2	7	2
	^{133}Xe	rCBF	2	7	3
PET	$[^{15}O]H_2O$	rCBF	0.5–1	5	15+
	$[^{11}C]$2-deoxyglucose	rCMRglu	15–30	5	2
	$[^{18}F]$FDG	rCMRglu	15–30	5	1
fMRI	Blood oxygen	Primarily rCBF	<1 s	2	100+

oxyglucose, forming [^{18}F]FDG, to permit the measurement of brain glucose metabolism. The fluorine isotope is used because it does not interfere with the physiological function of deoxyglucose, a glucose substitute. Deoxyglucose is useful as a substitute because, unlike glucose, it ceases in its metabolic path after the first metabolic step (phosphorylation), at which point it accumulates in the brain, permitting its measurement over the lengthy period of time that ^{18}F remains radioactive. Another common radionuclide used in PET is ^{15}O, which is incorporated into water and used to measure blood flow through the brain.

When positron-emitting radionuclides decay, they emit from the nucleus a positron, which has the mass of an electron and a positive electrical charge. The positron travels an average distance of 2 mm before striking an electron; this distance is known as the positron range.[1] When the positron collides with an electron, both particles are annihilated, and their combined mass is transformed into a pair of high-energy (511 thousand electron volts [keV]) gamma rays, referred to as photons. Although the event of interest is the radioactive decay, which fixes in space the positron of the radionuclide, only the annihilation event can be detected, thereby introducing a physical limitation on spatial resolution. Were the colliding positron and electron both at rest (an impossibility), the photons would be emitted at exactly 180° relative to each other.[2] Because the particles are in motion, however, the photons' flight only approximates a straight line. The deviation from a straight line places a second physical limitation on spatial resolution. The two photons rush away from each other at the speed of light and strike opposing detectors; the annihilation event, therefore, occurs somewhere along this coincidence line.[3]

[1]Positrons from different radionuclides have different energy levels and, as a result, different positron ranges: The higher the energy level, the farther the positron tends to travel before annihilation.

[2]The higher the particles' kinetic energy, the more the angle of flight differs from 180°. The positron usually has lost most of its kinetic energy before it strikes an electron, and, therefore, the photons' flight approximates a straight line.

[3]Rather than being strictly localized in space by the detector pair, the position of each coincidence event is characterized as a probability distribution described in a line spread function. The spatial resolution of the scanner is the distance at which two sources of radioactivity can be

In the most commonly used PET scanners, information regarding the position of the annihilation event along the coincidence line is absent.[4] Constructing a three-dimensional image from information limited in this way presents a significant problem. One widely used solution, adapted from X-ray CT, is filtered back-projection. Coincidence lines from each image are segregated into parallel groups to form profiles of radioactivity detected at different angles. Then, these profiles are combined to form a tomographic image (Herscovitch, 1988). A tomograph is an image slice through an organ—unlike a chest X ray, for instance, which images all of the tissues through which the X-rays penetrate.

PET Scanners

PET scanners for neuroimaging applications contain arrays of gamma-ray detectors, which are positioned around the subject's head; these are designed to acquire information concerning the spatial location of the annihilation events. The most common arrangement consists of rings of detectors placed serially next to one another in the axial plane (see Figure 2.1). Each detector interacts electronically with other detectors within its field of view to detect a photon pair that arrives within a short time frame, called the coincidence resolving time (usually 5–20 ns), which indicates a true annihilation event.[5] The detectors are scintillation crystals (i.e., light-emitting crystals) of sodium iodide or bismuth germinate that convert the energy of the gamma-ray photons into lower-energy photons. The lower size limit of the crystals places a third and final limitation on spatial resolution. Scintillation crystals are coupled to photomultiplier tubes that amplify the emitted light.

Spatial Resolution

The spatial resolution of the scanner is the distance at which two sources of radioactivity can be discerned as separate. A scanner's actual spatial resolution always is less than the theoretical spatial resolution imposed by the physics of the annihilation event and the size of the detectors (i.e., the three above-described physical limitations) be-

---

discerned as separate and is expressed in terms of this line spread function as equal to the full width at half maximum (FWHM) of this distribution. Finite spatial resolution results in blurring and partial volume effects. For small structures (i.e., those less than two times the FWHM of the line spread function), averaging occurs between the radioactivity concentration of the structure and surrounding tissue.

[4]One might surmise that knowing the speed at which the photons travel (i.e., the speed of light) and the time interval between detection of the photons, one could calculate the position of the annihilation event along the coincidence line. This generally is not so, however. Scanners are being developed that take the difference in arrival time of the photon pair into account; these so-called time-of-flight scanners are capable, based on their timing resolution, of placing the annihilation event within a radius of 9 cm from the center (Ter-Pogossian et al., 1982). This may seem to be a useless accomplishment, but even this degree of fixing of position allows tomographic reconstruction algorithms to improve signal-to-noise ratios (Politte, 1990).

[5]There are major differences in PET scanner designs and settings. In traditional PET scanners, called two-dimensional scanners, lead septa separate detector rings. This limits axial field of view (FOV) to the single ring adjacent to either side. Three-dimensional PET scanners permit retraction (removal) of these septa, which allows the FOV to be expanded axially over several rings. Although this increases sensitivity (i.e., detected events divided by all events), it also dramatically increases detection of false coincidences: The probability of true coincidences increases linearly with increase of radioactivity, whereas that of accidental coincidences, one source of false coincidences, increases with the square of radioactivity (Townsend et al., 1991). Nevertheless, the increase in sensitivity, by permitting lower radiation doses, justifies the use and further development of three-dimensional scanners.

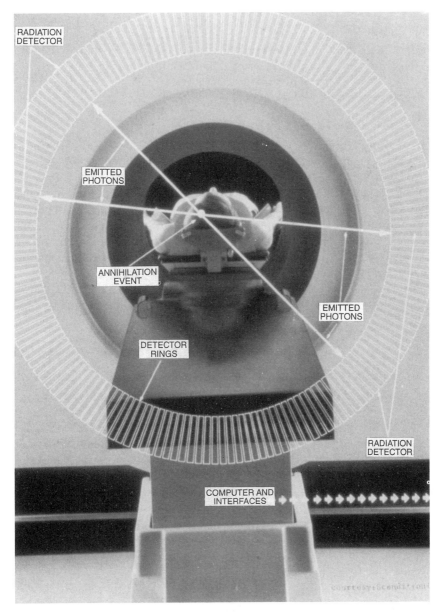

Figure 2.1. View of a PET scanner. Superimposed on the photograph is a schematic representation of an annihilation event, two pairs of emitted photons, and rings of detectors that are located in the scanner housing.

cause of additional sources of limitation. Finite spatial resolution results in blurring and partial volume effects. For small structures, averaging occurs between the radioactivity concentration of the structure and surrounding tissue. As a result, to obtain accurate functional measures in disease conditions that result in the shrinkage of brain structures, a correction for change in the structure's volume is required. For example, in patients who have diseases involving degeneration of the caudate nuclei, regions containing the nuclei may appear to be hypometabolic on PET as compared with those in control subjects, because the nuclei are surrounded by much less metabolically active white matter, the metabolism of which is averaged with the metabolism of the nuclei. The remaining tissue of the diseased, smaller caudate nuclei may or may not be as metabolically active as that of healthy caudate nuclei. Without correcting for size, this distinction cannot be made (Hayden et al., 1986).

Correcting for Sources of Error

As highlighted in Figure 2.2, failing to count true coincidences and counting false coincidences result in error. One source of lost coincidences, on which we focus because of its direct bearing on the study of special populations, is attenuation, the loss of true coincidences through tissue absorption.[6] Corrections for attenuation can be estimated on the basis of published normative data (calculated attenuation correction) or measured for each individual at the time of the PET scan (measured attenuation correction).[7] For individuals who belong to special populations, a measured correction is preferred because their cranial characteristics (e.g., thinner skulls, smaller brains), as in the case of patients with Down syndrome, may differ from those of the population on which calculated attenuation coefficient norms were based. An in-depth discussion of radioactivity quantification was presented by Hoffman and Phelps (1986).

Transforming Radioactivity Counts into Measures of Biological Function

Tracer Kinetics

Kinetic tracer models are mathematical models that transform radioactivity counts into measures of the physiological parameter of interest (e.g., cerebral glucose metabolism, blood flow). These models are simplified quantitative descriptions of the physiological behavior of tracer molecules in the brain. Several factors must be established for model development: the amount of radiotracer available in the blood for uptake during the period of scanning, formalized as the input function; the uptake and distribution of the tracer in the organ of interest, for example, the brain; the rate at which the tracer serves as a substrate in metabolic pathways; and the washout from and redistribution in the brain of the tracer throughout the course of scan acquisition.

For example, to transform radioactivity counts into regional cerebral metabolic rates of glucose utilization (rCMRglu), Sokoloff et al. (1977) devised a three-compart-

---

[6]Attenuation of a photon pair is constant anywhere along a coincidence line and is proportional to the photon pair's combined distance of travel through matter for the following reason: Because both photons must reach their detectors for a coincidence event to occur, the combined risk for the two photons remains constant. As risk increases for one, it decreases for the other. Attenuation, however, differs along different coincident lines. For instance, a photon pair has a higher probability of attenuation when traveling through the central portion of the cranium than when traveling through the vertex, which contains less tissue. Therefore, an attenuation coefficient is established individually for each detector pair.

[7]When a calculated attenuation correction is used, an elliptical outline is matched to the shape of the subject's head, and attenuation coefficients, derived from previous work, are set based on the thickness of tissue between each detector pair. When a measured attenuation correction is used, a transmission scan is obtained for each individual by using either a ring source of radioactivity or a point source that circles the head. Because the amount of radioactivity from the source is known, one can measure the degree to which it has been attenuated by the subject's head. Because the transmitted photon's traveled distance equals the combined traveled distance of the emitted photon pair, the attenuation measured by the transmitted photon equals the attenuation for the actual PET scan.

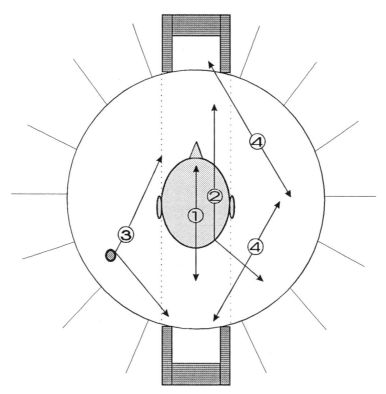

Figure 2.2.   Sources of error in PET scanning. Axial rings of detectors surround
the subject's head as represented by a single pair of detectors in a single ring
(not drawn to scale). The dashed lines represent the detector pair's field of view.
The numbered circles represent annihilation events that release paired photons. The photon pair of annihilation event 1 is correctly detected. The photons
of event 2 are not detected as a result of scatter of one of the photons. Interaction of a photon with an electron in intervening tissue causes, among other effects, deflection of the photon from its straight path (Compton scattering). The
photons of event 3 are falsely detected as a result of scatter of one of the photons
by interaction with tissue (represented by the unnumbered circle), causing mis-
placement of the annihilation event into this detector pair's field of view. The photons of two annihilation events (represented by 4) are falsely detected as a result
of the two photons arriving at this detector pair during the coincidence-resolving
time, despite the fact that the photons are from separate annihilation events.

ment model of tracer distribution for deoxyglucose, a glucose substitute, that addresses each of the above-mentioned factors.[8] This model was later adapted for PET by
labeling deoxyglucose with radioactive fluorine, thereby forming FDG (Huang et al.,
1980; Phelps et al., 1979; Reivich et al., 1979). The tracer kinetic model for $[^{15}O]H_2O$
studies of rCBF is simpler. Because the tracer is not metabolized and $[^{15}O]H_2O$ is freely
diffusible, a single-compartment physiological model is sufficient (Herscovitch et al.,
1983; Kety, 1951).

---

[8]The 2-deoxyglucose is distributed in plasma (compartment 1), in the free deoxyglucose
precursor pool (compartment 2), and in the phosphorylated pool (compartment 3). Rate con-
stants were established for tracer movement into and out of each compartment, and an additional constant, the lump constant, was derived to account for differences in the distribution and
metabolism of deoxyglucose, the analog, and glucose, the substrate of interest. Then, a formula
relating these factors was constructed.

The above-described tracer kinetic models transform regional radioactivity counts provided by the PET scanner into absolute, quantitative measures of rCMRglu or rCBF. Because this transformation requires an input function that indicates the amount of radiotracer available for uptake into the brain, arterial blood sampling is required. However, the primary interest may lie in relative, rather than absolute, regional activity and in differences in this relative activity across groups or tasks. In such situations, radioactivity counts may be analyzed directly without being transformed into measures of rCMRglu or rCBF, thereby eliminating the need for arterial (or arterialized venous) blood sampling and making the PET procedure less invasive and more comfortable.[9]

Relationship of rCMRglu and rCBF to Underlying Neuronal Activity

Although numerous activation studies show that both rCMRglu and rCBF increase in response to cognitive tasks, the mechanism underlying these changes remains unclear. More than a century ago, Roy and Sherrington (1890) proposed the homeostasis hypothesis. The updated hypothesis states that neuronal activity, by diminishing ionic gradients, leads to increases in metabolism that are needed to restore the gradients, which, in turn, lead to increases in blood flow to provide the necessary energy sources—oxygen and glucose (Mata et al., 1980). The mediating factors were hypothesized to be products of metabolism that altered blood flow in regions of increased neuronal activity. Lou et al. (1987) found, however, that ions and metabolites released by neuronal activity do not accumulate in the short time necessary for them to serve as mediating factors. Dynamic regulation, therefore, has been proposed: The brain may regulate blood flow by actively releasing mediator substances (Collins, 1987; Lou et al., 1987). One promising candidate as a mediator substance is nitric oxide, which, because of its ubiquity, rapid diffusion, high chemical reactivity, and known role as a vasodilator, meets the temporal and physiological constraints of change in blood flow as a function of neuronal activity (Gally et al., 1990; Iadecola, 1993). In 1994, however, studies by Iadecola et al. showed conflicting results regarding the role of nitric oxide, and, so, the search for a mediator substance continues.

An unwarranted inference that hypometabolism in a region reflects neuronal inhibition sometimes is made. Inhibition may be as energy demanding as activation, and, therefore, inhibited regions are as likely to be hypermetabolic as hypometabolic (Ackermann et al., 1984). If the energy expended to maintain a hyperpolarized postsynaptic membrane is greater than that saved as a result of inhibited output, the inhibited region will be hypermetabolic. The occurrence of hypometabolism is more consistent with a region receiving low total input, either excitatory or inhibitory (the hypothesis of Ackermann et al., 1984). This condition and the following discussions are, with minor variations, applicable to SPECT as well as to PET.

Coupling of Metabolism and Blood Flow

rCMRglu and rCBF appear to be closely coupled under both resting and task conditions (Baron et al., 1984; Sokoloff, 1981). For instance, Fox and Raichle (1986) found that, when somatosensory stimulation was used, both rCMRglu and rCBF increased

---

[9]Because, with the rCBF tracers used in PET, the radioactivity to rCBF function is approximately linear across a wide range of values (Herscovitch et al., 1983), a nearly constant proportional relationship between radioactivity counts and rCBF values is maintained. This proportional relationship permits the use of ratios of regional-to-global (whole brain) radioactivity counts as a good approximation of rCBF.

by more than 50% over resting states. The relationship of regional cerebral metabolism of oxygen (rCMRO$_2$) to rCBF is more complex. Although, under resting conditions, the coupling of oxidative metabolism to blood flow is excellent, this may not be the case when stimulation is present. When somatosensory stimulation was used, rCMRO$_2$ increased by only 5%, whereas rCBF increased by 29% (Fox & Raichle, 1986). Ackermann and Lear (1989) hypothesized, and confirmed with experiments in rats, that rCMRglu and rCBF increase dramatically with activation, but rCMRO$_2$ does not, because glucose undergoes significant nonoxidative metabolism in the brain, which is an inefficient path for releasing energy for useful work and results in the formation of lactate. Only later, when oxygen is plentiful, is the glucose re-formed from lactate and metabolized oxidatively.

Experimental Design

Resting Studies

When PET was in its infancy, most subjects were studied at rest; studies varied as to whether subjects' eyes were covered or uncovered and whether their ears were plugged or unplugged, but, uniformly, the room was quiet and darkened to minimize sensory stimulation. Groups of normal subjects were compared (e.g., men versus women, young versus old), and patient groups (e.g., Down syndrome, Alzheimer's disease) were compared with control groups. Although resting studies are a useful preliminary method, many PET studies now use cognitive tasks and/or pharmacological challenges to better appreciate the function and dysfunction of various brain regions and their interactions in complex networks. These brain regions and their interactions may not be active in resting conditions.

Cognitive Challenge

A cognitive challenge presumes several abilities. Subjects must have the cognitive resources to understand instructions and perform tasks adequately and the motivation to persevere throughout the task. For individuals with cognitive limitations, tasks that are minimally demanding must be presented. For example, in the Laboratory of Neurosciences, National Institute on Aging, National Institutes of Health, Bethesda, Maryland, visual pattern stimuli that demand only a minimum of attention and no effortful processing are presented to subjects with mental retardation and dementia (Mentis et al., 1996).

Tasks should be simple enough or the cognitive processing steps delineated thoroughly enough to support a reasonable expectation that subjects will use homogeneous cognitive strategies. For instance, in musical representation, subjects may use audiological representations of successive pitches, visual representations of musical notes, or kinesthetic representations of patterned limb movements that correspond to playing a particular instrument (Sergent, 1993). In studying tasks for which multiple strategies may be used, limiting a sample to individuals with similar musical backgrounds or skill levels and/or specifying and rehearsing specific approaches may limit the use of heterogeneous strategies.

In most paradigms, tasks must be performed over an adequate percentage of the total time of radiotracer uptake into the brain. This can be as short as 40 s for rCBF studies or as long as 30–45 min for rCMRglu studies. The change in a physiological parameter is influenced by the time taken to perform the task. A task that is brief relative to the uptake period may be repeated throughout the uptake period.

New approaches may, however, obviate this need for repetition. One group of investigators reported that the ability to discern regional brain activations with cognitive tasks of short duration centered on the time of the radiotracer's arrival to the brain (Hurtig et al., 1994). Another approach permits imaging mental events that are of short duration *and* occur randomly, such as hallucinations (Silbersweig et al., 1993; Silbersweig et al., 1994). In this paradigm, the subject signals the duration of the mental event by pressing a button for its entirety. With the use of differential equations, a score is calculated for each scan on the basis of the amount of radioactivity entering the brain during the mental event, thereby reflecting the contribution of the event to the image. A statistical analysis is then performed to identify those pixels in which the intensity covaries with the scan scores over a subject's scans (Silbersweig et al., 1994).

Task performance should be evaluated. In many instances, an objective, item-by-item measure of performance is possible. Subjects may, for example, push a button to indicate their response or read aloud. In cognitive challenge experiments that lack observable behavior responses and instead have strictly internal responses (e.g., thinking sad thoughts [Pardo et al., 1990]), task compliance through postexperimental self-ratings should be ascertained. The criticism remains that there is no external validator of the mental activity. Although they are impossible to address directly, physiological parameters, such as heart rate or galvanic skin response, may provide indirect validation of a subject's mental state or reactivity.

Pharmacological Challenge

Pharmacological agents may be used in conjunction with cognitive tasks to assess the effects of medications on overall activity and on specific task-related activity. The use of appropriate experimental designs that systematically alter both pharmacological and cognitive challenges permits the evaluation of interactions of such variables (Frackowiak & Friston, 1994). For example, the effects of a drug on memory performance may be determined by the systemic evaluation of the effects of the drug and of the memory task separately and in combination (Grasby, Friston, Bench, Cowen, et al., 1992; Grasby, Friston, Bench, Frith, et al., 1992).

Categorical versus Parametric Design

In categorical activation studies, a single categorical variable (e.g., doing versus not doing a cognitive task) is manipulated (Frackowiak & Friston, 1994). When images from the two conditions (doing versus not doing a task) are compared, the differences seen are presumed to reflect only the influence of the categorical variable (for a discussion of the problems with this assumption, see Horwitz, 1994). When a complex task (e.g., a complex language task demanding focused attention, reading, verbal generation, changes in categorical set, signaling with button presses) is compared with a resting state, it is not clear which variables or mental operations account for the differences in images. As a result, as experimental designs associated with brain imaging have become more sophisticated, the challenge has focused on methods for fractionating tasks into individual components that can be manipulated systematically one at a time (Posner et al., 1988).

Parametric designs manipulate a single variable along a quantitative continuum, so that task difficulty, medication blood level, or some other variable is studied at different levels in the same experiment (Frackowiak & Friston, 1994; Haxby et al., 1991;

Haxby et al., 1995). A mathematical function relating brain activation—as approximated by radioactivity counts transformed into rCMRglu or rCBF—to changes across values of this variable can then be constructed and displayed graphically.

Image Analysis

In this section, statistical image analysis techniques, a dynamic area of development in functional neuroimaging, are discussed. These techniques permit the quantification of changes in physiological parameters across groups of images. Image analysis consists of multiple steps involving preprocessing and data analysis. Preprocessing involves the preparation of data for analysis of change across the variable(s) of interest by normalizing extraneous or confounding variables, such as differences in brain shape or global blood flows in different individuals, to the same value across scans. Data analysis comprises the steps taken to localize and quantify remaining differences.

Global versus Regional Differences

Not only is rCBF coupled to local neuronal activity, it also is affected by global (whole brain) cerebral blood flow (gCBF) (Ramsay et al., 1993), which, in turn, is affected by changes in perfusion pressure and autoregulation that are dependent on factors extraneous to cognitive tasks, such as anxiety level and environmental condition.[10] Even within individuals, gCBF changes across time can be substantial (Bartlett et al., 1988). Through effects on gCBF, rCBF, therefore, is affected by factors other than that of primary interest, the local neuronal activation. To accurately measure changes in local neuronal activity, therefore, the confounding effects of gCBF must be factored out. A study of different methods for correcting rCBF for differences in gCBF in healthy subjects found great comparability in the answers the various methods yielded (McIntosh et al., 1995).[11]

Single-Subject versus Group Analysis

Single-subject analysis refers to the comparison of images from one individual under different experimental conditions, whereas group analysis refers to the comparison of images between groups of subjects with different characteristics (e.g., young versus old, men versus women) or different conditions or illnesses (e.g., children with autism versus normal control subjects) or between matched groups of subjects scanned under different experimental conditions (e.g., language task versus control task). In both analysis approaches, images from each experimental condition or group often are averaged.

Until the 1990s, PET studies were group studies. The enormous number of data points involved—each complete brain scan has 60,000 or more pixels—required a minimum of 6–20 subjects for a two-condition design to permit valid statistical comparison. New high-sensitivity scanners, coupled with short half-life isotopes (e.g., ^{15}O has a half-life of 2 min), have made single-subject analysis possible by enabling a researcher to take many (i.e., 15–30) scans of a single individual in closely spaced ses-

---

[10]Perfusion pressure and autoregulation are themselves affected by factors such as partial pressure of carbon dioxide (PCO_2) in capillaries and perivascular spaces, H^+ ion concentration, and cerebral tissue partial pressure of O_2 (Ramsay et al., 1993).

[11]The types of normalization of rCBF to gCBF include the following: ratio adjustments, in which each individual's rCBF is divided by that individual's gCBF; analyses of covariance based on a regression model; and transformation of each individual's pixel activity counts into within-subject z-scores (McIntosh et al., 1995).

sions. (The preprocessing steps described below permit image preparation for data analysis for both single-subject and group analysis approaches.)

What are the benefits of single-subject analysis? One benefit is that the issue of variability of brain damage among subjects who have diseases is eliminated (Frackowiak & Friston, 1994). A clear example of this issue is the variability in the perimeters of lesions caused by stroke. In cognitive studies of healthy individuals, variability in neuroanatomy (e.g., sulcal/gyral patterns), cognitive strategies, and brain function among subjects is avoided when single-subject analysis is used (Frackowiak & Friston, 1994; Steinmetz & Seitz, 1991).

Preprocessing

Preparation of data for analysis involves the following steps: 1) data normalization, 2) anatomical localization, and 3) combining data within and across subjects. These steps and their components are grouped conceptually and are not in mandatory order; although certain components have prerequisites, many are logically and mathematically independent.

Data Normalization   Because different PET scanners provide different numbers of image slices, images may be interpolated mathematically to provide a standard number of image slices for comparison with published brain atlases. Individual image slices are registered, or aligned, to one another to provide a well-formed three-dimensional brain. Roll-yaw corrections are then applied to align the now–well-formed brains in three-dimensional space relative to a standardized brain atlas. Regional values are corrected, or normalized, relative to gCBF. These steps are performed for both pixel-by-pixel and region-of-interest (ROI) approaches. However, in a pixel-by-pixel approach, an extra step is necessary: Data are smoothed, by averaging to a small number of surrounding pixels, to increase the signal-to-noise ratio and to decrease the influence of variable gyral/sulcal patterns across subjects.

Anatomical Localization   Anatomical localization differs depending on the image analysis method chosen. The underlying task is to define homologous brain regions across scans; this task is more difficult in multiple subject analysis because of the variability among individual brains. The ROI method entails defining regions on the PET image (image ROI) that correspond to brain anatomy (anatomical ROIs). For example, if a researcher is interested in blood flow to the caudate nuclei, he or she would attempt to place an image ROI, which usually is a small circle between 0.5 and 1.5 cm in diameter that defines this ROI, on the caudate nuclei to measure activity in that structure. Limited resolution may make it difficult to accurately and precisely identify anatomy, particularly in small structures such as caudate nuclei. Methods for anatomical localization, therefore, are necessary, and, in ROI analysis, the best method for localization is to register the PET image (a low-resolution functional image) to a higher-resolution anatomical image, such as an MRI of the brain. One then can more accurately define the boundaries of the structures on the PET image. However, even when MRI is used for localization, a major problem is the systematic identification of well-defined landmarks in the neocortex.

In the pixel-by-pixel approach, each pixel may be viewed as a tiny ROI.[12] To over-

---

[12]A pixel is the smallest discrete unit of value on an image. Because it is a term for a two-dimensional object, its use in this context is incorrect. Each pixel represents the radioactivity counts — or, in transformed images, physiological values — of a three-dimensional brain region. The correct term in this case is voxel, which is a three-dimensional object (i.e., a pixel with depth).

come normal variability in brain anatomy and ensure that each pixel represents the same anatomical region in each brain, individual images are warped (i.e., stereotactically normalized), or made to conform to a standardized brain space, before statistical tests are performed (Friston et al., 1991b; Mintun et al., 1989).[13] The assumption is that, after individual scans from different individuals are stereotactically normalized (and smoothed), each pixel across scans will represent homologous brain space. This assumption seems to be reasonably well founded for PET and SPECT data, except in severely atrophied or otherwise misshapen brains, because of the limited spatial resolution of these techniques. This assumption presents a greater problem for fMRI.

Combining Data within and across Subjects   After preprocessing, with each pixel or ROI across subjects now representing the same brain region, the scans in each experimental group are averaged. Then data analysis through subtraction or correlational techniques can be performed as described below.

Data Analysis

How is the method of analysis chosen? Subtraction techniques statistically assess the difference in activity in each pixel or ROI in one group or condition from the activity in homologous pixels or ROIs from another group or condition (Friston et al., 1991a). These techniques are useful in localizing neural activation. They also are useful in categorical experimental designs in which one wishes to localize the differential activation between control and experimental tasks (Horwitz & Sporns, 1994).

Most cognitive tasks, however, are presumed to activate anatomically distributed networks in complex ways. In such situations, subtraction techniques may be insufficient. Suppose brain region A is active in both a control and an experimental task. In these two tasks, region A may function as a component of different networks, playing different functional roles. By analogy, region B may be inactivated in both a control and an experimental task, but it may be inhibited by input from different nerve tracts. In both cases, simple subtraction analysis would not indicate the differential response of these regions to the two tasks (Horwitz, 1990; Horwitz & Sporns, 1994). To address these issues, covariance techniques that enable researchers to determine under which conditions individual brain regions may interact with other regions have been developed (Horwitz et al., 1992). In brief, covariance analysis permits a researcher to ascertain which distributed groups of pixels or ROIs act in concert, thereby suggesting a neuronal interaction between these brain regions. Covariance analysis demonstrates differences in the patterns of correlations in regions A and B under different conditions even when the values of the regions remain constant across these conditions.

To glean more and more information from the potentially vast store contained in functional neuroimages, researchers are developing approaches that combine the correlational analysis of data present within the images with that of data derived from other sources (e.g., anatomical data). For example, McIntosh and Gonzalez-Lima (1992) adapted a computational technique from genetics and the social sciences, called path analysis, that enables evaluation of the functional associations among multiple components of the brain. Path analysis combines anatomical data of the location of nodes and paths of a hypothesized network with the radioactivity counts of the nodes

---

[13]In a single-subject analysis, this step may be unnecessary because a single brain is being studied. However, when anatomical brain images are not available for localization, one still may stereotactically normalize to permit anatomical localization by assessing location in a standardized brain space. In addition, one may wish to relate one's results to results obtained by other investigators by using stereotactic coordinates as a common coordinate system.

(i.e., ROIs on the PET scan) that are obtained from a functional neuroimage, simultaneously quantifying the weights of a network's multiple internal connections during the particular cognitive task being studied (McIntosh et al., 1994).[14]

SPECT

In SPECT, radioisotopes decay by emitting a single gamma ray. Differences from PET in scanner design and functional capabilities correspond to this crucial difference. Although SPECT first became available in the 1980s, not until the early 1990s did improved instrumentation make this technique attractive for brain imaging.

The principal isotopes used with SPECT allow for measurements of rCBF. The long half-lives of the radioisotopes used in SPECT obviate the need for an on-site cyclotron or access to a radiochemistry laboratory. SPECT scanning, therefore, is less expensive and more widely available than is PET and yields nearly equal spatial and temporal resolution. Procedures for quantifying blood flow, however, are not well standardized, and, on a practical level, normative data frequently are inadequate.

Radioisotopes and Radiopharmaceuticals

The radioisotopes used in SPECT emit single photons that have lower energy than do the photons released during the positron/electron annihilation in PET. For instance, in SPECT, ^{99m}Tc emits a photon of 140 keV (compared to the two 511 keV photons released during positron annihilation in PET). Lower energy results in greater attenuation (lower sensitivity), which can be compensated for by scans of longer duration. More critical (and not easily compensated for) is that attenuation differs as a function of the distance that the photons travel through tissue. The deeper in the brain the isotope decays, the greater the attenuation. Deeper structures, therefore, may give artifactually low radioactivity counts. This dependence of attenuation on depth within tissue makes difficult the absolute quantification of physiological parameters (Gilardi et al., 1988).

The first radioisotope used in SPECT was ^{133}Xe, an inert, freely diffusible isotope that previously had been used in a nontomographic technique for measuring cortical blood flow by using a detector array fitted to the surface of a subject's head to form a two-dimensional image. Because ^{133}Xe, an inert gas, rapidly clears from the brain, multiple scans can be performed in the same session under differing experimental conditions. The low-energy photon (80 keV) emitted by ^{133}Xe results in high attenuation and scatter and thereby produces an image with relatively poor spatial resolution (Ring et al., 1991). Subsequently, other labeled radiopharmaceutical molecules were introduced, and the radioisotopes ^{123}I and ^{99m}Tc were used.

Radiopharmaceuticals, also called tracers, are molecules into which radioisotopes are incorporated. To accurately reflect rCBF, they must cross the blood–brain barrier easily, distribute proportionally to rCBF, remain trapped in the brain for sufficient lengths of time to allow scanning, and permit labeling with radioisotopes such as ^{123}I

---

[14]The stress on functional networks highlights the power of this technique: Changes in the network's connections can be analyzed as a function of sequentially and systematically altered experimental conditions. One set of theories of brain function postulates the distributed parallel nature of information processing (Farah, 1994; Mesulam, 1990). A corollary of these theories is that a change in experimental task would be expected to result in a change in interactions, not only in an isolated piece of the network, but in the entire network (Horwitz et al., 1992). Path analysis is particularly well suited to such analyses of entire networks.

or ^{99m}Tc (Holman & Devous, 1992). [^{123}I]isopropyl iodoamphetamine (IMP) (removed from the U.S. market in 1992), ^{99m}Tc-hexamethyl-propyleneamine oxime (HMPAO), and ^{99m}Tc-ethyl cysteinate dimer (ECD) are rCBF tracers.[15]

SPECT Scanners

In SPECT, as in PET, scintillation crystal arrays detect radioactivity. Because only single photons are released in SPECT, and because these travel in all directions (i.e., isotropically), their points of origin in space can be ascertained only with use of collimators. These collimators usually are made of lead septa and are placed in front of the crystal arrays that make up the camera to limit photon detection to photons traveling nearly perpendicular to the camera surface. Photons traveling at an obtuse angle strike the lead septa and are absorbed. Each square of detector surface, therefore, has a field of view that is restricted to a narrow pyramidal volume directly in front of it.

Although collimators are necessary to localize the source of radioactivity, they also are one of the main causes of nondetection of emitted photons. Collimators that emphasize resolution are even less sensitive because resolution and sensitivity are inversely related. (See Figure 2.2 for a review of sources of loss of sensitivity and resolution in SPECT.) Multiple head cameras were introduced into routine use in the 1990s. The detectors rotate around a patient's head, and the resultant SPECT images have significantly improved sensitivity and resolution (Links, 1993). Resolution also varies inversely with the distance of emission to the detector surface (see Figure 2.3). Deep brain structures (e.g., basal ganglia), therefore, because they are farthest from a rotating camera, are more poorly resolved than are cortical regions (Bushberg, 1994).

Brain Studies with SPECT

Although the long half-lives of ^{99m}Tc and ^{123}I and the slow washouts of [^{123}I]IMP, ^{99m}Tc-HMPAO, and ^{99m}Tc-ECD from the brain add to the convenience of scheduling and use of SPECT scanning, these factors diminish study design flexibility in other ways. In general, subjects' brains should not be rescanned until radiopharmaceutical washout and radioisotope decay are nearly complete (i.e., not until the next day). Although same-day test/retest protocols are available, they assume an equal rate of washout for all brain regions (Holm et al., 1994). Because this condition is not always met, especially when [^{123}I]IMP or ^{99m}Tc-ECD is used (Moretti et al., 1995), same-day multiple scanning could introduce error. Group designs in which each subject in the experimental group is scanned once and the mean of the experimental group is compared

---

[15]The strengths of ^{123}I-labeled IMP are its high extraction ratio and kinetics that maintain a nearly linear relationship between radioactivity counts and rCBF, thereby allowing for quantitative rCBF measurements (Moretti et al., 1995). Its weaknesses include fairly quick redistribution within the brain, which necessitates scanning within 60 min post-injection (Nishizawa et al., 1989; Rapin et al., 1983), and prelabeling with ^{123}I by the manufacturer, which decreases flexibility in scheduling emergent scans (Holman & Devous, 1992). The strengths of ^{99m}Tc-HMPAO are fast uptake and slow washout (approximately 2% per hour) from the brain, which permit scanning over a long time period after injection. It is unstable in vitro and is synthesized on site. The need for highly trained personnel for on-site labeling is balanced by the ability to produce labeled radiopharmaceutical emergently. Its drawbacks include a lower extraction ratio, which leads to underestimation of rCBF. ^{99m}Tc-ECD is stable in vitro, which allows for prelabeling, perhaps during regular working hours. Brain extraction and blood clearance are rapid, leading to a higher brain-to-background radioactivity ratio. Its drawbacks include the fact that only moderate brain extraction is possible, again leading to perfusion underestimation (Holman & Devous, 1992). In activation studies in which rCBF increases, ^{99m}Tc-HMPAO and ^{99m}Tc-ECD may underestimate high-flow regions (Moretti et al., 1995).

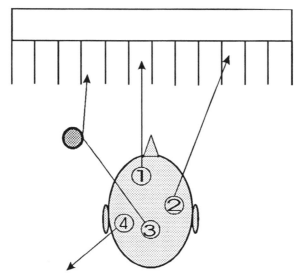

Figure 2.3.   Sources of error in SPECT scanning. A collimator is placed on the surface of the camera, as represented by the parallel lines (not drawn to scale). The numbered circles represent radioactive decay events with the release of a single photon. The photon of event 1 is correctly detected. The photon of event 2 is incorrectly detected as a result of its penetration of a collimator septum. The photon of event 3 is incorrectly detected as a result of scatter caused by interaction with tissue (as represented by the unnumbered circle). The photon of event 4 travels away from the camera and is not detected.

with that of a control group, therefore, are the norm. (For a review of SPECT activation methods, see Ring et al., 1991.)

An innovative technique, called dual-isotope imaging, may permit a group of subjects to serve as their own controls by undergoing two back-to-back scans in which different isotopes are used for each scan. Different radioisotopes release photons with different energy peaks, just as different colors of visible light are made up of photons of different energy levels. This approach can be used, for example, to assess vascular brain reserves (to evaluate for risk of stroke): ^{99m}Tc-HMPAO is injected into subjects, followed by pharmacological vasodilation of brain vessels with acetazolamide, and, finally, by injection of [^{123}I]IMP. Certain high-resolution, multidetector SPECT cameras, which can separate the energy peaks of the two isotopes, can then be used to obtain two images, one of ^{99m}Tc-HMPAO, which shows resting rCBF, and one of [^{123}I]IMP, which shows rCBF after vasodilation. Those regions that do not show increased blood flow in the postvasodilation scan are presumed to be supplied by vessels with no reserve capacity to increase flow (Devous, 1995). Dual-isotope imaging probably is too insensitive, however, to be used for cognitive experiments.

The SPECT radiopharmaceuticals permit absolute quantification of rCBF.[16] Frequently, however, just as in PET, radioactivity counts are not transformed into absolute

[16]As in PET, this requires kinetic tracer models, which calls for establishing an input function through arterial blood sampling, correcting for incomplete radiotracer extraction into the brain, diffusion back into the bloodstream, and radionuclide decay. As in PET, simplifications are made. The microsphere model assumes that the radiotracer is freely diffusible into the brain, completely extracted from the vascular compartment, and trapped in the brain without redistribution into the bloodstream (Kuhl et al., 1982). No assumption is met completely. Other models, based on a compartment approach, are available (Greenberg et al., 1990; Iida et al., 1994).

rCBF measures. Instead, relative measures of rCBF are obtained, and ROIs are referenced to a particular ROI least affected by the disorder being studied. Some studies use the cerebellum, some use the occipital or calcarine cortex, and some use global activity to reference the ROI. This lack of a standard reference makes it difficult to make comparisons across studies. Additional problems are suggested by the finding of Gemmel et al. (1990) that cerebellar perfusion, for instance, may vary independently across subjects, thereby decreasing its value as a reference region.

One clinical use of brain SPECT is in the evaluation of cerebrovascular disease states, such as transient ischemic attacks, strokes in progress, arteriovenous malformations, and decreased vascular reserves. Other clinical uses include localization of epileptic foci (the brain regions from which seizures originate) that are frequently hyperperfused during seizures and hypoperfused between seizures; evaluation of brain tumors, in which tumor recurrence and tissue necrosis from radiation treatment can be differentiated with the use of ^{201}Tl; and evaluation of dementia subtypes. Research areas include rCBF evaluation of psychiatric illnesses, in particular, their differential diagnoses and prognosis. A separate research area is based on studies of neuroreceptors (density, distribution, and receptor binding characteristics) (Holman & Devous, 1992).

Data Analysis

Most rCBF SPECT studies are group studies in which averaged values of predetermined ROIs are compared. Although a SPECT image is equivalent to a PET image, and image analysis software is commercially available, pixel-by-pixel approaches are not used as frequently in SPECT studies as they are in PET studies. Although many SPECT studies lag PET studies in quality of image analysis, sophisticated approaches are being used (for an example, see Chan et al., 1994).

MRI

Nuclear magnetic resonance has given rise to the following two neuroimaging methods: MRI, for the study of anatomy, and fMRI, for the study of blood flow and volume through the brain and, indirectly, of brain activation. MRI includes specialized methods, which are not discussed in this chapter; these include magnetic resonance angiography for the study of blood flow in major vessels and magnetic resonance spectroscopy for the study of concentrations of specific organic chemicals.

MRI, which became widely available in the mid-1980s, has rapidly become the preferred modality for both clinical and research anatomical imaging applications. Unlike CT, MRI scans can be obtained in various imaging planes (i.e., axial, coronal, sagittal) without repositioning the patient or subject. MRI produces highly resolute (1 mm–2 mm) images and is more flexible than is CT. By using different pulsing sequences (or parameters) for image acquisition, contrasts among gray matter, white matter, and cerebrospinal fluid (CSF) can be manipulated to yield images that are optimal for specific and diverse purposes, such as anatomical definition and examining for pathology. Unlike CT, MRI is not susceptible to artifacts created by bone (bone-hardening artifacts) and, as a result, brain tissue near the bone and its boundaries are delimited clearly. This definition permits accurate imaging of posterior fossa structures, such as the cerebellum. The lack of ionizing radiation makes it safe for repeated scanning of a single individual and for scanning of children. Most children older than 6 years of age can cooperate with the requirement to remain still, but younger children may need to be sedated.

Physics of MRI

The protons and neutrons found in atomic nuclei have a property called spin, which results in their having a magnetic moment. If a nucleus has unpaired spins, it will then have a net magnetic moment. The most commonly evaluated element is hydrogen, the nucleus of which has no neutron 99.98% of the time and instead has only a single proton, which identifies it as hydrogen. This proton has the largest magnetic moment of any nucleus and is the most abundant physiologically; all anatomical MRIs, therefore, are based on its resonating properties. Most hydrogen protons are found in H_2O, which is the source of greatest signal (Bushberg, 1994). Each cubic centimeter of tissue contains 10^{21} (H) protons and, under normal circumstances (i.e., not influenced by strong magnetic fields), the direction of each proton's magnetic moment is random, causing individual magnetic moments to cancel one another.

Taken as a whole, therefore, tissue does not display a magnetic moment. However, in an MRI scanner, which typically has a magnetic field strength of 0.5–2.5 teslas (i.e., 10,000–50,000 times the magnitude of Earth's magnetic field), a percentage of protons align in reference to this magnetic field. Of the protons that align, a small majority aligns parallel to the field, a lower energy state, whereas the remainder aligns antiparallel to the field, a higher energy state.

No proton, however, spins exactly on its longitudinal axis. Instead, a proton's magnetic moment precesses about it. Nuclei of a particular element in a given magnetic field strength have a specific precessional frequency, the Larmor frequency. Selective excitation of protons into higher energy states is accomplished by choosing the radiofrequency (RF) pulse emitted by the MRI scanner to which the protons resonate (their Larmor frequency). When this excitatory RF signal ceases, the protons return to their lower energy state and emit an RF signal equal to their Larmor frequency. This emitted RF signal, the free induction decay signal, is detected by the receiver coil (antenna) of the MRI scanner (Bushberg, 1994).

When protons absorb energy from the appropriate excitatory RF pulse, they flip from the parallel to the antiparallel position. This flip takes a finite amount of time, and the pulse duration can be varied to result in a specific flip angle, commonly 90°, which is halfway between the parallel and antiparallel positions and which brings the spins into the transverse plane.[17] The protons begin a process of relaxation as soon as the RF pulse terminates. There are two types of relaxation: T2 relaxation and T1 relaxation. First, the protons dephase from alignment from their particular transverse axis but remain in the transverse plane (imagine the spreading ribs of an opening fan). This loss of phase coherence is T2 relaxation.[18] Large molecules have short T2 relaxation times, whereas small molecules have long T2 relaxation times. Second, the protons begin to relax out of the transverse plane, termed T1 relaxation, back onto the longitudinal axis, their original parallel orientation.[19] Both small and large molecules tend to be

---

[17]This orientation causes the magnetic moment to be oriented perpendicular to the external field, thereby making the longitudinal magnetization, that part of the magnetic moment oriented along the longitudinal axis, equal to zero. The protons all flip in the same direction, combining to form transverse magnetization, that part of the magnetic moment oriented along a transverse axis.

[18]T2 relaxation causes decay of transverse magnetization. T2 relaxation time depends on spin–spin interactions. The greater the local (on the level of molecules) magnetic inhomogeneity, the shorter the T2 relaxation time.

[19]T1 relaxation causes recovery of longitudinal magnetization. T1 relaxation time depends on spin–lattice interactions. The greater the ability of the surrounding lattice to absorb the energy emitted by the relaxing nucleus, the shorter the T1 relaxation time.

Table 2.2.   Representative MRI sequence settings and signal intensities of tissue

Contrast weighting	T1	Proton density	T2
Sequence settings	TR=200 TE=20	TR=2000 TE=10–20	TR=2000 TE=80
Signal intensity[a]	Fat White matter Gray matter CSF	Fat Gray matter White matter CSF	CSF Gray matter White matter Fat

[a]Signal intensity is listed vertically from highest to lowest.

poor energy acceptors from the relaxing nuclei and, as a result, have long T1 relaxation times. Intermediate-size molecules are the best energy acceptors and have short T1 relaxation times (Bushberg, 1994).

RF Pulse Sequences

T1 and T2 relaxations and proton density are physical properties of a tissue being studied. Certain pulse parameter settings are effective in detecting small differences in these physical properties, thereby heightening the contrast among them. The repetition time (TR) (i.e., the time interval between the beginning of two sequential excitatory pulse sequence cycles) can be manipulated. Tissues with short T1 relaxation times are farther along in recovery of longitudinal magnetization before the next pulse. Tissues with short T1 times emit higher RF signals. The echo time (TE) is the time interval between an initial excitatory pulse and a particular emitted signal, termed an echo.[20] The TE also is an experimental parameter that can be manipulated. The echo amplitude depends on the tissue's proton density and T2 relaxation time. The shorter the T2, the lower the resultant echo amplitude (Bushberg, 1994). In structural MRI results, variously weighted images are provided. For example, in T1-weighted images, CSF is dark, and in T2-weighted images, CSF is bright (see Table 2.2). Altering pulse sequence parameters, such as flip angle, TR, and TE, therefore, enables one to emphasize proton density, T1, or T2.

Image Construction in Three Dimensions

How are these signals localized spatially? The use of linear magnetic field gradients (i.e., variation in the magnetic field strength as a function of position along a dimension in space, applied in each of the three dimensions) permits localization of signal. These linear field gradients are small, approximately 0.1%–1% of the main field strength.[21]

---

[20]After the initial excitatory pulse, a second excitatory pulse 180° out of phase of the initial pulse is generated by the RF coils. This pulse has the effect of inverting the direction of the dephasing individual transverse magnetic moments (i.e., magnetic moments undergoing T2 relaxation). This inversion of direction causes the individual transverse moments to regain phase coherence. When these transverse moments have rephased, an RF signal, called an echo, is emitted by the tissue. The TE is the time interval between the initial 90° pulse and the echo's appearance. The 180° pulse arrived at the midpoint of the interval, at TE/2.

[21]In addition to the large external magnetic field, which is as nearly uniform as possible, small magnetic gradients are superimposed. Along the longitudinal (z) axis, the slice select gradient causes protons at different longitudinal positions to have slightly different Larmor frequencies. (Recall that Larmor frequencies vary by element and by magnetic field strength.) When an

Data Analysis

A well-characterized research method for comparing structural MRI results is volu-metrics, the evaluation of selected brain volumes across subject groups or across time in a single group. Working with image analysis software, an investigator can trace the outline of the brain or brain region on consecutive image slices and generate a volume by adding the areas across slices. If necessary, brain images can be resliced to stan-dardize alignment across individual scans using MRI software. Because brains differ in size, a total cranial volume (or comparable measure) usually is obtained to allow spe-cific regional volumes to be normalized by dividing the specific region by the total cra-nial volume (or comparable measure).

For particular brain structures, such as the corpus callosum, volumetric measures are difficult to obtain. In this case, a cross-sectional area measurement of the corpus callosum through the midsagittal slice gives an accurate measure of the number and health of the long axons connecting regions of the two hemispheres. When image analysis capabilities are not available to researchers, brain area or linear measures can be obtained by conducting measurements on a single slice directly on the MRI scan-ner console.

Alternatively, ordinal scores (e.g., absent, mild, moderate, severe) can be obtained through subjective ratings of morphological or signal intensity abnormalities. Many parameters can be assessed by using such ratings, while maintaining adequate relia-bility, through direct comparison to a template of predefined levels of abnormality. One can assess, for example, micro- or macrogyral abnormalities, sulcal widening in-dicative of atrophy, or white matter hyperintensities indicative of a demyelinating pro-cess, such as that which occurs in multiple sclerosis or microvascular disease. These volumetric, planar, linear, and ordinal measurements have been used in assessing var-ious degenerative and neurodevelopmental disorders such as autism and Down syn-drome (Wang & Jernigan, 1994).

fMRI

fMRI, also known as real-time, fast, or dynamic MRI, represents the most recent ad-vancement in neuroimaging, having become available in the 1990s. fMRI uses conven-

RF signal with a given frequency is applied, only those protons with equivalent Larmor frequen-cies will resonate. Therefore, only one predetermined tissue slice will be excited with each pulse. To excite adjacent slices, the RF pulse frequency is altered. To localize proton signals along a transverse (x) axis, a frequency encode gradient is applied along the x-axis at the time of echo for-mation. The echo signal, therefore, is composed of multiple frequencies. This complex wave-form, when received by the MRI receiver coil, must be Fourier transformed for the individual fre-quencies to be distinguished. Each individual frequency signal, now localized along the x-axis, can be analyzed for proton density and relaxation characteristics as described above. The slice select gradient and frequency encode gradient localize the signal along the z- and x-axes in a sin-gle pulse sequence cycle. The y-axis localization, however, occurs with sequential pulse se-quences. With each pulse sequence, the amplitude of the gradient along the y-axis, called the phase encode gradient, is incremented. The protons along the y-axis take on a specific phase as a function of the magnetic field strength, which, of course, varies linearly because of the gradi-ent. With each pulse sequence, the amplitude of the y gradient is incremented, which causes variations in phase of the protons as a function of position along the y-axis: The further peripher-ally the signal is located, the greater the phase variations that will occur with the series of gradi-ent amplitude alterations. The complex waveform formed from each x column in each z slice is then Fourier transformed to give the individual contributions of the voxels in the y-axis (Bush-berg, 1994).

tional MRI scanners with fast imaging techniques to detect alterations in blood flow and blood volume in activated tissue, thereby permitting the study of brain function. Major advantages over other functional techniques include the lack of radiation and lack of invasiveness (no needles or injections); these advantages make this the first functional technique with potential for wide application to children, including those with subtle cognitive disorders and healthy, normal control subjects. Furthermore, fMRI data do not need to be averaged across subjects, but rather are interpretable for each individual, thus providing an opening to the study of individual differences. The temporal resolution of fMRI is superior to that of PET and permits finer discriminations to be made among stages of cognitive processing. In addition, spatial resolution is superior, and the ability to obtain an anatomical scan and functional images in a single scanning session allows for easier matching of function to structure (i.e., better structural and functional image registration).

Limitations of fMRI include significant susceptibility to artifacts, such as those from draining veins and from head motion. Considerable subject cooperation in remaining still and performing a task is required. Quantitative measures of blood flow cannot be obtained with this technique, and methods frequently limit functional mapping to selected image slices rather than permitting whole-brain exploration. For surveying the entire brain and for validating fMRI methods, PET remains the gold standard.

fMRI Based on BOLD Contrast

If one injects a magnetic contrast agent into the vascular space, changes in rCBF and regional cerebral blood volume (rCBV) cause changes in concentration of agent in those regions. Because the agent's concentration affects signal strength from surrounding tissue, the change in contrast agent concentration can be detected by subtracting resting from activated scans (Prichard & Rosen, 1994). An ingenious technique based on the differing signal characteristics of blood in activated versus resting brain regions permits imaging based on blood oxygenation level–dependent (BOLD) contrast, in which the blood itself becomes a contrast agent.

The paradox on which the BOLD contrast method is based is that venous blood oxygenation is greater in neuronally activated regions than in resting regions. Hemoglobin, the iron-containing macromolecule in red blood cells that transports oxygen to the body's tissues, is found as oxyhemoglobin, which contains oxygen, and deoxyhemoglobin, which does not contain oxygen. When blood flow increases by more than the increase of oxygen extraction from the blood by the tissue, as happens in neuronally activated brain regions, the ratio of oxyhemoglobin to deoxyhemoglobin increases in the postcapillary blood vessels (Ogawa et al., 1990). Oxy- and deoxyhemoglobin differ in magnetic susceptibility, which is the degree of their response to a magnetic field. The degree of magnetic susceptibility affects the signal strength from that area: Greater susceptibility causes weaker signal. Signal strength, therefore, depends on the ratio of oxy- to deoxyhemoglobin in the region's blood vessels.[22]

---

[22]The greater the magnetic susceptibility, the higher the degree to which the material becomes magnetized. Oxyhemoglobin, like most substances, is a diamagnetic material and interacts only weakly with the applied magnetic field, whereas deoxyhemoglobin, a paramagnetic material, interacts more strongly. This paramagnetic property causes local magnetic field gradients (inhomogeneities) to form, thereby causing faster relaxations, which translate into a weaker signal. Because magnetic susceptibility–based signal changes extend from blood vessels to brain tissue several (blood vessel) diameters away, the lower the deoxyhemoglobin concentration in blood, as found in activated regions, the stronger the emitted RF signal from surrounding brain tissue (Ogawa et al., 1990; Rosen et al., 1989).

In echoplanar imaging, a technique common in fMRI, the entire planar image (slice) is acquired during each excitation sequence—in traditional techniques, in contrast, each transverse row of voxels is obtained sequentially—thereby allowing whole image slice formation in 30–100 ms (Stehling et al., 1991). At such speeds, however, spatial resolution is limited, and artifacts may be substantial (Edelman et al., 1994).

Capabilities and Their Impact on Experimental Design

The breathtaking speed of image acquisition in fMRI dramatically expands experimental horizons. The most direct result is that temporal resolution is markedly improved. fMRI signal strength is dependent on blood oxygenation levels, which are directly related to rCBF and rCBV. Neuronal activation itself is not measured. fMRI, therefore, is limited by the brain's vascular response time to neuronal activation. As summarized by Bandettini et al. (1993), the RF signal emitted from the brain takes 5–8 s after stimulus onset to reach 90% of maximum and 5–9 s after stimulus termination to return to 10% above baseline.

What is the point of having temporal resolution on the order of tenths of a second if vascular response and consequent signal change are on the order of seconds? Such temporal resolution may permit the formation of sequential images of evolving changes in rCBF and rCBV in response to experimental tasks that may involve multiple cognitive operations. It may be possible to form "motion pictures" of activated brain regions, differentiating, to some degree, those regions activated concurrently from those activated sequentially. For example, in a study of working (short-term) memory, one can image the perception component of the task and the retention component separately (Courtney et al., 1995).

Because the BOLD contrast mechanism is less sensitive to rCBF and rCBV changes than are exogenous contrast agents (or exogenous radionuclides in PET and SPECT), studies using the BOLD mechanism use tasks, such as motor tasks and primary sensory tasks, that cause large, spatially limited, vascular changes (Binder & Rao, 1994). Signal increases in motor, visual, and auditory cortices in response to activation tasks are between 1.5% and 5% when 1.5-tesla scanners of the sort commonly available in medical settings are used (Bandettini et al., 1993). The association cortex has less dramatic vascular response parameters and, consequently, smaller signal increases. To detect the smaller vascular changes of the association cortex, the experimental design must be optimized. Binder and Rao (1994) report that their group was able to discriminate signal changes as small as 1%. The averaging of perhaps dozens of images acquired under one experimental condition permits increased sensitivity to activation changes by decreasing variance (Binder & Rao, 1994).

Data Analysis Methods

In fMRI, data are not analyzed as absolute changes in a physiological parameter, such as rCBF or rCBV, but rather as relative changes in signal strength. Statistical significances of change across experimental variables often are expressed as z-scores, which are normalized difference scores (i.e., expressed in the number of standard deviations from the mean) (Binder & Rao, 1994). Of course, interest in developing methods for absolute measurements of physiological parameters is high.

In fMRI, the approach often is a single-subject analysis. The several dozen images available from a single subject within an experimental condition are averaged and normalized to a global mean across conditions. In the subtraction technique, which is the most commonly used image analysis method in fMRI and is analogous to subtraction

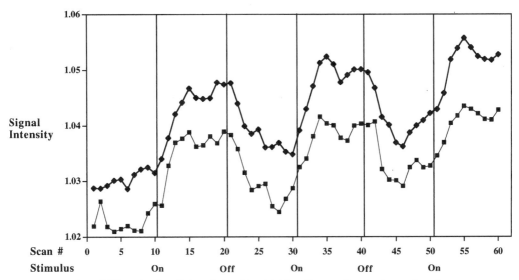

Figure 2.4.   In an fMRI study, signal intensity in left and right auditory cortices is shown changing across scans with auditory stimulation. The *x*-axis shows scan number; the *y*-axis, signal intensity in relative terms. *On* indicates the onset of auditory stimulation; *Off*, the onset of silence. The signal intensity is higher during auditory stimulation than during silence. The plateaus of increased signal intensity during stimulation are shifted to the right of the stimulus onset by approximately one scan (3 s) because vascular response lags behind neuronal activation. (–■– = left; –◆– = right.)

techniques used in PET and SPECT image analysis, the averaged image from one experimental condition is subtracted from the averaged image from another condition. Only voxels that differ by a predetermined z-score are regarded as significantly changed. The resultant difference image is superimposed onto a high-resolution structural MRI that is obtained in the same session.

fMRI generates hundreds of sequential images that may be analyzed for change across time. A preliminary fMRI study of selective attention to auditory stimuli (word presentations) undertaken at the Laboratory of Neurosciences, National Institute on Aging, illustrates this point (Grady et al., 1995). At one point in the study, subjects were presented with spoken lists of words for 30 s, alternating with 30 s of silence. Figure 2.4 shows how signal intensity in ROIs in the left and right auditory cortices changes with experimental condition. The signal intensity of the ROIs during the 10 scans (3 s/scan) obtained during stimulation was higher than that of the ROIs during the 10 scans obtained during silence.

Binder and Rao (1994) reviewed data analysis approaches that took into account the dimension of time. For example, in experimental designs with repetitive activations of a given frequency, such as motor responses or stimulus presentations, each voxel's signal across images (time) can be Fourier transformed. (Fourier analysis allows for the transformation of a complex waveform into constituent waveforms of particular frequencies.) In this way, those voxels with signal peaks at the frequency corresponding to the frequency of the activation are identified. For example, if each auditory stimulation/silence cycle lasted 2 s, those voxels with frequency peaks at 0.5 Hz could be identified.

This and related approaches have the added benefit of differentiating experimentally induced from artifactually induced signal changes, thereby increasing sensitivity to small, experimentally induced signal changes. fMRI, like PET, is sensitive to changes in rCBF, rCBV, and regional blood oxygenation levels caused by factors other than changes in experimental conditions. In fMRI, these artifacts are temporal and include physiological rhythms, such as subject motion, pulsatile brain motion, and pulsatile blood and CSF flows (Bandettini et al., 1993).

To summarize, fMRI has several advantages. One is that it is noninvasive. It does not require injection of radioisotopes or exogenous contrast agents, thus permitting repeated studies on a single subject without the limit of maintaining radiation dose or contrast load within safe levels. The single-subject approach, by avoiding the variability in structure among individuals, has the advantage of not losing detail of anatomical localization through group averaging of signal or through warping of brains into a common brain space. fMRI has better spatial resolution than does either PET or SPECT, which means that fMRI also has improved localization of activation. Another important advantage of fMRI is its temporal resolution, which is better than is the brain's vascular response, thus permitting imaging of the evolving vascular response in response to neuronal activation.

fMRI has attendant disadvantages as well. First, the sensitivity of fMRI techniques to changes in rCBF is lower than is that in PET or SPECT, which keeps changes in signal strength in response to neuronal activation low, at times so low that it is swamped by artifacts and confounding biological rhythms. Second, fMRI primarily is based on changes in rCBF; it shares with PET and SPECT the inability to image neuronal activity directly. Third, the greatest change in oxy- to deoxyhemoglobin concentration appears to take place in the postcapillary venules, thereby somewhat distorting or misplacing the region of greatest neuronal activation (Turner & Jezzard, 1994).

CONCLUSIONS AND FUTURE DIRECTIONS

Since the mid-1970s, neuroimaging technology has provided increasingly precise and diverse methods for exploring brain structure and function, allowing clinicians and scientists to examine the brains of children and adults with developmental disorders. In the anatomical domain, the arrival of X-ray CT in the 1970s was superseded by MRI in the 1990s. The exquisite resolution, flexibility, and safety of MRI have stimulated numerous studies of normal and anomalous development. In the functional domain, first PET and then SPECT have yielded reliable, quantitative determinations of regional brain metabolism and blood flow, thus helping to localize the neural pathways involved in cognitive activity and dysfunction associated with neuropsychological impairments in individuals with developmental disorders. fMRI, with its improved safety and spatial and temporal resolution, promises to further advance our understanding of normal and abnormal brain development and important individual differences.

As is evident from this discussion, these advancements have resulted from the collaborative, multidisciplinary efforts of physicists, radiochemists, physicians, neuroscientists, computer scientists, and psychologists, among others. In addition to the technology, experimental methods and controls (e.g., accurate diagnoses, careful sampling, thoughtful task selection and design) have been and continue to be essential to advancing our knowledge of brain–behavior relationships in healthy individuals and in those with developmental disorders. No longer limited to lesion methods, human neuropsychology can develop a new, more refined body of knowledge of normal brain–behavior relationships, their development, and their subtle deviations. Together, these methods and technologies may allow for earlier and more precise diagnosis, assessment of risk factors and prognosis, development of more useful nosologies with known biological correlates, and improved ability to assess the effects of interventions (educational, behavioral, and medical) on brain development.

REFERENCES

Ackermann, R.F., Finch, D.M., Babb, T.L., & Engel, J., Jr. (1984). Increased glucose metabolism during long-term duration recurrent inhibition of hippocampal pyramidal cells. *Journal of Neuroscience, 4*, 251–264.

Ackermann, R.F., & Lear, J.L. (1989). Glycolysis-induced discordance between glucose metabolic rates measured with radiolabeled fluorodeoxyglucose and glucose. *Journal of Cerebral Blood Flow and Metabolism, 9*, 774–785.

Bandettini, P.A., Jesmanowicz, A., Wong, E.C., & Hyde, J.S. (1993). Processing strategies for time-course data sets in functional MRI of the human brain. *Magnetic Resonance in Medicine, 30*, 161–173.

Baron, J.C., Rougement, D., Soussaline, F., Bustany, P., Crouzel, C., Bousser, M.G., & Comar, D. (1984). Local interrelationships of cerebral oxygen consumption and glucose utilization in normal subjects and in ischemic stroke patients: A positron emission tomographic study. *Journal of Cerebral Blood Flow and Metabolism, 4*, 140–149.

Bartlett, E.J., Brodie, J.D., Wolf, A.P., Christman, D.R., Laska, E., & Meissner, M. (1988). Reproducibility of cerebral glucose metabolic measurements in resting human subjects. *Journal of Cerebral Blood Flow and Metabolism, 8*, 502–512.

Binder, J.R., & Rao, S.M. (1994). Human brain mapping with functional magnetic resonance imaging. In A. Kertesz (Ed.), *Localization and neuroimaging in neuropsychology* (pp. 185–213). New York: Academic Press.

Bushberg, J.T. (1994). Magnetic resonance imaging. In *The essential physics of medical imaging* (pp. 291–366). Baltimore: Williams & Wilkins.

Chan, K.H., Johnson, K.A., Becker, J.A., Satlin, A., Mendelson, J., & Garada, B. (1994). A neural network classifier for cerebral perfusion imaging. *Journal of Nuclear Medicine, 35*, 771–774.

Collins, R.C. (1987). Physiology–metabolism–blood-flow couples in brain. In M.E. Raichle & W.J. Powers (Eds.), *Cerebrovascular diseases* (pp. 149–162). New York: Raven Press.

Courtney, S.M., Ungerleider, L.G., Keil, K., & Haxby, J.V. (1995). Identification of cortical areas for perception and working memory through analysis of FMRI time series. *Human Brain Mapping, Suppl. 1*, 332.

Devous, M.D., Sr. (1995). Instrumentation, radiopharmaceuticals, and technical factors. In R.L. Van Heertum & R.S. Tikofsky (Eds.), *Cerebral SPECT imaging* (2nd ed., pp. 3–29). New York: Raven Press.

Edelman, R.R., Wielopolski, P., & Schmitt, F. (1994). Echo-planar MR imaging. *Radiology, 192*, 600–612.

Farah, M.J. (1994). Neuropsychological inference with an interactive brain: A critique of the locality assumption. *Behavioral Brain Science, 17*, 43–104.

Fox, P.T., & Raichle, M.E. (1986). Focal physiological uncoupling of cerebral blood flow and oxidative metabolism during somatosensory stimulation in human subjects. *Proceedings of the National Academy of Sciences of the United States of America, 83*, 1140–1144.

Frackowiak, R.S.J., & Friston, K.J. (1994). Functional neuroanatomy of the human brain: Positron emission tomography—A new neuronatomical technique. *Journal of Anatomy, 184*, 211–225.

Friston, K.J., Frith, C.D., Liddle, P.F., & Frackowiak, R.S.J. (1991a). Comparing functional (PET) images: The assessment of significant change. *Journal of Cerebral Blood Flow and Metabolism, 11*, 690–699.

Friston, K.J., Frith, C.D., Liddle, P.F., & Frackowiak, R.S.J. (1991b). Plastic transformation of PET images. *Journal of Computer Assisted Tomography, 15*, 634–639.

Gally, J.A., Montague, P.R., Reeke, G.N.J., & Edelman, G.M. (1990). The NO hypothesis: Possible effects of a short-lived, rapidly diffusible signal in the development and function of the nervous system. *Proceedings of the National Academy of Science of the United States of America, 87*, 3547–3551.

Gemmell, H.G., Evans, N.T.S., Besson, J.A.O., Roeda, D., Davidson, J., Dodd, M.G., Sharp, P.F., Smith, F.W., Crawford, J.R., Newton, R.H., Kulkarni, V., & Mallard, J.R. (1990). Regional cerebral blood flow imaging: A quantitative comparison of technetium-99m-HMPAO SPECT with C^{15}O$_2$ PET. *Journal of Nuclear Medicine, 31,* 1595–1600.

Gilardi, M.C., Bettinardi, V., Todd-Pokropek, A., Milanesi, L., & Fazio, F. (1988). Assessment and comparison of three scatter correction techniques in single photon emission computed tomography. *Journal of Nuclear Medicine, 29,* 1971–1979.

Grady, C.L., VanMeter, J.W., Maisog, J.M., Pietrini, P., Krasuski, J., & Rauscheker, J.P. (1995). Changes in auditory cortex activation during selective attention. *Society for Neuroscience Abstracts, 21,* 1988.

Grasby, P.M., Friston, K.J., Bench, C., Cowen, P.J., Frith, C.D., Liddle, P.F., Frackowiak, R.S.J., & Dolan, R.J. (1992). Effect of the 5-HT$_{1A}$ partial agonist buspirone on regional cerebral blood flow in man. *Psychopharmacology, 108,* 308–386.

Grasby, P.M., Friston, K.J., Bench, C., Frith, C.D., Paulescu, E., Cowen, P.J., Liddle, P.F., Frackowiak, R.S.J., & Dolan, R.J. (1992). The effect of apomorphine and buspirone on regional cerebral blood flow during their performance of a cognitive task: Measuring neuromodulatory effects of psychotropic drugs in man. *European Journal of Neuroscience, 4,* 1203–1212.

Greenberg, J.H., Kushner, M., Rango, M., Alavi, A., & Reivich, M. (1990). Validation studies of iodine-123-iodoamphetamine as a cerebral blood flow tracer using emission tomography. *Journal of Nuclear Medicine, 31,* 1364–1369.

Haxby, J.V., Grady, C.L., Ungerleider, L.G., & Horwitz, B. (1991). Mapping the functional neuroanatomy of the intact human brain with brain work imaging. *Neuropsychologia, 29,* 539–555.

Haxby, J.V., Ungerleider, L.G., Horwitz, B., Rapoport, S.I., & Grady, C.L. (1995). Hemispheric differences in neural systems for face working memory: A PET rCBF study. *Human Brain Mapping, 3,* 68–82.

Hayden, M.R., Martin, W.R.W., & Stoessel, A.J. (1986). Positron emission tomography in the early diagnosis of Huntington's disease. *Neurology, 36,* 888–894.

Herscovitch, P. (1988). Measurement of regional cerebral hemodynamics and metabolism by positron emission tomography. In A.A. Boulton & G.B. Baker (Eds.), *Neuromethods: Neurochemistry* (Vol. 8, pp. 179–231). Totowa, NJ: Humana Press.

Herscovitch, P., Markham, J., & Raichle, M.E. (1983). Brain blood flow measured with intravenous H$_2$^{15}O. I. Theory and error analysis. *Journal of Nuclear Medicine, 24,* 782–789.

Hoffman, E.J., & Phelps, M.E. (1986). Positron emission tomography: Principles and quantitation. In M. Phelps, J. Mazziotta, & H. Schelbert (Eds.), *Positron emission tomography and autoradiography* (pp. 237–286). New York: Raven Press.

Holm, S., Madsen, P.L., Sperling, B., & Lassen, N.A. (1994). Use of ^{99m}Tc-bicisate in activation studies by split dose technique. *Journal of Cerebral Blood Flow and Metabolism, 14*(Suppl. 1), S115–S120.

Holman, B.L., & Devous, M.D., Sr. (1992). Functional brain SPECT: The emergence of a powerful clinical method. *Journal of Nuclear Medicine, 33,* 1888–1904.

Horwitz, B. (1990). Quantification and analysis of positron emission tomography metabolic data. In R. Duara (Ed.), *Emission tomography in dementia* (pp. 13–70). New York: Wiley-Liss.

Horwitz, B. (1994). Data analysis paradigms for metabolic-flow data: Combining neural modeling and functional neuroimaging. *Human Brain Mapping, 1,* 112–122.

Horwitz, B., Soncrant, T.T., & Haxby, J.V. (1992). Covariance analysis of functional interactions in the brain using metabolic and blood flow data. In F. Gonzalez-Lima, T. Finkenstädt, & H. Scherch (Eds.), *Advances in metabolic mapping techniques for brain imaging of behavioral and learning functions* (pp. 189–217). Dordrecht, The Netherlands: Kluwer Academic Publishers.

Horwitz, B., & Sporns, O. (1994). Neural modeling and functional neuroimaging. *Human Brain Mapping, 1,* 269–283.

Huang, S.C., Phelps, M.E., Hoffman, E.J., Sideris, K., Selin, C.J., & Kuhl, D.E. (1980). Noninvasive determination of local cerebral metabolic rate of glucose in man. *American Journal of Physiology, 238,* E69–E82.

Hurtig, R.R., Hichwa, R.D., O'Leary, D.S., Boles Ponto, L.L., Narayana, S., Watkins, G.L., & Andreason, N.C. (1994). Effects of timing and duration of cognitive activation in [^{15}O]water PET studies. *Journal of Cerebral Blood Flow and Metabolism, 14,* 423–430.

Iadecola, C. (1993). Regulation of the cerebral microvasculature during neural activity: Is nitric oxide the missing link? *Trends in Neuroscience, 16,* 206–214.

Iadecola, C., Pelligrino, D.A., Moskowitz, M.A., & Lassen, N.A. (1994). Nitric oxide synthase inhibition and cerebrovascular regulation. *Journal of Cerebral Blood Flow and Metabolism, 14,* 175–192.

Iida, H., Itoh, H., Bloomfield, P.M., Munaka, M., Higano, S., Murakami, M., Inugami, A., Eberl, S., Aizawa, Y., Kanno, I., & Uemura, K. (1994). A method to quantitate cerebral blood flow using a rotating gamma camera and iodine-123 iodoamphetamine with one blood sampling. *European Journal of Nuclear Medicine, 21,* 1072–1084.

Kety, S.S. (1951). The theory and applications of the exchange of inert gas at the lungs and tissues. *Pharmacological Reviews, 3,* 1–41.

Kuhl, D.E., Barrio, J.R., Huang, S.C., Selin, C., Ackermann, R.F., Lear, J.L., Wu, J.L., Lin, T.H., & Phelps, M.E. (1982). Quantifying local cerebral blood flow by N-isopropyl-p(I-123) iodoamphetamine tomography. *Journal of Nuclear Medicine, 23,* 196–203.

Links, J.M. (1993). Multidetector single-photon emission tomography: Are two (or three or four) heads really better than one? *European Journal of Nuclear Medicine, 20,* 440–447.

Lou, H.C., Edvinsson, L., & MacKenzie, E.T. (1987). The concept of coupling blood flow to brain function: Revision required? *Annals of Neurology, 22,* 289–297.

Mata, M., Fink, D.J., Gainer, H., Smith, C.B., Davidsen, L., Savaki, H., Schwartz, W.J., & Sokoloff, L. (1980). Activity-dependent energy metabolism in rat posterior pituitary primarily reflects sodium pump activity. *Journal of Neurochemistry, 34,* 213–218.

McIntosh, A.R., & Gonzalez-Lima, F. (1992). The application of structural modeling to metabolic mapping of functional neural systems. In F. Gonzalez-Lima, T. Finkenstädt, & H. Scherch (Eds.), *Advances in metabolic mapping techniques for brain imaging of behavioral and learning functions.* Dordrecht, The Netherlands: Kluwer Academic Publishers.

McIntosh, A.R., Grady, C.L., Haxby, J.V., Maisog, J.M., Horwitz, B., & Clark, C.M. (1995). *Within-subject transformations of PET regional cerebral blood flow data: ANCOVA, ratio and Z-score adjustments on empirical data.* Manuscript submitted for publication.

McIntosh, A.R., Grady, C.L., Ungerleider, L.G., Haxby, J.V., Rapoport, S.I., & Horwitz, B. (1994). Network analysis of cortical visual pathways mapped with PET. *Journal of Neuroscience, 14,* 655–666.

Mentis, M.J., Horwitz, B., Grady, C., Alexander, G.E., VanMeter, J.W., Maisog, J.M., Pietrini, P., Schapiro, M.B., & Rapoport, S.I. (1996). Visual cortical dysfunction in Alzheimer's disease evaluated using a temporally graded "stress-test" during PET. *American Journal of Psychiatry, 153,* 32–40.

Mesulam, M.M. (1990). Large-scale neurocognitive networks and distributed processing for attention, language, and memory. *Annals of Neurology, 28,* 597–613.

Mintun, M.A., Fox, P.T., & Raichle, M.E. (1989). A highly accurate method of localizing regions of neuronal activation in the human brain with positron emission tomographic data. *Journal of Cerebral Blood Flow and Metabolism, 9,* 96–103.

Moretti, J.L., Caglar, M., & Weinmean, P. (1995). Cerebral perfusion imaging tracers for SPECT: Which one to choose? *Journal of Nuclear Medicine, 36,* 359–363.

Nishizawa, S., Tanada, S., Yonekura, Y., Fujita, T., Mukai, T., & Saji, H. (1989). Regional dynamics of N-isotropyl-(I-123)-iodo-amphetamine in human brain. *Journal of Cerebral Blood Flow and Metabolism, 30,* 150–156.

Ogawa, S., Lee, T.M., Kay, A.R., & Tank, D.W. (1990). Brain magnetic resonance imaging with contrast dependent on blood oxygenation. *Proceedings of the National Academy of Sciences of the United States of America, 87,* 9868–9872.

Pardo, J.V., Pardo, P.J., & Raichle, M.E. (1990). Neural correlates of self-induced dysphoria. *American Journal of Psychiatry, 150,* 713–719.

Phelps, M.E., Huang, S.C., Hoffman, E.J., Selin, C.J., Sokoloff, L., & Kuhl, D.E. (1979). Tomographic measurement of local glucose metabolic rate in humans with [F-18] 2-fluoro-2-deoxy-D-glucose: Validation of method. *Annals of Neurology, 6,* 371.

Politte, D. (1990). Image improvements in positron-emission tomography due to measuring differential time-of-flight and using maximum-likelihood estimation. *IEEE Transactions on Nuclear Science, 37,* 737–742.

Posner, M.I., Petersen, S.E., Fox, P.T., & Raichle, M.E. (1988). Localization of cognitive operations in the human brain. *Science, 240,* 1627–1631.

Prichard, J.W., & Rosen, B.R. (1994). Functional study of the brain by NMR. *Journal of Cerebral Blood Flow and Metabolism, 14,* 365–372.

Ramsay, S.C., Murphy, K., Shea, S.A., Friston, K.J., Lammerstma, A.A., Clark, J.C., Adams, L., Guz, A., & Frackowiak, R.S.J. (1993). Changes in global cerebral blood flow in humans: Effects on regional cerebral blood flow during a neural activation task. *Journal of Physiology, 471,* 521–534.

Rapin, J.R., Duterte, D., Le Poncin-Lafitte, M., Lageron, A., Monmaur, P., Rips, R., & Lassen, N.A. (1983). Iodoamphetamine derivatives as tracers for cerebral blood flow or not? Autoradiography and autochistodiographic studies. *Journal of Cerebral Blood Flow and Metabolism*, 3(Suppl. 1), S105–S106.

Reivich, M., Kuhl, D., Wolf, A., Greenberg, J., Phelps, M., Ido, T., Casella, V., Fowler, J., Hoffman, E., Alavi, A., Som, P., & Sokoloff, L. (1979). The [18F]fluorodeoxyglucose method for the measurement of local cerebral glucose utilization in man. *Circulation Research*, 44, 127–137.

Ring, H.A., George, M., Costa, D.C., & Ell, P.J. (1991). The use of cerebral activation procedures with single photon emission tomography. *European Journal of Nuclear Medicine*, 18, 133–141.

Rosen, B.R., Belliveau, J.W., & Chien, D. (1989). Perfusion imaging by nuclear magnetic resonance. *Magnetic Resonance Quarterly*, 5, 263–281.

Roy, C.W., & Sherrington, C.S. (1890). On the regulation of the blood-supply of the brain. *Journal of Physiology (London)*, 11, 85–108.

Sergent, J. (1993). Mapping the musician brain. *Human Brain Mapping*, 1, 20–38.

Silbersweig, D.A., Stern, E., Frith, C.D., Cahill, C., Schnorr, L., Grootoonk, S., Spinks, T., Clark, J., Frackowiak, R.S.J., & Jones, T. (1993). Detection of thirty-second cognitive activations in single subjects with positron emission tomography: A new low-dose $H_2^{15}O$ regional cerebral blood flow three-dimensional imaging technique. *Journal of Cerebral Blood Flow and Metabolism*, 13, 617–629.

Silbersweig, D.A., Stern, E., Schnorr, L., Frith, C.D., Ashburner, J., Cahill, C., Frackowiak, R.S.J., & Jones, T. (1994). Imaging transient, randomly occurring neuropsychological events in single subjects with positron emission tomography: An event-related count rate correlational analysis. *Journal of Cerebral Blood Flow and Metabolism*, 14, 771–782.

Sokoloff, L. (1981). Relationship among local functional activity, energy metabolism, and blood flow in the central nervous system. *Federation Proceedings*, 40, 2311–2316.

Sokoloff, L., Reivich, M., Kennedy, C., Des Rosiers, M.H., Patlak, C.S., Pettigrew, K.D., Sakurada, O., & Shinohara, M. (1977). The [14C]deoxyglucose method for the measurement of local cerebral glucose utilization: Theory, procedure, and normal values in the conscious and anesthetized albino rat. *Journal of Neurochemistry*, 28, 897–916.

Stehling, M.K., Turner, R., & Mansfield, P. (1991). Echo-planar imaging: Magnetic resonance imaging in a fraction of a second. *Science*, 254, 43–50.

Steinmetz, H., & Seitz, R.J. (1991). Functional anatomy of language processing: Neuroimaging and the problem of individual variability. *Neuropsychologia*, 12, 1149–1161.

Ter-Pogossian, M.M., Ficke, D.C., & Yamamoto, M. (1982). A positron emission tomograph utilizing photon time-of-flight information. *IEEE Transactions on Medical Imaging MI-1*, 179–187.

Townsend, D.W., Geissbuhler, A., Defrise, M., Hoffman, E.J., Spinks, T.J., Bailey, D.L., Gilardi, M.C., & Jones, T. (1991). Fully three-dimensional reconstruction for a *PET* camera with retractable septa. *IEEE Transactions on Medical Imaging*, 10, 505–512.

Turner, R., & Jezzard, P. (1994). Magnetic resonance studies of brain functional activation using echo-planar imaging. In R.W. Thatcher, M. Hallet, T. Zeffiro, E.R. John, & M. Huerta (Eds.), *Functional neuroimaging technical foundations* (pp. 69–78). San Diego, CA: Academic Press.

Wang, P.P., & Jernigan, T.L. (1994). Morphometric studies using neuroimaging. *Neurologic Clinics*, 12, 789–802.

II

Application of Neuroimaging Methods to the Understanding of Childhood Disorders

Children with medical illnesses and developmental disorders face an agonizing array of difficulties and challenges as they grow up. Difficulties in learning how to read, write, and calculate; deficits in the ability to pay attention in school; problems in developing social relationships; difficulties in understanding what constitutes appropriate behavior in different settings; and deficits in language and cognitive development can reduce a child's self-esteem and severely limit his or her potential to achieve academically and occupationally, not to mention his or her happiness in life. It is clear that, to protect children from these deleterious outcomes, we must develop a full understanding of the effects of medical illnesses; the types of developmental disorders that exist; and the biological, psychological, and educational reasons for their occurrence. Without a detailed and comprehensive grasp of the biological substrates and etiologies for learning and behavioral deficits in children, our ability to develop early identification methods, apply early interventions, and understand the developmental course and outcome of a particular disorder or illness will be hampered significantly.

In this section of the book, a range of specific disorders and conditions that affect children is discussed in detail, with an eye toward identifying their neurobiological origins via the application of neuroimaging methods. In these chapters, significant advances in our understanding of how brain development and neural processing relate to learning and behavior are highlighted and explored. For example, two chapters are devoted to discussing the cognitive and neurobiological underpinnings of dyslexia. This reading disorder warrants two chapters for a number of reasons. First, dyslexia is much more prevalent than was initially thought, and its impact on school learning, self-esteem, and vocational and occupational success is extremely negative. As such, it is imperative that we develop a clear understanding of this disorder. Second, the relatively large number of neuroimaging studies conducted with children and adults who have dyslexia since the mid-1980s attests to its scientific and clinical importance, and the range of investigative methods used requires two chapters to provide the necessary breadth and depth of coverage of the topic. In Chapter 3, therefore, Dr. Judith M. Rumsey provides a comprehensive review of the nature and types of structural and functional neuroimaging studies that have sought to determine whether individuals with reading disorders differ from their counterparts who read normally in the development of specific neuroanatomical structures and in the functional processing of information within these brain structures. In this context, Dr. Rumsey discusses how anatomical information has been obtained from children and adults with dyslexia by using magnetic resonance imaging (MRI) and how information about the processing of information in the brain has been obtained via studies of regional cerebral blood flow (rCBF) and positron emission tomography (PET). In Chapter 4, Dr. Sally E. Shaywitz and her coauthors provide a critical discussion of the need to identify the core cognitive deficits in dyslexia before applying neuroimaging methods. This discussion is followed by a review of functional neuroimaging studies using functional MRI (fMRI), which allows researchers to characterize the activation of specific neural systems that are involved in the developmental reading process. Chapters 3 and 4 provide the reader with the most current information available about the cognitive and linguistic mechanisms involved in dyslexia and their neurobiological origins.

In Chapter 5, Dr. Monique Ernst provides an excellent discussion of the construct of attention-deficit/hyperactivity disorder (ADHD) and of the conceptual and methodological factors that must be considered when interpreting neuroimaging data obtained from children with ADHD. Her subsequent discussion of the neuroanatomical substrate involved in the modulation of attention and her analysis and interpretation of neuroimaging data derived from structural (CT and MRI) studies of these regions are valuable for their insights on structural variation in ADHD. Likewise, Dr. Ernst's analysis of functional neuroimaging data derived from PET studies of cerebral glucose metabolism illustrates the difficulties that must be recognized when interpreting information obtained from functional studies using this methodology and highlights the importance of sample definition and activation task development.

Autism is a rare and severe behavioral syndrome that impairs, among other skills, the abilities to communicate verbally and nonverbally and to interact socially. In Chapter 6, Dr. Judith M. Rumsey provides an informative and compelling discussion of the core behavioral features of, and diagnostic criteria for, autism and addresses the complex issues associated with etiology and comorbidity. Dr. Rumsey then provides a review and an analysis of both structural and functional neuroimaging studies conducted in individuals with autism. The information presented in this chapter is critical to both clinicians and scientists because of its emphasis on diagnostic criteria, the need to define samples for research in an operational manner, and the factors to consider when attempting to link biology and behavior in autism via the interpretation of neuroimaging data.

In Chapter 7, Drs. Allan L. Reiss and Martha Bridge Denckla provide a much-needed synthesis and analysis of research in the areas of fragile X syndrome, Turner syndrome, and neurofibromatosis-1. In this context, the authors trace the neurobiological pathways through which genetic factors produce abnormalities of brain development and neurobehavioral function in children. In addition, a discussion of state-of-the-art applications of both CT and MRI to the study of each of these three disorders is provided.

Epilepsy in its different forms is the topic of Chapter 8. In this chapter, Dr. William D. Gaillard brings his wealth of clinical and research expertise to a discussion of which types of neuroimaging modalities are best suited for different types of neuroimaging studies of children with epilepsy. An overview of CT and MRI procedures is provided within the context of an analysis of studies of brain anatomical structures, and studies involving the use of PET and single photon emission computed tomography (SPECT) are discussed vis-à-vis their application to the study of neurophysiological functions.

Pediatric acquired immunodeficiency syndrome and human immunodeficiency virus, the virus that causes the syndrome, have obvious, devastating effects on children's longevity and quality of life. In Chapter 9, Drs. Pim Brouwers, Charles DeCarli, and Lucy A. Civitello provide an elegant and insightful review of neuroimaging studies of HIV-related diseases of the central nervous system in infants and young children. A critically important feature of this chapter lies in the authors' review of the relationships that exist among measures of brain structure (CT and MRI) and brain function (PET and SPECT) and aspects of clinical neurological, neuropsychological, and pathological findings and outcomes.

In the final chapter of this section, critical issues relevant to the early identification and prediction of a range of developmental disorders are discussed. Specifically, in Chapter 10, Drs. Rachelle Tyler and Judy Howard provide an excellent analysis of the types of behavioral and neuroimaging measures that can help portend long-term neurological, cognitive, and school-related outcomes for infants and children who are at risk. Emphasis is placed on assessing the relative predictive power of electrophysiological data, findings from ultrasonography, and data derived from CT, MRI, and PET to predict outcomes in children.

3

Neuroimaging in Developmental Dyslexia
A Review and Conceptualization
Judith M. Rumsey

NEUROIMAGING AS A TOOL
FOR UNDERSTANDING DYSLEXIA

With the advent of X-ray computed tomography (CT) scanning in the 1970s, neuro-imaging studies began to explore anatomical deviations associated with developmental dyslexia. Functional neuroimaging studies of dyslexia began in the late 1980s with the availability of xenon-inhalation techniques for studying regional cerebral blood flow. Magnetic resonance imaging (MRI) and positron emission tomography (PET) soon offered improved technology for studying brain structure and function in developmental and other disorders. As of late 1995, 13 anatomical and 8 functional neuroimaging studies of dyslexia using these methods had been published, and additional work was in progress in this exciting area.

The neuroimaging literature indicates that developmental dyslexia is not associated with macroscopic lesions imageable with anatomical techniques, such as CT and MRI. The great majority of physically healthy children with dyslexia are expected to have clinically normal CT and MRI scans, and dyslexia alone is not an indication for an MRI or a CT scan. The value of neuroimaging in dyslexia at this time lies primarily in its research applications, that is, as a tool for exploring brain anatomy and function and for testing hypotheses about deviations in structure and/or function. For anatomical research, MRI is the method of choice given its superiority over CT in resolution, flexibility, and safety (i.e., lack of ionizing radiation). Research methods that appear to be useful are quantitative. Brain structures are imaged in a variety of planes, and their areas or volumes are measured. Children or adults with dyslexia are compared with normal control subjects to determine deviations in the size, shape, or symmetry of certain structures.

Functional techniques, such as PET and, more recently, functional MRI (fMRI), permit the examination of brain activity under a variety of cognitive challenges. Structures that are difficult to quantify anatomically because of unclear boundaries and the difficulties associated with measuring three-dimensional structures on and across two-dimensional slices may be involved in dyslexia and may contribute to alterations of brain function. Structures with normal gross anatomy may contain microscopic anomalies too small to be imaged in vivo with anatomical methods, but these may affect brain function nonetheless.

This chapter reviews nearly 20 years of neuroimaging research (both anatomical and functional) on dyslexia. In addition, it provides a brief overview of what is known

The author thanks Brian Donohue for preparing the figures that appear in this chapter.

about developmental dyslexia from a variety of perspectives, including those of epidemiology, genetics, and neuropsychology. Also included is an overview of what is known and hypothesized about the functional neuroanatomy of normal reading based on both lesion studies and functional neuroimaging of healthy brains. Autopsy studies of dyslexia also are reviewed because they permit the most direct look at the brain possible, thereby providing an invaluable basis for generating hypotheses that can, to a limited extent, be tested in larger, better characterized samples using neuroimaging techniques.

DEVELOPMENTAL DYSLEXIA AND ITS NEUROPSYCHOLOGICAL CORRELATES

According to the *Diagnostic and Statistical Manual of Mental Disorders* (4th ed.) (DSM-IV) (American Psychiatric Association, 1994), developmental dyslexia, or reading disorder, is defined by a significant impairment in individually measured reading achievement (either accuracy or comprehension) relative to that expected on the basis of an individual's age, intelligence, and education. The impairment must be clinically significant; that is, it must interfere with academic achievement or activities of daily living that require reading skill, and sensory impairments cannot account for the reading impairment.

Although the imaging studies reviewed in this chapter have relied on such a discrepancy-based definition of dyslexia, the specific operationalization of this definition has varied among researchers. Most biologically oriented researchers have focused on deficits in word recognition or reading decoding (accuracy and rate) rather than reading comprehension. The size of the deficit that is considered significant has varied in these studies and will vary with age, the tests used, and IQ level (e.g., greater discrepancies may be required for individuals with high IQs).

Discrepancy-based definitions have been challenged by several investigators who have argued for definitions based on absolute, rather than IQ-relative, reading deficits (Siegel, 1992; Stanovich, 1994; Stanovich & Siegel, 1994). The essential argument is that reading (decoding) deficits result from more basic or core phonological deficits (discussed later in this chapter) regardless of an individual's IQ level. Indeed, Siegel (1992) suggests that IQ is irrelevant to the definition of learning disabilities. In considering such arguments, it is important to recognize that factors such as IQ may be relevant for some purposes and irrelevant for others; for example, IQ may be differentially relevant for educational intervention and biological research (Lyon, 1989).

For purposes of neuroimaging research, brain-based correlates of dyslexia may differ in children with selective versus generalized cognitive or learning deficits, and IQ may be relevant to variations in brain structure and function (Andreasen et al., 1993). Decades of neuropsychological research support the value of well-defined syndromes (involving clusters of symptoms) in the search for brain–behavior relationships. For example, acquired brain lesions underlying selective reading disorder (i.e., alexia without agraphia, acquired reading disorder with intact writing and spoken language) differ in their localization from those causing alexia in the context of aphasia (i.e., acquired language impairment).

Prevalence estimates for reading disorders in school-age children in the United States range from 4% to 9% when discrepancy-based definitions are used (American Psychiatric Association, 1994; Shaywitz et al., 1990). In contrast, estimates based on absolute, rather than IQ-relative, deficits fall in the 17%–20% range (Shaywitz et al.,

1994). One epidemiological study (Shaywitz et al., 1992) suggests that dyslexia exists on a continuum with normal reading ability, making the boundaries between normal reading and dyslexia fuzzy. Approximately 60%–80% of affected individuals are male, although disruptive behaviors more common in males may result in a higher identification rate for boys than for girls (Pennington, 1995; Shaywitz et al., 1992).

Genetic studies reviewed by Pennington (1995) suggest that both dyslexia and normal reading ability are influenced significantly by heredity, although the mode of genetic transmission may vary from family to family. Approximately 27%–49% of parents and 40% of siblings of children with dyslexia also are affected. A child with an affected parent has an approximately eightfold increase in risk compared with the approximate 5% risk found in the general population. Genes on chromosomes 15 and 6 are candidates for influencing reading ability.

Decades of research, which included developmental studies and family genetic studies (Olson et al., 1991; Wagner & Torgeson, 1987), have linked developmental dyslexia to core deficits in phonological processing, which underlie deficits in word recognition, or decoding (i.e., reading accuracy and rate; see Lyon, 1995). Phonological processing involves the application of rules for translating letters and their sequences into their speech-sound equivalents (i.e., sounding out words). This type of processing builds on phonological awareness (i.e., the explicit awareness of individual phonemes, or speech sounds, in words). Phonological awareness develops at around the age at which children learn to read and is an important predictor of success in learning to read (Liberman & Shankweiler, 1985; Wagner & Torgeson, 1987). Phonological awareness frequently is measured with auditory rhyme detection tasks, which do not require reading.

Although reading ability improves with age in many children with dyslexia, severe dyslexia persists into adolescence and adulthood (Scarborough, 1984). Adults with dyslexia, even those with good outcomes, still show phonological processing deficits, as manifested in poor nonword reading (e.g., surke, pyte) and spelling (Pennington et al., 1987). Phonological deficits appear to span the clinical course of the disorder, making it possible to explore their neural correlates in adults.

Although phonological deficits appear to be specifically linked to deficits in word recognition or decoding (i.e., reading accuracy and rate), children with dyslexia frequently show additional neuropsychological deficits. These include subtle deficits in spoken language that involve syntax, naming, verbal memory, digit span, differing degrees of developmental language disorder, and, in rarer instances, visuospatial deficits (Brady, 1986; Mann & Brady, 1988; Mann et al., 1980; Satz & Morris, 1981). Reading problems in children with developmental language disorders may parallel their spoken language problems, resulting in reading comprehension being more affected than reading decoding (Bishop & Adams, 1990). Children without histories of significant preschool language problems, who first experience clinically significant problems when learning to read, are more likely to show disproportionate deficits in reading decoding and better reading comprehension (Conners & Olson, 1990). Children with dyslexia frequently have comorbid academic skill deficits involving spelling, writing, and mathematics (American Psychiatric Association, 1994). In addition, perhaps 20%–40% of children with dyslexia have a comorbid attention deficit disorder (Lambert & Sandoval, 1980).

Although past research has indicated that deficient visual memory and learning are unlikely to contribute to dyslexia (Hulme, 1988; Willows, 1991), reports of difficulties with rapid visual processing (Lovegrove et al., 1986; Martin & Lovegrove, 1988)

have led to the hypothesis that a portion of the visual system (the large-celled, or magnocellular, system) is affected in dyslexia. The cells of this system are most sensitive to
stimuli at low spatial frequencies and low contrasts. At low spatial frequencies and low
contrasts, individuals with dyslexia may show a slowed flicker fusion rate (defined as
the fastest rate at which a contrast reversal of a stimulus can be seen) and decreased
contrast sensitivity (Martin & Lovegrove, 1988). Flicker fusion rate is determined by
asking subjects to adjust the contrast level of a grating stimulus (alternating black and
white bars, the thickness of which is determined by their spatial frequency) until they
see it flicker or see a striped pattern (Martin & Lovegrove, 1988). This is done at different rates of flicker to characterize the transient properties of the visual system. Visual
persistence (measured by the temporal separation needed to distinguish two stimuli)
also may be prolonged (Lovegrove et al., 1986). However, unlike the case with phonological deficits, deficits in rapid visual processing have not been causally linked to poor
reading (Hulme, 1988).

Other hypotheses include Tallal et al.'s (1993) hypothesis of a general deficit in
rapid temporal (i.e., sequential) processing across sensory modalities (e.g., auditory,
visual, tactile) in individuals with dyslexia. Additional studies are needed to clarify the
nature of such deficits and their role in reading. Work by Studdert-Kennedy and Mody
(in press) attributes the deficits observed by Tallal et al. (1993) to difficulty in discriminating highly similar stimuli (e.g., syllables, tones) rapidly rather than to difficulties
in judging the order of such stimuli. Studdert-Kennedy and Mody (in press) challenge
the notion that the phonological deficits of individuals with reading impairments are
linked to any co-occurring nonspeech deficits and conclude that the full nature, origin,
and extent of the phonological deficits of individuals with reading impairments have
yet to be determined.

NEUROANATOMY AND MODELS OF READING

Reviewing the literature on lesions that disrupt reading, Henderson (1986) described
the posterior pathways involved in reading: A simplified view is that print (written
language) is processed in striate and visual association cortex in the occipital lobe. Ipsilateral and contralateral pathways from visual association cortex in the inferior occipital lobe ascend to portions of the left angular gyrus, which is linked to Wernicke's area
in the posterior superior temporal gyrus. Fibers from the right occipital cortex cross in
the splenium of the corpus callosum. The angular gyrus is thought to be involved in
translating visual information into phonological representations (speech sounds),
whereas Wernicke's area is thought to mediate semantic processing or the linking of
these representations to meaning. The angular gyrus also may contribute to associations with meanings. In addition, the inferior temporal cortex receives input from visual association cortex and projects to the superior temporal lobe and inferior parietal
lobe (see Figure 3.1).

PET studies using ^{15}O as a tracer to measure changes in regional cerebral blood
flow (as a reflection of neuronal activity) have sought to refine models of reading based
on patients with acquired lesions by studying reading in individuals with healthy, intact brains. Conceptualizing single word recognition as a serial (i.e., sequential) process involving elemental operations, the landmark studies of Petersen et al. (1988a,
1988b) employed stepwise, hierarchical subtraction methods to localize these operations. Subjects underwent PET scans while 1) fixating their vision on a blank screen,
2) passively viewing nouns, 3) reading nouns aloud, and 4) viewing nouns while gen-

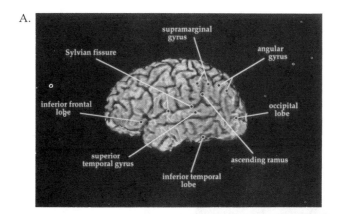

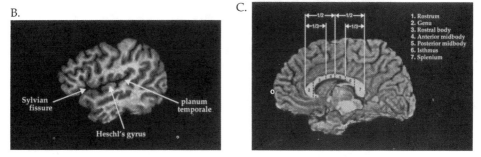

Figure 3.1   Regions involved in reading as seen on anatomical MRI. A) Lateral view of the left hemisphere of the brain, as reconstructed (or "surface rendered") from axial slices. B) Parasagittal slice through the left hemisphere illustrating Heschl's gyrus and the planum temporale. C) Midsagittal slice showing the corpus callosum and one approach to its segmentation for purposes of quantification.

erating a semantic association (i.e., a use) for each of them (e.g., cake–eat). To determine which brain regions were involved in each stage of processing, images were subtracted from one another sequentially. To identify regions involved in semantic association, scans obtained while subjects read aloud were subtracted from those obtained while subjects generated a semantic association; to identify regions involved in reading aloud, scans obtained while subjects passively viewed a word were subtracted from those obtained while subjects read aloud; and so on. The extrastriate cortex (in the occipital lobe) was shown to be involved in the processing of visual word forms; the left temporoparietal cortex, in phonological processing; and the left prefrontal cortex, in semantic association. Missing was an expected activation in the left posterior temporal cortex while subjects read aloud, which subsequently was demonstrated in later studies of word reading (Howard et al., 1992; Price et al., 1994).

Recent work has demonstrated that many factors may contribute to such inconsistent findings. These factors include, but are not limited to, the nature of the baseline task subtracted from the task of primary theoretical interest and secondary factors, such as the rate of stimulation and practice effects (Demonet et al., 1993). When one compares patients and control subjects, differences in difficulty and performance also may affect brain activations. For studies of reading, *what* one is reading (the nature of the material) may affect findings. Words vary in many linguistic parameters (e.g., frequency, regularity, concreteness, imagery, part of speech) that potentially are relevant to how and where language is processed in the brain (Fiez et al., 1993).

Other [15]O PET work has implicated the left posterior superior temporal cortex in single-word recognition as well (Rumsey et al., 1995) and left frontal regions near Broca's area in certain types of acoustic, phonological, and articulatory processing in receptive language function (Fiez et al., 1995). Although left-sided activations, in general, are more extensive, right-sided homologous regions frequently are activated as well, which suggests that they, too, play a role in language and reading. Figure 3.2 illustrates activations elicited in normal readers (right-handed men) while they read single words aloud (Rumsey et al., unpublished data, 1996).

Demonet et al. (1993) have discussed the limitations of hierarchical subtractions as applied to functional imaging studies of language and reading. Although such models may be appropriate for the study of brain activations related to peripheral neural activities, such as sensory input or motor output, hierarchical models are inadequate for studying more central, elaborate processes, such as levels of language processing. Even simple tasks involve many cognitive components. Should the baseline task activate processing similar to that in the experimental task, a failure to identify activation in neural structures involved in that process will result. For example, passively viewing a word may affect word recognition, thereby resulting in a failure to identify activation in neural structures (e.g., temporal lobe) involved in reading aloud when passive viewing of a word is used as a control task. In other words, it may be difficult to view a word without recognizing it. In addition, reading aloud, used as a control for semantic association, may activate semantic networks. Indeed, Wise et al. (1991) demonstrated activation of the temporal cortex with semantic tasks when compared with a resting baseline. Because it is difficult, if not impossible, to completely segregate single components of language processing, it is more appropriate to conceptualize language tasks in terms of variations in the weight and the attentional resources allocated to various aspects of language processing.

The basic assumptions that underlie hierarchical subtraction methods (e.g., serial processing) also have been challenged. Sergent et al. (1992) have discussed the need for task designs to rely on theoretical models that specify the nature and order of the

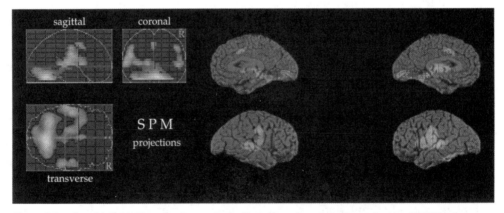

Figure 3.2.   Graphic illustration of regions activated by oral reading of single words using PET. The four projection maps on the right depict the regions activated relative to a visual fixation control condition (viewing a crosshair at the center of a screen) on maps of the left and right lateral and medial hemispheres. The three "see-through" maps on the left depict all regions activated as seen from a sagittal, a coronal, and a transverse view. Activated were regions in the occipital lobe (related to visual processing); the superior temporal gyrus (related to language processing), with a more extensive activation seen on the left than on the right for this structure; and the perirolandic area (related to motor aspects of reading aloud).

processing steps required for the performance of those tasks. Different aspects of information processing may proceed in parallel or in cascade rather than serially. Processing may not be unidirectional but may influence earlier operations retroactively. Processing that is not essential to the task at hand nonetheless may occur; for example, in deciding whether a string of letters constitutes a real word, visual, lexical, orthographic, semantic, and phonetic codes all may be activated (Sergent et al., 1992).

Connectionist models of reading have been proposed as an alternative to serial models of reading (Seidenberg & McClelland, 1989; Waters & Seidenberg, 1985). Connectionist models assume that different processes involved in reading proceed simultaneously and interactively in distributed neural networks. More congruent with such models than are hierarchical subtractions are designs that employ a common baseline to compare different aspects of reading and language, such as that used by Bookheimer et al. (1995) to compare oral and silent reading. Bookheimer et al. (1995) found that oral, but not silent, reading activated the superior temporal and angular/supramarginal gyri, regions implicated in phonological processing by other functional imaging studies. In contrast, the inferior frontal gyrus was significantly more active in silent reading.

NEUROPATHOLOGICAL FINDINGS IN DYSLEXIA

Few neuropathological studies of dyslexia have been completed because of the low availability of brains with subtle, non–life-threatening developmental disorders. The major work in this area is that of Galaburda and his colleagues, who have reported anomalies in brains from four men and three women with dyslexia (Galaburda et al., 1985; Humphreys et al., 1990). Comorbidities in the males included significant developmental language delays in three and seizures in one; in the females, these included attentional disorders, psychiatric disturbances, and brain injury.

All seven brains showed unusual symmetry (i.e., a loss of typical leftward [left larger than right] asymmetry) in the planum temporale. The planum temporale, which lies on the superior surface of the superior temporal gyrus inside the Sylvian fissure (see Figure 3.1A and 3.1B), shows a prominent leftward asymmetry in approximately 70% of brains and a rightward (right larger than left) asymmetry in approximately 10% of brains (Geschwind & Levitsky, 1968), thereby making the symmetry seen in the dyslexic brains a statistically significant finding and one that may constitute a risk factor for reading and/or subtle language disorder. Galaburda et al. (1985) and Galaburda et al. (1987) noted that an increase in size on the right, rather than a decrease on the left, appeared to account for the unusual symmetry found in the dyslexic brains. This finding was hypothesized to reflect an increased survival of neurons during corticogenesis (i.e., a reduction of normal cell death) and an increase in their synaptic targets.

In addition, neuronal ectopias (small loci of abnormally placed neurons) and dysplasias (focally distorted cortical architecture), most or all of which are too small to be seen on MRI, were reported in the cerebral cortex of the dyslexic brains. These cortical anomalies likely were of prenatal origin, most probably occurring during midgestation—a peak time for neuronal migration from germinal zones to the cerebral cortex. These anomalies were distributed bilaterally in the males' brains, with the greatest numbers being located along the left Sylvian fissure. These brains also showed anomalies in the inferior frontal cortex, an area that is connectionally related to the temporal and parietal language cortices. Galaburda et al. (1985) speculated that exuberant planum-related synaptic targets may include ectopic neurons in the inferior frontal gyrus and connectionally related ectopic cells in other cortical and subcortical locations.

Such improper connections and/or abnormal electrical properties of such lesions might interfere with normal function.

The females' brains also showed symmetrical plana temporale and cortical anomalies similar to those seen in the males' brains, except that the cortical anomalies were more variably distributed in the females' brains. Multiple foci of cerebrocortical glial scarring, thought to be of late prenatal or early postnatal origin, also were seen in two of the three females' brains. The distribution of these glial scars was primarily left perisylvian, with portions of the vascular border zone of the temporal cortex being involved in one brain and the border zone of the major cerebral arteries being involved symmetrically in the other (Humphreys et al., 1990).

Other findings have involved the thalamus. A case study (Galaburda & Eidelberg, 1982) reported bilateral disruption of the cytoarchitecture of the medial geniculate nucleus (part of the auditory system) and of the lateral posterior nucleus of the thalamus, which connectionally relates to the inferior parietal lobule.

Livingstone et al. (1991) reported anomalies (disorganization, unusually small cell bodies) of the magnocellular layers of the lateral geniculate nucleus of the thalamus in five of the brains previously reported by Galaburda et al. (1985). Parallel magnocellular (large cell) and parvocellular (small cell) visual pathways are thought to subserve transient (rapid) processing of low-contrast visual stimuli and sustained (slower) high-contrast stimuli, respectively. Although these subdivisions begin at the level of the retina and may continue through higher association cortex, their segregation is most apparent in the lateral geniculate nucleus of the thalamus. Because small cell bodies are likely to have thinner axons, their conduction velocities (their ability to transmit information rapidly) may be slower. Transient visual processing may be impaired as a result of anomalies of the magnocellular system.

NEUROANATOMICAL IMAGING OF DYSLEXIA

Cerebral Asymmetries

Viewing dyslexia as a language disorder, several researchers have examined features thought to reflect the predilection of the left hemisphere to preferentially subserve language function. Several anatomical asymmetries characterize most (but not all) normal brains: The Sylvian fissure slopes upward more markedly on the right than on the left, which results in the right temporal lobe being greater in volume when measured on coronal MRI scans (Jack et al., 1988). There is a tendency for the left hemisphere to protrude farther posteriorly and for the right frontal lobe to extend farther anteriorly. Although little significance has been attributed to the anterior rightward asymmetry, this and other left posterior asymmetries are thought to provide a substrate for the lateralization of language function.

One of the most dramatic anatomical asymmetries of the human brain is that of the planum temporale. The planum temporale lies on the supratemporal plane within the depths of the sylvian fissure and generally is defined as extending from the posterior border of Heschl's transverse gyrus to the bifurcation of the Sylvian fissure into an ascending ramus and a descending ramus (or branch) (see Figure 3.1A and 3.1B). Frequently there are two Heschl's gyri on the right side of the brain and one Heschl's gyrus on the left. When more than one Heschl's gyrus is present, the anterior boundary of the planum temporale usually is taken as the posterior border of the first (most anterior) Heschl's gyrus.

Geschwind and Levitsky (1968) demonstrated a highly significant leftward asymmetry in approximately 65% of 100 autopsied brains and the reverse asymmetry in only 11%. This asymmetry, which is present prenatally (Chi et al., 1977; Wada et al., 1975; Witelson & Pallie, 1973), is less pronounced in left-handed than in right-handed individuals (Steinmetz et al., 1991). The close proximity of Heschl's gyrus, the planum temporale, and Wernicke's area suggests a relationship between planum asymmetry and functional asymmetry in the superior temporal cortex (Karbe et al., 1995), which has close interhemispheric connections through the isthmus of the corpus callosum (Witelson, 1989) with corresponding areas on the right.

Because planum asymmetry and the size (i.e., midsagittal area) of the corpus callosum have been reported to vary with handedness, with strongly right-handed individuals showing greater leftward asymmetry and smaller callosal areas than nonconsistent right-handed or left-handed individuals (Steinmetz et al., 1991; Witelson, 1989), it is important to control for handedness in imaging studies. Although most studies do not find an increased incidence of left-handedness in dyslexia (Bishop, 1990), some investigators (Eglinton & Annett, 1994) report a small increase in non–right-handedness in this disorder. Handedness is related to the degree to which language function is lateralized to the left hemisphere, with left-handed individuals generally showing less strongly lateralized language function (i.e., greater bihemispheric sharing of language function) than right-handed individuals (Benton, 1981). Failures to control for handedness in anatomical and/or functional imaging studies should be considered a methodological weakness.

Early CT studies reported alterations (either reductions or reversals) of the usual leftward asymmetry of the parieto-occipital region (characteristic of the general population) in dyslexia (Haslam et al., 1981; Hier et al., 1978; Leisman & Ashkenazi, 1980; Rosenberger & Hier, 1980). Reversed asymmetry in this region was linked to histories of language delay and low verbal IQs by Hier et al. (1978) and Rosenberger and Hier (1980). The only CT study that examined frontal asymmetry in dyslexia failed to find any deviation here (Haslam et al., 1981).

MRI studies have examined a variety of anatomical asymmetries relating to language function, as well as to the topography of the corpus callosum, which subserves interhemispheric communication, inhibition, and integration. In an early uncontrolled study of men with severe dyslexia, Rumsey et al. (1986) reported a high incidence of symmetry of temporal lobe volumes and mild reversals of the usual left-predominant ventricular asymmetry on the basis of qualitative evaluations by two radiologists. Neuronal ectopias and dysplasias described in autopsy studies were not seen, possibly because of limitations in the resolution of MRI.

Two studies have examined hemispheric widths and areas on axial slices at the level of the planum temporale. Duara et al. (1991) reported normal rightward frontal asymmetries of hemispheric area on axial slices at the level of the planum temporale in familial dyslexics but a reversal of the normal leftward asymmetry in a segment of brain containing the angular gyrus. This reversal primarily was due to an increase in area on the right. The extent of the reversed asymmetry and the size of the area on the right correlated with the severity of the dyslexia. No unusual asymmetries were noted for the segment containing the planum. Hynd et al. (1990) reported bilaterally smaller and symmetrical frontal cortices in children with dyslexia without attention deficit disorders as a result of differences on the right. Other measures on lateral sagittal slices indicated bilaterally shorter insula in children with dyslexia. Of 10 children with dyslexia, 3 were left-handed, whereas all control subjects were right-handed.

Few studies (Larsen et al., 1990; Leonard et al., 1993) have used slices thin enough to identify and use Heschl's gyrus, the anterior boundary of the planum temporale, as an anatomical landmark. Using coronal slices, Larsen et al. (1990) measured the planum temporale in adolescents with dyslexia. Adolescents with dyslexia showed greater symmetry (i.e., a loss of normal leftward asymmetry) than did normal readers, and deficits in phonological decoding were strongly related to this symmetry. Differences in handedness were associated with this finding, however, because dyslexics were less consistently right-handed than were control subjects, and those with greater left-handedness had symmetrical plana temporale.

Two additional studies used coronal slices for measures of the supratemporal plane or portions of it on slices that were too thick to permit the identification of the anatomical boundaries of the planum temporale. Kushch et al. (1993) measured the entire supratemporal plane, whereas Schultz et al. (1994) measured the portion of the supratemporal plane posterior to the insula. Individuals with dyslexia (ages 8–53 years) studied by Kushch et al. (1993) showed increased symmetry, particularly for the posterior half of this plane (more closely related to the planum temporale), relative to control subjects, who showed leftward asymmetries for both the anterior and posterior portions. The groups differed more for left-sided measures than for right-sided measures. Dyslexic individuals with better reading skills showed more normal asymmetry. Again, differences in handedness contributed to the findings. With good controls for handedness, sex, and IQ, Schultz et al. (1994) found no differences in asymmetry of the supratemporal plane posterior to the insula. A leftward asymmetry for 70%–75% of both dyslexic and control subjects was noted.

Finally, Leonard et al. (1993) measured the planum temporale, as well as its extension into the parietal lobe, on several thin parasagittal slices in 9 dyslexic individuals, 10 of their unaffected relatives, and 12 control subjects (see Figure 3.1B). Good word attack (decoding) skills in nearly all of the dyslexic subjects characterized them as "recovered." The planum was subdivided into its temporal bank, which began at the posterior border of Heschl's gyrus and terminated at the bifurcation of the Sylvian fissure into a posterior ascending and a posterior descending ramus, or branch (see Figure 3.1A). The parietal planum was measured along the ascending ramus. Nearly all subjects across groups showed a leftward asymmetry of the temporal bank and a rightward asymmetry of the parietal bank. Unexpectedly, the dyslexic subjects showed an exaggerated leftward asymmetry of the temporal bank. In addition, on the right side of the brain, a larger proportion of the planum was devoted to the parietal bank relative to the temporal bank in dyslexic subjects. Given the involvement of the right parietal lobe in visuospatial function, Leonard et al. (1993) hypothesized that this might provide a substrate for enhanced visuospatial function at the expense of phonological or other language skills in dyslexia. Subjects with dyslexia also showed more cerebral anomalies, such as missing or duplicated gyri bilaterally, a finding that might result from disordered cellular migration during brain development. The unaffected relatives of the dyslexic subjects showed more anomalies than did control subjects but fewer anomalies than did the dyslexic subjects.

Studies of the Corpus Callosum

The corpus callosum, which is easily seen and measured on midsagittal MRI slices (see Figure 3.1C), is the largest mass of connecting fibers in the brain. Fibers enter it from nearly every part of the cortex and cross the midline of the brain to synapse on corresponding areas of the other hemisphere, providing a substrate for interhemispheric communication. The genu and anterior third of the body of the corpus callosum contain fibers from the frontal lobes; the middle third of the body contains fibers from the frontal, parietal, and temporal areas; the posterior third of the body contains fibers from the parietal, temporal, and occipital lobes; and the splenium contains fibers from the occipital regions. Most fibers from the superior temporal and posterior parietal cortex cross in the isthmus, whereas most from the occipital cortex cross in the splenium (Witelson, 1989).

Given reports of increased symmetry of the planum temporale and other posterior language regions in dyslexia, several investigators have hypothesized alterations in the size of posterior portions of the corpus callosum. Much easier to image in a single plane (midsagittal) than the planum temporale, the corpus callosum has been segmented and measured using a variety of approaches.

Both Duara et al. (1991) and Larsen et al. (1992) measured the area of the splenium, defined as the posterior fifth of the corpus callosum on a midsagittal slice (see Figure 3.1C). Duara et al. (1991) reported that right-handed familial dyslexics (e.g., dyslexic individuals with family histories of dyslexia) showed a larger splenium, on average, than did control subjects. This finding was, however, primarily attributable to female, rather than male, subjects. Using similar measures, Larsen et al. (1992) found no difference in total callosal area or the area of the splenium in a sample of adolescents with dyslexia, most of whom were male.

Using a different method, Hynd et al. (1995) also found no difference in the splenium in a sample of children with dyslexia; instead they found a reduction in the size of the genu, or anterior fifth, of the corpus callosum. Despite the lack of a group difference in the splenium, reading scores showed a significant correlation with the size of the splenium and the genu, such that smaller areas were associated with poorer reading. Some of the children with dyslexia had comorbid psychiatric disorders—in particular, attention deficit disorders. In other studies, Hynd and his colleagues (Hynd et al., 1991; Semrud-Clikeman et al., 1994) reported reductions of area in posterior portions of the corpus callosum in children with attention deficit disorder. The issue of comorbid attention deficit disorders, not adequately addressed in any of the abovementioned studies, therefore, may represent a significant confounding factor for studies of brain structure in dyslexia.

In a study that addressed this issue, Rumsey et al. (1996) segmented and measured the corpus callosum in 21 men with dyslexia, only 2 of whom had received childhood diagnoses of attention deficit disorders. Retrospective ratings for childhood symptoms of attention deficit disorders were used to further identify patients in whom attention deficit disorders may have gone undiagnosed. Because most of the fibers from the superior temporal and posterior parietal cortex cross in the isthmus, the isthmus was included, together with the splenium, in a measure of the posterior segment, which was hypothesized to differ in dyslexia. Although no difference was seen in the total corpus callosal area or in the anterior or middle third, the posterior third (containing the isthmus and splenium) was larger in dyslexic men than in control subjects as was predicted. This finding retained significance after the five subjects with suspected or diagnosed childhood attention deficit disorders were removed from the data set. The increase in size could reflect a greater number of fibers crossing in this region, greater myelination, thicker fibers, or greater packing density of fibers (Witelson, 1989). Such histological changes theoretically might result in increased communication between the two hemispheres, with either decreased lateralization of language functions related to reading or increased inhibition of one hemisphere by the other.

One other study of the corpus callosum in a large sample of children with varied learning disorders (Njiokiktjien et al., 1994) measured only the total midsagittal area of the corpus callosum. Of the 110 children studied, 39 had specific developmental dysphasia and dyslexia (with full-scale and performance IQs greater than 84); 24 had mild, mixed learning disabilities, which included reading (full-scale IQs greater than 84 with no significant verbal/performance discrepancies); and 47 had low IQs (full-scale IQs of 50–85). These three groups were compared with control children who had been scanned clinically for headaches, seizures, mild head trauma, and precocious puberty. Total corpus callosum size in the dysphasia/dyslexia and mild learning disability subgroups was normal. However, children with familial dysphasia/dyslexia had thicker corpora callosa, presumably influenced by genetic mechanisms. Children with learning disabilities who had experienced adverse perinatal events had smaller corpora callosa than did the familial cases, suggesting damage to this structure.

FUNCTIONAL NEUROIMAGING OF DYSLEXIA

The first functional neuroimaging studies of dyslexia made use of [133]xenon-inhalation techniques for measuring (primarily cortical) regional cerebral blood flow and were followed by PET studies of glucose utilization and regional cerebral blood flow. Both glucose utilization and blood flow changes reflect underlying neuronal activity. Because these techniques involve low-dose radiation, adults, rather than children, have been studied.

Xenon-Inhalation Studies

Examining right-handed dyslexic men during their performance of tasks designed to preferentially activate either the left or right hemisphere, Rumsey et al. (1987) found exaggerated asymmetries in both directions, depending on the demands of the task. Subjects completed a series of three tasks, all of which involved visual input and a simple motor response (pressing one of four numbered buttons to indicate one's answer). A number-matching task served as an attentional baseline: The subject saw a number from 1 to 4 and pressed one of four numbered buttons to match his answer. A semantic classification task involved reading a series of easy (low grade level) concrete nouns and classifying each as 1) animal, 2) body part, 3) food, or 4) tool, again by pressing one of four numbered buttons. Finally, in a task involving judgment of line orientation, the subject was presented with two angled lines and required to select one of four numbered lines to match the angle of one of the stimulus lines. Control subjects showed greater blood flow on the left side of the brain during semantic classification and greater blood flow on the right side of the brain during line orientation. Dyslexic men showed an exaggerated leftward asymmetry of blood flow during semantic classification and a trend toward an exaggerated rightward asymmetry during line orientation, differences that suggested difficulties with bihemispheric integration or an inefficient allocation of cognitive resources. In addition, lower frontal flows were seen, particularly on the difficult line orientation task.

In another study that used xenon-inhalation methods, Flowers et al. (1991) measured regional cerebral blood flow in a large sample of adults, including many with childhood histories of reading impairment, while they listened to concrete nouns and identified those containing four letters. Accuracy of performance was correlated positively with blood flow only at Wernicke's area (the higher the flow, the better the performance). This result was true for both a nonclinical sample and for a group of individuals whose childhood reading ability ranged from severely impaired to normal. Poor readers showed reduced blood flow at Wernicke's area in accordance with their poor performance. In contrast, childhood reading level (known from preserved childhood records) was inversely correlated with a more posterior focus of activation at the temporoparietal juncture. Adults with poorer childhood reading levels showed greater blood flow in this region, independent of task performance. The investigators hypothesized that these findings may reflect atypical connectivity, in which axons normally targeted for Wernicke's area instead synapse in temporoparietal cortex, thereby resulting in inefficiency related to reading. Alternatively, these findings may reflect different cognitive strategies on the parts of dyslexic and normal readers.

PET Studies of Glucose Utilization

Two PET studies have used [^{18}F]fluorodeoxyglucose to study regional cerebral glucose metabolism in adults with dyslexia. Gross-Glenn et al. (1991) examined right-handed dyslexic men with family histories of reading disorder while they read single words aloud. Compared with control subjects, the men with dyslexia showed focal increases in glucose utilization (possibly reflecting inefficient processing) in the lingual (inferior occipital) cortex (part of the ventral pathway from the occipital to the temporal cortex) and greater symmetry in prefrontal and lingual regions.

Hagman et al. (1992) studied dyslexic adults, primarily men, while they performed a speech discrimination task, modeled after Tallal's (Tallal & Piercy, 1975) hypothesis that language-impaired dyslexic children have difficulty processing speech sounds characterized by rapidly changing acoustic spectra critical for speech perception, specifically consonant-vowel syllables. The task required the detection of a target syllable (*da*) from among six stop consonant-vowel syllables (e.g., *a*, *da*, *ga*), degraded with cocktail party speech background noise. Dyslexic subjects showed higher metabolism in the medial temporal lobe bilaterally, which was hypothesized to reflect either inefficient processing or the activation of compensatory pathways.

^{15}O PET Studies of Regional Cerebral Blood Flow

Limitations of the above-described studies included the poor temporal resolution of glucose studies, imposed by the long half-life of the tracer (scans reflected activity over 30–45 min), and the use of a single state, precluding the identification of brain regions activated when a task was performed. In contrast, studies using the short-lived tracer ^{15}O to measure blood flow permit repeated scanning of an individual subject in a single session. Tasks generally are performed for relatively brief periods of time (1–5 min) with equal temporal resolution.

Using ^{15}O to measure regional cerebral blood flow, Rumsey and colleagues studied right-handed, severely dyslexic men and well-matched control subjects during their performance of several neuropsychological tasks designed to activate posterior and anterior language regions in the left hemisphere, as well as homologous regions in the right hemisphere (Rumsey et al., 1992; Rumsey, Andreason, et al., 1994; Rumsey, Zametkin, et al., 1994). All tasks involved auditory stimuli and a button-press response. These patients had clear childhood histories of developmental reading disorder without clinically significant spoken language deficits in their histories or in adulthood. All patients showed persistent reading deficits, both on an absolute basis and relative to their verbal IQs.

Physiological correlates for neuropsychological deficits thought to underlie or contribute to their reading disorder were sought with tasks that did not require reading.

Although phonological awareness provides an important, perhaps critical, foundation for reading, reading itself may increase phonological awareness (i.e., the two may enhance each other interactively). Reading also may facilitate the development of other language skills. Therefore, although, the use of nonreading tasks may not entirely eliminate the impact of reading failure in imaging studies, it at least minimizes the influence of reading failure.

Because deficient phonological awareness is thought to play a key causal role in dyslexia and because these patients remained severely reading impaired, a very easy phonological awareness task was used to probe left posterior language cortex: Rhyme detection, which is an early (preschool) predictor of the ability to learn to read, was used. Subjects listened to paired words and indicated with a button press which pairs rhymed.

Left anterior language regions were probed with an auditory syntax task. This task required subjects to listen to paired sentences that differed in grammatical structure and to indicate which paired sentences had the same meaning (e.g., "I'll go if you need me"; "If you need me, I'll go"). In addition to phonological deficits, syntactic deficits have been documented in dyslexia, even in adulthood. Furthermore, autopsy studies have reported cortical anomalies in these anterior, as well as posterior, language regions. Many individuals with dyslexia have subtle spoken language deficits (involving syntax) in addition to their written language disorder. The boundary between dyslexia and developmental language disorder is fuzzy, and it is further obscured by the tendency of many investigators to speak of the two interchangeably.

Right homologous regions also were of interest. If dyslexia were solely a language disorder, few differences in patterns of activation might be expected on nonlanguage tasks designed to activate right-sided cortex. Alternatively, given that neuropathological findings include bilateral cortical anomalies and an enlarged right planum temporale, unusual patterns of activation also might be expected on tasks designed to preferentially activate right temporal cortex. Furthermore, adults who continue to have significant reading impairments (uncompensated) may fail to compensate on the basis of bilateral brain dysfunction, given that many children with dyslexia improve substantially (compensate) over time. Tonal memory tasks are preferentially sensitive to right hemisphere lesions and have been shown previously to activate right temporal cortex in healthy subjects. A tonal memory task, therefore, was designed. Paired sequences of three to four tones were presented, and subjects indicated which paired sequences were identical.

All tasks were compared with a common resting baseline. When a region of interest approach was used for data analysis (see Chapter 2), dyslexic subjects, relative to control subjects, showed a small reduction in blood flow (approximately -8%) at rest in a single region near the left angular/supramarginal gyri. This finding was comparable in magnitude to changes elicited by the tasks and, therefore, may reflect a purely functional abnormality, as the resting state is not devoid of cognitive activity. Alternatively, this finding may be consistent with disordered cytoarchitecture or other structural abnormalities in the region near the left angular/supramarginal gyri.

As expected, in control men (normal readers), the various tasks activated the following regions: Rhyme detection activated the left temporoparietal region near the angular gyrus and a left posterior temporal region near Wernicke's area, consistent with earlier findings using a rhyme detection task in which words were presented visually (Petersen et al., 1988a); the right temporal and parietal cortices were activated to a lesser extent. The syntactic, sentence comprehension task activated left middle to anterior temporal and inferior frontal cortex. Tonal memory activated right frontotemporal, as well as left temporal, cortex.

Compared with control subjects, dyslexic subjects showed abnormal patterns of activation in left posterior language regions during rhyme detection, as illustrated in Figure 3.3. The dyslexic group failed to activate the left temporoparietal cortex (near the angular gyrus) and the left posterior temporal region (near Wernicke's area) activated by control subjects. Dyslexic subjects showed only mild performance deficits on the very easy task of rhyme detection. Within the dyslexic group, those with higher verbal IQs showed greater (more normal) activation of the left parietal cortex. These findings are compatible with dysfunction of the left temporoparietal and posterior temporal regions.

During the syntactic, sentence comprehension task, dyslexic subjects showed normal patterns of activation of left middle to anterior temporal and inferior frontal cortex, despite showing mild performance deficits. This suggests that the most common or consistent dysfunction of language cortex resides in left posterior language regions involved in reading. Although multifaceted language-related deficits have been documented in dyslexia, these may emanate from more basic deficits in phonological representation. Developmental dyslexia without language disorder may result from more restricted dysfunction involving regions in the left posterior temporal and temporoparietal cortex, with the core deficits involving decoding and phonological processing

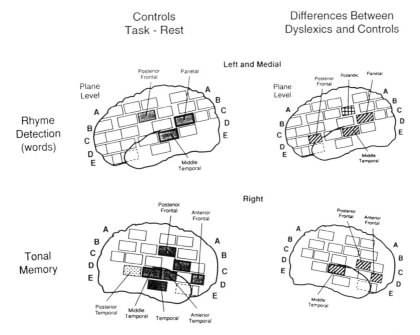

Figure 3.3. Activation patterns and differences between dyslexic men and control subjects associated with auditory rhyme detection and tonal memory tasks. Rhyme detection activated (relative to a resting baseline) the temporoparietal region (containing the angular gyrus) and midportion (from front to back) of the superior temporal lobe (labeled middle temporal to indicate its position along an anterior-posterior axis) more on the left than on the right, in normal readers. The tonal memory task activated the right frontotemporal and left temporal cortex in normal readers. Dyslexic men failed to activate left temporoparietal cortex during rhyme detection and activated fewer right frontotemporal regions during tonal memory testing. ($\blacksquare$ = activated by task, $p < 0.01$; $\blacksquare$ = activated by task, $p < 0.05$; $\blacksquare$ = deactivated by task, $p < 0.05$) ($\boxed{//}$ = dyslexics < controls, $p < 0.01$; $//$ = dyslexic < controls, $p < 0.05$; $\#\#\#$ = dyslexics > controls, $p < 0.05$)

(Rumsey, Zametkin, et al., 1994). Because these findings reflect group data (averaged across individuals), more extensive or variable involvement is possible in individual cases.

Finally, the tonal memory task elicited activation of fewer right frontotemporal regions in dyslexic subjects relative to control subjects (Rumsey, Andreason, et al., 1994) (see Figure 3.3). Furthermore, dyslexic subjects showed highly significant impairments in performance. A rapid stimulus rate was employed and contributed to this task being quite demanding for both groups and more difficult than either of the two language tasks. These findings suggest that neuropsychological deficits in severe cases of dyslexia are unlikely to be limited to phonological deficits. Corresponding to this premise is the hypothesis that severe, uncompensated dyslexia is associated with involvement of widely distributed neural circuits, affecting bilateral temporal and, possibly, other brain regions.

CONCLUSIONS AND FUTURE DIRECTIONS

Although varying methods and controls have yielded discrepant findings, the above-cited studies, taken as a whole, suggest that both anatomical and physiological signatures of dyslexia exist. Imaging of language-related brain regions has yielded positive, although sometimes conflicting, results. Asymmetries of the planum temporale and other language-related regions, noted both in neuropathological and neuroimaging studies, warrant further study with available improved methods. Most existing studies have been limited severely by thick slices, which have precluded precise anatomical definitions, and by the failure of curved structures, such as the planum temporale, to conform to a flat surface, which has made accurate measurement difficult. Neuroimaging technology, however, continues to improve at a rapid rate. Current imaging and image analytic techniques now allow rapid acquisition of thin slices and three-dimensional reconstruction of structure surfaces (surface rendering). When such features are well measured, relationships among various anatomical asymmetries (e.g., planum temporale, angular gyrus) and other brain structures (e.g., posterior segments of the corpus callosum) also can be explored. Such studies are under way at the National Institutes of Health, Bethesda, Maryland.

Functional studies have demonstrated a variety of differences in activation in left posterior language regions shown to be involved in reading. These differences include PET scan findings of decreased activation of the left temporoparietal and superior temporal cortex during phonological processing. The left temporoparietal region also was highlighted as a marker of childhood reading disability in earlier xenon studies. Together, these findings suggest an aberrant organization of language function in left posterior regions, possibly due to a functional lesion in this region. It is also noteworthy that differences seen in functional neuroimaging studies of dyslexia have not been confined to the left hemisphere; rather, differences have been demonstrated bilaterally in medial and lateral temporal cortex under a variety of conditions.

Motivated by a clinical interest in dyslexia, these studies used tasks selected for their neuropsychological relevance to dyslexia and/or their ability to activate in control subjects regions of theoretical interest in dyslexia. Rather than attempting to localize specific elementary cognitive operations, these studies have focused on the ability of dyslexic individuals to activate certain brain regions under various task conditions. Although single-state studies and the use of a common resting state baseline in ^{15}O PET studies do not permit the localization of specific elementary cognitive operations, the differential patterns of activation seen have been consistent with a wide body of neuropsychological knowledge. Additional studies are needed to better understand the neural networks involved in reading and the function and organization of these networks in dyslexia. PET studies designed to localize networks subserving phonological and other components of reading (Rumsey et al., 1995) and fMRI studies designed to localize pathways involved in motion processing (one aspect of transient visual processing [Eden et al., 1995]) in the brains of normal readers and those of dyslexic individuals are in progress at the National Institute of Mental Health, National Institutes of Health, Bethesda, Maryland. Other fMRI work in progress is described in Chapter 4.

The variable findings noted above also may reflect heterogeneity in the neuropsychological deficits associated with dyslexia and variability in the small samples studied. In addition to core phonological deficits, children with dyslexia frequently show associated multifaceted language and other deficits, comorbid academic skill deficits in spelling, writing, and mathematics, and comorbid attentional disorders. These findings, together with available neuropathological evidence, are compatible with the notion that the subtle developmental anomalies that may constitute the substrate of this disorder are not localized strictly to any small portion of the cortex. Rather, cortical anomalies may be variably distributed, and additional subcortical structures (e.g., thalamus) may be affected. Study of these additional comorbid disorders and deficits in isolation and in association with one another may, in the future, enrich our understanding of the full spectrum of developmental learning disorders.

REFERENCES

American Psychiatric Association. (1994). *Diagnostic and statistical manual of mental disorders* (4th ed.). Washington, DC: Author.

Andreasen, N.C., Flaum, M., Swayze, V., II, O'Leary, D.S., Alliger, R., Cohen, G., Ehrhardt, J., & Yuh, W.T. (1993). Intelligence and brain structure in normal individuals. *American Journal of Psychiatry, 150*, 130–134.

Benton, A. (1981). Aphasia: Historical perspectives. In M.T. Sarno (Ed.), *Acquired aphasia* (pp. 1–25). New York: Academic Press.

Bishop, D.V.M. (1990). Specific reading retardation (developmental dyslexia). In *Handedness and developmental disorder* (pp. 122–125). Philadelphia: Oxford University Press.

Bishop, D.V.M., & Adams, C. (1990). A prospective study of the relationship between specific language impairment, phonological disorders and reading retardation. *Journal of Child Psychology and Psychiatry, 31*, 1027–1050.

Bookheimer, S.Y., Zeffiro, T.A., Blaxton, T., Gaillard, W., & Theodore, W. (1995). Regional cerebral blood flow during object naming and word reading. *Human Brain Mapping, 3*, 93–106.

Brady, S. (1986). Short-term memory, phonological processing and reading ability. *Annals of Dyslexia, 36*, 138–153.

Chi, J.G., Dooling, E., & Gilles, F.M. (1977). Left–right asymmetries of the temporal speech areas of the human fetus. *Archives of Neurology, 34*, 346–348.

Conners, F., & Olson, R. (1990). Reading comprehension in dyslexic and normal readers: A component skills analysis. In D.A. Balota, G.B. Flores d'Arcais, & K. Rayner (Eds.), *Comprehension processes in reading* (pp. 557–579). Hillsdale, NJ: Lawrence Erlbaum Associates.

Demonet, J.F., Wise, R., & Frackowiak, R.S.K. (1993). Language functions explored in normal subjects by positron emission tomography: A critical review. *Human Brain Mapping, 1*, 39–47.

Duara, R., Kushch, A., Gross-Glenn, K., Barker, W.W., Jallad, B., Pascal, S., Loewenstein, D.A., Sheldon, J., Rabin, M., Levin, B., & Lubs, H. (1991). Neuroanatomic differences between dyslexic and normal readers on magnetic resonance imaging scans. *Archives of Neurology, 48*, 410–416.

Eden, G.F., Van Meter, J.W., Maisog, J.M., Rumsey, J., & Zeffiro, T.A. (1995). Abnormal visual motion processing in dyslexic subjects demonstrated with functional magnetic resonance imaging. *Society for Neuroscience Abstracts, 21*, 268.1.

Eglinton, E., & Annett, M. (1994). Handedness and dyslexia: A meta-analysis. *Perceptual and Motor Skills, 79,* 1611–1616.

Fiez, J.A., Balota, D.A., Raichle, M.E., & Petersen, S.E. (1993). The effects of word frequency and spelling-to-sound regularity on the functional anatomy of reading. *Society for Neuroscience Abstracts, 19,* 1808.

Fiez, J.A., Tallal, P., Raichle, M.E., Katz, W.F., Miezin, F.M., & Petersen, S.E. (1995). PET studies of auditory and phonological processing: Effects of stimulus type and task condition. *Journal of Cognitive Neuroscience, 7,* 357–375.

Flowers, D.L., Wood, F.B., & Naylor, C.E. (1991). Regional cerebral blood flow correlates of language processes in reading disability. *Archives of Neurology, 48,* 637–643.

Galaburda, A.M., Corsiglia, J., Rosen, G.D., & Sherman, G.F. (1987). Planum temporale asymmetry, reappraisal since Geschwind and Levitsky. *Neuropsychologia, 25,* 853–868.

Galaburda, A.M., & Eidelberg, D. (1982). Symmetry and asymmetry in the human posterior thalamus. II. Thalamic lesions in a case of developmental dyslexia. *Archives of Neurology, 39,* 333–336.

Galaburda, A.M., Sherman, G.F., Rosen, G.D., Aboitiz, F., & Geschwind, N. (1985). Developmental dyslexia: Four consecutive patients with cortical anomalies. *Annals of Neurology, 18,* 222–233.

Geschwind, N., & Levitsky, W. (1968). Human brain: Left–right asymmetries in temporal speech region. *Science, 161,* 186–187.

Gross-Glenn, K., Duara, R., Barker, W.W., Loewenstein, D., Chang, J.Y., Yoshii, F., Apicella, A.M., Pascal, S., Boothe, T., Sevush, S., Jallad, B.J., Novoa, L., & Lubs, H.A. (1991). Positron emission tomographic studies during serial word-reading by normal and dyslexic adults. *Journal of Clinical and Experimental Neuropsychology, 13,* 531–544.

Hagman, J.O., Wood, F., Buchsbaum, M.S., Tallal, P., Flowers, L., & Katz, W. (1992). Cerebral brain metabolism in adult dyslexic subjects assessed with PET during performance of an auditory task. *Archives of Neurology, 49,* 734–739.

Haslam, R.H.A., Dalby, J.T., Johns, R.D., & Rademaker, A.W. (1981). Cerebral asymmetry in developmental dyslexia. *Archives of Neurology, 38,* 679–682.

Henderson, V.W. (1986). Anatomy of posterior pathways in reading: A reassessment. *Brain and Language, 29,* 119–133.

Hier, D.B., LeMay, M., Rosenberger, P.B., & Perlo, V.P. (1978). Developmental dyslexia: Evidence for a subgroup with a reversal of cerebral asymmetry. *Archives of Neurology, 35,* 90–92.

Howard, D., Patterson, K., Wise, R., Brown, D., Friston, K., Weiller, C., & Frackowiak, R.S.J. (1992). The cortical localization of the lexicons. *Brain, 115,* 1769–1782.

Hulme, C. (1988). The implausibility of low-level visual deficits as a cause of children's reading difficulties. *Cognitive Neuropsychology, 5,* 369–374.

Humphreys, P., Kaufmann, W.E., & Galaburda, A.M. (1990). Developmental dyslexia in women: Neuropathological findings in three patients. *Annals of Neurology, 28,* 727–738.

Hynd, G.W., Hall, J., Novey, E.S., Eliopulos, D., Black, K., Gonzalez, J.J., Edmonds, J.E., Riccio, C., & Cohen, M. (1995). Dyslexia and corpus callosum morphology. *Archives of Neurology, 52,* 32–38.

Hynd, G.W., Semrud-Clikeman, M., Lorys, A.R., Novey, E.S., & Eliopulos, D. (1990). Brain morphology in developmental dyslexia and attention deficit disorder/hyperactivity. *Archives of Neurology, 47,* 919–926.

Hynd, G.W., Semrud-Clikeman, M., Lorys, A.R., Novey, E.D., & Eliopulos, D. (1991). Corpus callosum morphology in attention deficit-hyperactivity disorder (ADHD): Morphometric analysis of MRI. *Journal of Learning Disabilities, 24,* 141–146.

Jack, C.R., Gehring, D.G., Sharbrough, F.W., Felmlee, J.P., Forbes, G., Hench, V.S., & Zinsmeister, A.R. (1988). Temporal lobe volume measurement from MR images: Accuracy and left–right asymmetry in normal persons. *Journal of Computer Assisted Tomography, 12,* 21–29.

Karbe, H., Wurker, M., Herholz, K., Ghaemi, M., Pietrzyk, U., Kessler, J., & Heiss, W.D. (1995). Planum temporale and Brodmann's area 22: Magnetic resonance imaging and high-resolution positron emission tomography demonstrate functional left–right asymmetry. *Archives of Neurology, 52,* 869–874.

Kushch, A., Gross-Glenn, K., Jallad, B., Lubs, H., Rabin, M., Feldman, E., & Duara, R. (1993). Temporal lobe surface area measurements on MRI in normal and dyslexic readers. *Neuropsychologia, 31,* 811–821.

Lambert, N.M., & Sandoval, J. (1980). The prevalence of learning disabilities in a sample of children considered hyperactive. *Journal of Abnormal Child Psychology, 8,* 33–50.

Larsen, J.P., Hoien, T., Lundberg, I., & Odegaard, H. (1990). MRI evaluation of the size and symmetry of the planum temporale in adolescents with developmental dyslexia. *Brain and Language, 39,* 289–301.

Larsen, J.P., Hoien, T., & Odegaard, H. (1992). Magnetic resonance imaging of the corpus callosum in developmental dyslexia. *Cognitive Neuropsychology, 9,* 123–134.

Leisman, G., & Ashkenazi, M. (1980). Aetiological factors in dyslexia. IV. Cerebral hemispheres are functionally equivalent. *International Journal of Neuroscience, 11,* 157–164.

Leonard, C.M., Voeller, K.K.S., Lombardino, L.J., Morris, M.K., Hynd, G.W., Alexander, A.W., Andersen, H.G., Garofalakis, M., Honeyman, J.C., Mao, J., Agee, O.F., & Staab, E.V. (1993). Anomalous cerebral structure in dyslexia revealed with magnetic resonance imaging. *Archives of Neurology, 50,* 461–469.

Liberman, I.Y., & Shankweiler, D. (1985). Phonology and the problems of learning to read and write. *Remedial and Special Education, 6,* 8–17.

Livingstone, M.S., Rosen, C.D., Drislane, F.W., & Galaburda, A.M. (1991). Physiological and anatomical evidence for a magnocellular defect in developmental dyslexia. *Proceedings of the National Academy of Sciences of the United States of America, 88,* 7943–7947.

Lovegrove, W., Martin, F., & Slaghuis, W. (1986). A theoretical and experimental case for a visual deficit in specific reading disability. *Cognitive Neuropsychology, 3,* 225–267.

Lyon, G.R. (1989). IQ is irrelevant to the definition of learning disabilities: A position in search of logic and data. *Journal of Learning Disabilities, 22,* 504–512.

Lyon, G.R. (1995). Toward a definition of dyslexia. *Annals of Dyslexia, 45,* 3–27.

Mann, V.A., & Brady, S. (1988). Reading disability: The role of language deficiencies. *Journal of Consulting and Clinical Psychology, 56,* 811–816.

Mann, V.A., Liberman, I.Y., & Shankweiler, D. (1980). Children's memory for sentences and word strings in relation to reading ability. *Memory and Cognition, 8,* 329–335.

Martin, F., & Lovegrove, W. (1988). Uniform field flicker masking in control and specifically-disabled readers. *Perception, 17,* 203–214.

Njiokiktjien, C., de Sonneville, L., & Vaal, J. (1994). Callosal size in children with learning disabilities. *Behavioral Brain Research, 64,* 213–218.

Olson, R.K., Gillis, J.J., Rack, J.P., DeFries, J.C., & Fulker, D.W. (1991). Confirmatory factor analysis of word recognition and process measures in the Colorado Reading Project. *Reading and Writing, 3,* 235–248.

Pennington, B.F. (1995). Genetics of learning disabilities. *Journal of Child Neurology, 10,* S69–S77.

Pennington, B.F., Lefly, D.L., Van Orden, G.C., Bookman, M.O., & Smith, S.D. (1987). Is phonology bypassed in normal or dyslexic development? *Annals of Dyslexia, 37,* 62–89.

Petersen, S.E., Fox, P.T., Posner, M.I., Mintun, M., & Raichle, M.E. (1988a). Positron emission tomographic studies of the cortical anatomy of single-word processing. *Nature, 331,* 585–589.

Petersen, S.E., Fox, P.T., Posner, M.I., Mintun, M., & Raichle, M.E. (1988b). Positron emission tomographic studies of the processing of single words. *Journal of Cognitive Neuroscience, 1,* 153–170.

Price, C.J., Wise, R.J.S., Watson, J.D.G., Patterson, K., Howard, D., & Frackowiak, R.S.J. (1994). Brain activity during reading: The effects of exposure duration and task. *Brain, 117,* 1255–1269.

Rosenberger, P.B., & Hier, D.B. (1980). Cerebral asymmetry and verbal intellectual deficits. *Annals of Neurology, 8,* 300–304.

Rumsey, J.M., Andreason, P., Zametkin, A.J., Aquino, T., King, A.C., Hamburger, S.D., Pikus, A., Rapoport, J.L., & Cohen, R.M. (1992). Failure to activate the left temporoparietal cortex in dyslexia. *Archives of Neurology, 49,* 527–534.

Rumsey, J.M., Andreason, P., Zametkin, A.J., King, A.C., Hamburger, S.D., Aquino, T., Hanahan, A.P., Pikus, A., & Cohen, R.M. (1994). Right frontotemporal activation by tonal memory in dyslexia, an O^{15} PET study. *Biological Psychiatry, 36,* 171–180.

Rumsey, J.M., Berman, K.F., Denckla, M.B., Hamburger, S.D., Kruesi, M.J., & Weinberger, D.R. (1987). Regional cerebral blood flow in severe developmental dyslexia. *Archives of Neurology, 44,* 1144–1150.

Rumsey, J.M., Casanova, M., Mannheim, G.B., Patronas, N., DeVaughn, N., Hamburger, S.D., & Aquino, T. (1996). Corpus callosum morphology, as measured with MRI, in dyslexic men. *Biological Psychiatry, 39,* 769–775.

Rumsey, J.M., Dorwart, R., Vermess, M., Denckla, M.B., Kruesi, M.J.P., & Rapoport, J.L. (1986). Magnetic resonance imaging of brain anatomy in severe developmental dyslexia. *Archives of Neurology, 43,* 1045–1046.

Rumsey, J.M., Nace, K., & Andreason, P. (1995). Phonologic and orthographic components of reading imaged with PET. *Journal of the International Neuropsychological Society, 1,* 180.

Rumsey, J.M., Nace, K., & Andreason, P. (1996). [Regions activated by oral reading of single words using PET.] Unpublished raw data.

Rumsey, J.M., Zametkin, A.J., Andreason, P., Hanahan, A.P., Hamburger, S.D., Aquino, T., King, A.C., Pikus, A., & Cohen, R.M. (1994). Normal activation of frontotemporal language cortex in dyslexia, as measured with oxygen 15 positron emission tomography. *Archives of Neurology, 51,* 27–38.

Satz, P., & Morris, R. (1981). Learning disability subtypes: A review. In F.J. Pirozzolo & M.C. Wittrock (Eds.), *Neuropsychological and cognitive processes in reading* (pp. 109–141). New York: Academic Press.

Scarborough, H.S. (1984). Continuity between childhood dyslexia and adult reading. *British Journal of Psychiatry, 75,* 329–348.

Schultz, R.T., Cho, N.K., Staib, L.H., Kier, L.E., Fletcher, J.M., Shaywitz, S.E., Shankweiler, D.P., Katz, L., Gore, J.C., Duncan, J.S., & Shaywitz, B.A. (1994). Brain morphology in normal and dyslexic children: The influence of sex and age. *Annals of Neurology, 35,* 732–742.

Seidenberg, M.S., & McClelland, J.L. (1989). Visual word recognition and pronunciation: A computational model of acquisition, skilled performance, and dyslexia. In A.M. Galaburda (Ed.), *From reading to neurons* (pp. 255–303). Cambridge, MA: MIT Press.

Semrud-Clikeman, M., Filipek, P.A., Biederman, J., Steingard, R., Kennedy, D., Renshaw, P., & Bekken, K. (1994). Attention-deficit hyperactivity disorder: Magnetic resonance imaging morphometric analysis of the corpus callosum. *Journal of the American Academy of Child and Adolescent Psychiatry, 33,* 875–881.

Sergent, J., Zuck, E., Levesque, M., & MacDonald, B. (1992). Positron emission tomography study of letter and object processing: Empirical findings and methodological considerations. *Cerebral Cortex, 2,* 68–80.

Shaywitz, S.E., Escobar, M.D., Shaywitz, B.A., Fletcher, J.M., & Makuch, R. (1992). Evidence that dyslexia may represent the lower tail of a normal distribution of reading ability. *New England Journal of Medicine, 326,* 145–150.

Shaywitz, S.E., Fletcher, J.M., & Shaywitz, B.A. (1994). A conceptual framework for learning disabilities and attention deficit-hyperactivity disorder. *Canadian Journal of Special Education, 9,* 1–32.

Shaywitz, S.E., Shaywitz, B.A., Fletcher, J.M., & Escobar, M.D. (1990). Prevalence of reading disability in boys and girls. *Journal of the American Medical Association, 264,* 998–1002.

Siegel, L.S. (1992). An evaluation of the discrepancy definition of dyslexia. *Journal of Learning Disabilities, 25,* 618–629.

Stanovich, K.E. (1994). Annotation: Does dyslexia exist? *Journal of Child Psychology and Psychiatry, 35,* 579–595.

Stanovich, K.E., & Siegel, L.S. (1994). Phenotypic performance profile of children with reading disabilities: A regression-based test of the phonological-core variable-difference model. *Journal of Educational Psychology, 86,* 24–53.

Steinmetz, H., Volkmann, J., Jancke, L., & Freund, H.J. (1991). Anatomical left–right asymmetry of language-related temporal cortex is different in left and right-handers. *Annals of Neurology, 29,* 315–318.

Studdert-Kennedy, M., & Mody, M. (in press). Auditory temporal perception deficits in the reading-impaired: A critical review of the evidence. *Psychonomic Bulletin & Review.*

Tallal, P., Miller, S., & Fitch, R.H. (1993). Neurobiological basis of the case for the preeminence of temporal processing. In P. Tallal, A.M. Galaburda, R.R. Linas, & C. von Euler (Eds.), *Temporal information processing in the nervous system: Special reference to dyslexia and dysphasia* (pp. 27–47). New York: The New York Academy of Sciences.

Tallal, P., & Piercy, M. (1975). Developmental aphasia: The perception of brief vowels and extended step consonants. *Neuropsychologia, 13,* 69–75.

Wada, J.A., Clarke, R., & Hamm, A. (1975). Cerebral hemisphere asymmetry in humans: Cortical speech zones in 100 adult and 100 infant brains. *Archives of Neurology, 32,* 239–246.

Wagner, R.K., & Torgeson, J.K. (1987). The nature of phonological processing and its causal role in the acquisition of reading skills. *Psychological Bulletin, 101,* 193–212.

Waters, G.S., & Seidenberg, M.S. (1985). Spelling-sound effects in reading: Time-course and decision criteria. *Memory and Cognition, 13,* 557–572.

Willows, D.M. (1991). Visual processes in learning disabilities. In B.Y.L. Wong (Ed.), *Learning about learning disabilities* (pp. 163–193). San Diego, CA: Academic Press.

Wise, R.J., Chollet, F., Hadar, U., Friston, K., Hoffner, E., & Frackowiak, R. (1991). Distribution of cortical neural networks involved in word comprehension and word retrieval. *Brain, 114,* 1803–1817.

Witelson, S.F. (1989). Hand and sex differences in the isthmus and genu of the human corpus callosum: A postmortem morphological study. *Brain, 112,* 799–835.

Witelson, S.F., & Pallie, W. (1973). Left hemisphere specialisation for language in the newborn: Neuroanatomical evidence of asymmetry. *Brain, 96,* 641–646.

4

The Neurobiology of Developmental Dyslexia as Viewed Through the Lens of Functional Magnetic Resonance Imaging Technology

Sally E. Shaywitz, Bennett A. Shaywitz,
Kenneth R. Pugh, Pawel Skudlarski, Robert K. Fulbright,
R. Todd Constable, Richard A. Bronen, Jack M. Fletcher,
Alvin M. Liberman, Donald P. Shankweiler, Leonard Katz,
_ *Cheryl Lacadie, Karen E. Marchione, and John C. Gore* _

Developmental dyslexia was first reported in the *British Medical Journal* in 1896 (Morgan, 1896). A century later, in 1996, we stand at the threshold of understanding the neural basis of dyslexia. The progress made in understanding dyslexia provides a model of scientific accomplishment; dyslexia has evolved from a puzzling and often poorly understood entity to a disorder for which the basic cognitive deficit has been identified and localization of the disorder in the brain itself is within reach. The study of dyslexia can be considered the true Cinderella of the scientific world, going from an often poorly tolerated and patronized discipline to one that is at the cutting edge of scientific discovery in cognitive neuroscience. This transformation reflects two major scientific accomplishments—one theoretical, the other technological.

Contributing first and foremost to the advance of the discipline was the development and validation of a theory of reading and reading disability (Goswami & Bryant, 1992; Gough et al., 1992; Gough & Tunmer, 1986; Liberman, 1971; Liberman et al., 1989; Perfetti, 1985). The elaboration of this theory brought the concept of dyslexia forward and allowed it to be considered within the framework of a cognitive model of brain function. The development of such a conceptual model was a necessary, but not sufficient, contribution to understanding dyslexia at the level of the brain. This cognitive model allowed dyslexia to be considered at the level of the brain, but an additional advance, this time in technology, was required to allow dyslexia to be considered from the perspective of brain organization and function: Revolutionary advances in imaging technology make it possible literally to view dyslexia from within the brain itself. This step required the development of methods necessary to conduct what essentially are in vivo studies of higher cognitive function, that is, studies of brain function in intact individuals while they are reading.

This chapter describes the evolution of the study of dyslexia. The first step of this journey was the discovery of the core deficit underlying reading disability: phonological processing. This discovery, isolating phonological processing as the core cognitive deficit in dyslexia, was an essential prerequisite to the study of the neural basis of the

The work at the Yale Center for the Study of Learning and Attention described in this chapter was supported by National Institute of Child Health and Human Development Grants HD21888 and HD25802. The authors thank Carmel Lepore and Hedi Sarofin for assistance.

disorder. Once phonological processing had been identified, scientists knew just *what* to study; they knew on which particular cognitive system (linguistic) and on which component of that system (phonological processing) to focus in their search for the neural locus of dyslexia. Rather than simply and broadly studying reading, scientists had defined the basic functional cognitive unit underlying reading and reading disability; they knew the precise cognitive component on which to focus within the brain. Armed with the knowledge that phonological processing was the critical variable to study, scientists needed to take the next step: developing a methodology appropriate to investigating phonological processing at the level of brain structure and function. The second major step in this journey relates to the evolution of procedures and technologies for studying and relating cognition and brain function. The development of imaging technology and, more recently, functional magnetic resonance imaging (fMRI), provided the technological tools with which to study the major component processes of reading (i.e., orthographic, phonological, semantic processing) in the brain while individuals read.

THE COGNITIVE BASIS OF DYSLEXIA

Epidemiology and Developmental Course

This remarkable journey has come about as the result of a targeted program of research in learning disabilities (Kavale, 1987; Lyon, 1987). A critical component of this research strategy has been the appreciation of the need for developmental longitudinal studies "where the same subjects are repeatedly observed and studied" (Lyon, 1987, p. 74). Such studies, particularly when they are based on representative samples, address questions relating to the epidemiology and developmental course of dyslexia: How many children are affected, and what happens to these children over the course of development?

The Connecticut Longitudinal Study

The Connecticut Longitudinal Study (CLS) is an epidemiological study of learning that is conducted within a developmental framework. More specifically, the CLS is a longitudinal study of a probabilistic sample of Connecticut children. Selected upon kindergarten entry, these children have been monitored for the entire span of their schooling; in 1996, when this book went to press, the children were at the brink of young adulthood—they were, on average, 18 years old and completing 12th grade. This cohort has been studied annually within their school setting. Ability and achievement are measured by direct individual assessments; behavior and school performance are evaluated by parent, teacher, and school rating forms specifically designed for the CLS. The CLS children and families are extraordinarily committed to the study, and more than 90% of the original subjects continued to participate, despite the fact that, as of 1996, they lived in 26 different states (Shaywitz & Shaywitz, 1996).

The systematic examination of the ontogeny of reading and reading disability in this virtually intact sample has provided new insights into both the prevalence and persistence of dyslexia over time. Results from the CLS indicate the scope of the problem—that many children in grades 1–9 have reading disability. The data indicate that reading disability is a very common disorder that affects at least 10 million children, or approximately 1 child in 5. Data from the CLS indicate not only that reading disability is common, but also that it is persistent. For example, of the children who had reading disability in third grade, 74% still had reading disability in ninth grade (Figure 4.1). Reading disability does not go away. This pernicious nature of reading disability to take hold and persist is observed when actual growth rates of reading are measured over time and compared in children with reading disability and children without reading disability. Data from the longitudinal study indicate that reading disability represents a persistent impairment—a discrepancy between children with reading disability and those without reading disability that is maintained over time. Rather than a simple lag in development that the children will outgrow, reading disability, therefore, represents an enduring deficit that remains with the child throughout his or her school years and perhaps beyond (Francis et al., 1994; Shaywitz & Shaywitz, 1994).

One fundamental issue to emerge from the CLS concerns the conceptual model within which reading disability should be considered. In other words, does reading disability represent the extreme of a normal distribution of reading ability, so that there is an unbroken continuum from reading ability to reading disability, or, conversely, should reading disability be considered an isolated entity that is qualitatively separate from normal reading ability? The issue is an important one, and, for many years, reading disability was conceptualized as a categorical entity distinct from the normal distribution of reading. The categorical model of reading disability had important ramifications for the field, because it served both as the basis for scientific investigations into the biology of the disorder and as the scientific rationale for common clinical practices relating to dyslexia, including the identification of and provision of services to children. The subsequent finding that reading disability is part of the continuum of reading ability placed the disorder in the context of most other biologically based disorders, such as hypertension and obesity (Shaywitz et al., 1992). Reading ability is distributed along a continuum in which individuals vary by degree from one another; this finding indicates that all that has been learned about reading can be applied to further our understanding of reading disability. In addition, awareness that reading disability is part of the continuum of reading ability suggests that any differences in brain function and

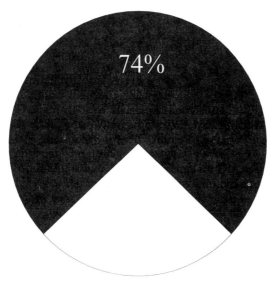

Figure 4.1.   Data from the CLS showing the percentage of children diagnosed with dyslexia in third grade who were still diagnosed with dyslexia in ninth grade.

organization between individuals with and without reading disability are quantitative and not qualitative. Just as reading performance in individuals with reading disability differs from that in individuals without reading disability by degree, but not in kind, the authors hypothesize that any difference emerging in the functional organization of the brain between individuals with reading disability and those without reading disability is dimensional rather than categorical. The following section discusses current conceptualizations of the cognitive mechanisms responsible for reading disability.

Neurolinguistic and Cognitive Mechanisms

The establishment of the persistent nature of reading disability raises the next consideration: Just what is it that persists? What is it that remains with the child and prevents him or her from learning to read? Evidence from several lines of investigation has converged to identify and isolate phonological processing as the specific cognitive deficit responsible for reading disability (see reviews by Liberman & Shankweiler, 1991; Stanovich, 1988; Wagner & Torgesen, 1987). Evidence from two large, well-studied populations of children with reading disability (Fletcher et al., 1994; Shankweiler et al., 1995; Stanovich & Siegel, 1994) has confirmed that a deficit in phonological processing represents the most robust correlate of reading disability. Studies in young adults, furthermore, support the notion that phonological processing deficits persist (Bell & Perfetti, 1994; Bruck, 1990, 1992). Phonological processing deficits most often are demonstrated by difficulties (i.e., lack of automaticity) in word identification, particularly in pseudoword reading. Not only does reading disability persist, but evidence indicates that difficulties in reading across the full span of development are unified, as reflected by a common deficit—phonological processing. An impairment in phonological processing, therefore, characterizes both young and older poor readers.

Nature and Definition of Reading Disability

Deficits in Phonological Processing Define Reading Disability

What should be the definition of reading disability? For too many years, the road to identifying a reading disability had been littered with artificial barriers that required children (and adults) to meet arbitrarily imposed criteria, such as the requirement of an ability–achievement discrepancy. Moreover, and of greatest concern, it is clear that definitions served administrative needs more often than they reflected valid biological underpinnings (Fletcher et al., 1994; Lyon, 1995; Shaywitz et al., 1992; Stanovich & Siegel, 1994). When little was known about the nature of reading disability, there was little choice: Definitions reflected the state of the art and, therefore, were removed from and unrelated to the fundamental processes responsible for creating the condition of disability in reading. Given the overwhelming consensus that exists in the 1990s that reading disability is related to reading and, furthermore, that reading reflects language, the opportunity exists for the development of a definition of reading disability that reflects the core deficit affecting individuals with reading disabilities: phonological processing. As a result of this lower-level deficit within the language system, individuals who are affected experience a predictable range of difficulties in both written and oral language. The effects of the phonological deficit, therefore, travel up through the language system and may affect such diverse but phonologically based linguistic processes as decoding, spelling, writing, word naming and retrieval, and speech perception and speech production.

In the 1990s, the astute diagnostician's approach to dyslexia will reflect that first described by Critchley (1981): to search for the signs of a language disorder in all of its forms. Indications of a history of a language disorder, particularly one reflecting an impairment in phonological processing, are much more informative than are any statistical gyrations that must be invoked involving a child's scores on reading and IQ tests. The following definition of dyslexia developed by a group of investigators, clinicians, representatives of advocacy groups, and representatives of the National Institutes of Health, Bethesda, Maryland, avoids the inadequacies and arbitrary nature of the discrepancy-based definition while incorporating newer knowledge about the basic or core deficit underlying reading disability:

> Dyslexia is one of several distinct learning disabilities. It is a specific language-based disorder of constitutional origin characterized by difficulties in single word decoding, usually reflecting insufficient phonological processing. These difficulties in single word decoding are often unexpected in relation to age and other cognitive and academic abilities; they are not the result of generalized developmental delay or sensory impairment. Dyslexia is manifest by variable difficulty with different forms of language, often including, in addition to problems with reading, a conspicuous problem with acquiring proficiency in writing and spelling (Operational definition of the Orton Dyslexia Society Research Committee, April 18, 1994). (Lyon, 1995, p. 9)

Importance of the History in the Diagnosis of Reading Disability

Although there is a tendency to focus on measures rather than the actuality of an individual's life history, for reading disability, a developmental history of difficulties with language, particularly phonologically based components of language, often provides the clearest and most reliable indication of a reading disorder (Shaywitz & Shaywitz, 1994). Phonological processing has been conceptualized as encompassing at least three different components: phonological awareness, phonological recoding in lexical access, and phonetic recoding in working memory (for a comprehensive review, see Wagner & Torgesen, 1987). The direct measurement of each of these components represents a rational goal of assessment for reading disability. Although progress is being made, particularly for the assessment of specific phonological components in younger children (Torgesen et al., 1992), the availability of a standardized and reliable test of phonological processing that is appropriate for older children, young adults, and very intelligent individuals remains more a goal than a reality. It is young adults, who often are intelligent and have worked extremely hard to compensate for their phonological impairments, for whom standardized testing and assessment procedures tend to be inadequate. Such individuals will often compensate for their impairment so that they are accurate in identifying words, but this accuracy comes at a cost—their decoding skills lack automaticity and, as a result, they decode and read very slowly (Lefly & Pennington, 1991). For these individuals, especially, the history is paramount; a history of early and continuing difficulties in oral language (e.g., in pronouncing words), reading new or unfamiliar words, spelling, and writing will provide the distinct diagnostic signature of an individual's reading disability. Speech punctuated by hesitancies and dysfluencies, spelling difficulties, and slow and laborious reading and writing represent rich historical data that provide evidence of a core deficit in phonological processing that results in the expression of a reading disability. The requirement of excessive amounts of time in relation to the relatively high level of competency achieved is the hallmark of a reading disability in an individual with compensated dyslexia.

Pending the development of appropriate and sensitive measures of phonological processing applicable to readers of all ages and levels of intelligence, the history, for

clinical purposes, represents the most sensitive and accurate indicator of reading disability in older children and adults. In younger children, the finding of either a discrepancy or low achievement in reading supports the diagnosis of a reading disability. As
children mature, however, those who are more intelligent will learn to compensate,
and simple reading tests will not be adequate to demonstrate the difficulties that such
individuals have in decoding or the effort that accurate decoding demands. For these
reasons, a history of phonologically based language difficulties, laborious reading and
writing, poor spelling, and additional time required in reading and taking tests provides indisputable evidence of an impairment in phonological processing, which, in
turn, serves as the basis for, and signature of, dyslexia.

In children and adults with dyslexia, therefore, there is incontrovertible evidence
that the first step in the reading pathway—decoding—is affected and that a basic and
persistent deficit in phonological processing is responsible. Studies indicate clearly
that deficits in phonological processing represent the most severe, consistent, and enduring deficit in children with reading disability. For example, data from the CLS indicate that phonological processing continues to make a critical contribution to reading
even in children as old as 15 years. In this population, the component of language or
reading that best predicts reading accuracy, reading speed, reading comprehension,
and spelling remains phonological processing, a deficit that is manifest as early as the
preschool period and continues through adolescence and into adulthood.

NEUROBIOLOGICAL MECHANISMS
IN READING AND READING DISABILITY

Given that the basic cognitive lesion in reading disability has been identified, it is possible to begin to address, at the most elemental level, the underlying neural substrate
of phonological processing and reading disability. In the mid-1990s, we are poised to
enter a new and extraordinary era in the study of reading disability. A powerful and,
indeed, revolutionary technology emerged to allow scientists to image the working
brain. This remarkable new technology, fMRI, captures the physiological changes that
take place when brain activation occurs.

Strategies for the Cerebral Localization of Reading

Studies of Subjects with Brain Injuries

Reading can be studied only in people; there can be no animal models of reading. In
contrast with other basic physiological processes that humans share with other species, higher cognitive processes, such as language and reading, can be studied only in
humans, a fact that significantly limits the range of scientific investigation. Given this
fundamental limitation, it is not surprising that studies of the cerebral localization of
cognitive functions in humans began only in the late 1700s. Not until the beginning of
the 19th century did Gall propose that mental functions were localized in the cerebral
hemispheres rather than in other organs, such as the liver or spleen (see Young, 1990).
After Gall's theories were advanced, others began to localize cognitive functions, including language, by studying the brains of individuals who had sustained brain lesions as a result of strokes or traumatic injury and began to relate the loss of particular
cognitive functions to damage to specific brain regions. The concept of the cerebral localization of motor and sensory functions was first mentioned by a German physician,
Baader, in 1763. Of the cognitive functions, language functions were the first to be

characterized. On the basis of a study of an individual with a large lesion in the region of the inferior frontal gyrus of the left hemisphere, Broca (Young, 1990) proposed that this brain region was responsible for speech production. Other investigations followed, relating a range of cognitive functions to specific brain regions on the basis of descriptions of patients with brain lesions; by the close of the 19th century, brain maps of the localization of cerebral function had become quite detailed (Figure 4.2; Ferrier, 1890; Young, 1990).

Much has been learned from studies of cerebral localization of cognitive function in individuals with brain damage, and such studies continue to provide important information, particularly given the emergence of modern imaging methods that allow very fine-grain anatomical resolution (Damasio & Damasio, 1992). Studies of individuals with brain damage, however, cannot address the question of brain function and organization in individuals without brain injuries; it is clear that dyslexia in children is not the result of an injury but represents a subtle developmental disorder with effects that emanate through the language module. Ideally, therefore, to study and understand dyslexia, researchers must measure brain function in individuals without brain damage.

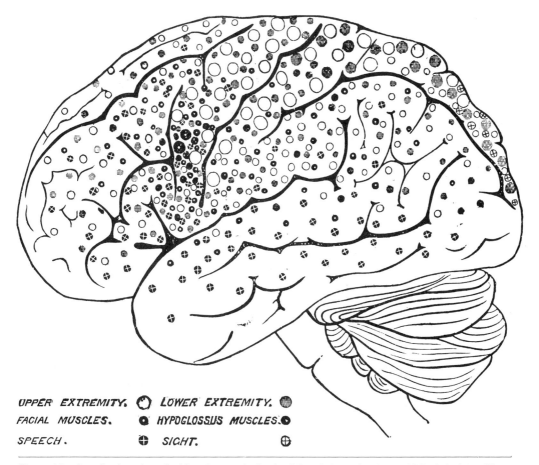

UPPER EXTREMITY. ● LOWER EXTREMITY. ●
FACIAL MUSCLES. ● HYPOGLOSSUS MUSCLES.●
SPEECH. ● SIGHT. ⊕

Figure 4.2.   Localization of cerebral functions on the basis of descriptions of patients with brain lesions. (From Ferrier, D. [1890]. *The Croonian lectures on cerebral localisation*, p. 16. London: Smith, Elder and Co.)

Studies localizing cerebral function on the basis of damage to specific brain regions in individuals with brain injuries provide a static picture of brain anatomy rather than a dynamic picture of brain function while individuals perform cognitive tasks. What is necessary is to be able to image and then identify the functional units of the working nervous system, that is, the neural networks that are engaged by specific cognitive functions. Functional imaging, the ability to measure brain function during performance of a cognitive task, meets this requirement and became available in the early 1980s. For the first time, rather than being limited to examining the brain in an autopsy specimen or measuring the size of brain regions with the use of static morphometric indices based on computed tomography (CT) or magnetic resonance imaging (MRI), scientists were able to study brain metabolism while individuals performed specific cognitive tasks. (See Chapter 2 for an overview of different types of neuroimaging procedures, and see Chapter 3 for an overview of several types of neuroimaging investigations used in studies of dyslexia, including positron emission tomography [PET] and MRI.)

Studies that Use Functional Imaging

The rationale of functional imaging is straightforward. When an individual performs a discrete cognitive task, that task places processing demands on particular neural systems in the brain. To meet those demands, neural systems in particular brain regions are activated, and those changes in neural activity, in turn, are reflected by changes in brain metabolic activity and accompanying changes in cerebral blood flow. It is possible to measure such changes in specific brain regions while subjects are engaged in cognitive tasks.

SPECT and PET   The first studies of this kind used [133]xenon single photon emission computed tomography (SPECT) (Lou et al., 1984, 1990) to measure cerebral blood flow, but more recent studies have used PET. In practice, PET requires the intravenous administration of a radioactive isotope to the subject, so that cerebral blood flow or cerebral utilization of glucose can be determined while a subject performs a task. To minimize the risks to the subject, isotopes with very short biological half-lives are synthesized in a cyclotron immediately before testing, which mandates that the time course of the experiment conform to the half-life of the radioisotope. Although much has been learned about language by using PET technology (for reviews, see Demonet et al., 1994; Frackowiak, 1994; Petersen & Fiez, 1993), the radiation involved and the logistics of generating short-lived isotopes limit the utility of the procedure, particularly in children (see Chapter 2).

fMRI

Since 1994, fMRI has emerged to allow scientists to determine the activation of specific neural systems in the brain while individuals perform cognitive tasks (see Chapter 2). In contrast with PET, fMRI does not require the administration of any radioactive isotope. Because no radiation is involved, numerous scans (100+, see Table 2.1) can be acquired with fMRI to achieve an adequate signal-to-noise ratio. fMRI studies can be repeated frequently without concern for radiation. The strategy used in fMRI parallels that developed for PET studies, a strategy termed *subtraction*, which depends on measuring differences in brain activity during a series of tasks. Differences in fMRI signal are determined by measuring differences in the magnetic properties of oxygenated and unoxygenated blood.

In practice, fMRI has proved to be a very user-friendly technology (Figure 4.3). The subject simply lies in the MRI machine and holds a response bulb in his or her hand, so that investigators can determine whether his or her responses are correct and how quickly he or she responds. The tasks, which are described below, are projected on a screen that the subject views through a periscope. Few contraindications exist to the procedure; the only significant one is that artifacts may be produced by objects that cause interference in the magnetic field. So, instead of the question commonly asked of adults—"Do you have a metal plate in your head?"—investigators ask children, "Do you wear braces on your teeth?"

The Tasks   The selection of specific tasks used in functional imaging studies is critical; the task must result in the isolation of a specific cognitive process. The function of task design is to develop tasks that reflect the response to a single, specific cognitive demand. For example, for studies of reading, the tasks used in fMRI studies are designed to examine the major components of the reading process: orthography, phonology, and semantics. The underlying rationale involves the subtraction strategy, a strategy designed to isolate specific brain–cognitive function relations (Friston et al., 1993; Petersen & Fiez, 1993; Sergent, 1994). The goal is to develop a series of hierarchical tasks such that each succeeding task differs from the previous one by a single cognitive demand. Both modalities and response demands should be equal, so that, for example, the tasks are all presented visually and responses are all made by pressing a response bulb. Activation patterns (i.e., patterns of metabolic activity) are monitored while subjects perform cognitive tasks that involve a given process (e.g., process X) among others. A control task is designed that, in principle, shares all cognitive operations with the experimental task, except for process X. By subtracting the activation produced in the control task from the activation produced in the experimental task, regions associated with process X can be isolated. The subtraction methods are the best available approach, but, to ensure sound results, care must be used in task design to 1) use a carefully constructed hierarchical set of tasks, which should tap language processes differentially while sharing as many secondary operations as possible; and 2) use a variety of subtractions to converge on a conclusion about the function of a given cortical region. (See Chapter 2 for a more detailed explanation of task design.)

Recent Progress Using fMRI to Study Reading

At the Yale Center for the Study of Learning and Attention, New Haven, Connecticut, in collaboration with the Yale Nuclear Magnetic Resonance Research Group, a systematic program of research focused on elucidating basic neurobiological mechanisms underlying reading and attention has been instituted. To investigate the reading process, a set of tasks based on the subtraction strategy was developed to isolate orthographic, phonological, and lexical–semantic foci. In these experiments, subjects perform four distinct same–different tasks. The decisions (same versus different) and response components (press a response bulb for same pairs) of these tasks are comparable, although, in each, the type of linguistic information engaged differs. In a line judgment task, subjects view two sets of four lines with either right or left orientation, one above the other, and determine whether the upper and lower displays have the same pattern of left-right alternation (Table 4.1). This task should primarily engage visuospatial information processing. In a letter case judgment task, two sets of consonant strings are displayed, and subjects determine whether they contain the same pattern of case (upper and lower) alternation. This task engages both visuospatial and orthographic (letter) processing. In a rhyme judgment task, subjects determine whether two non-

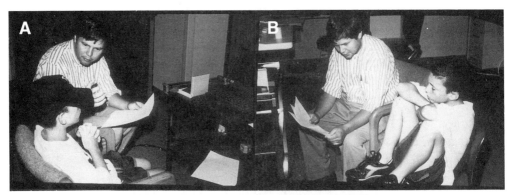

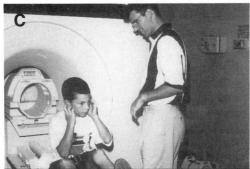

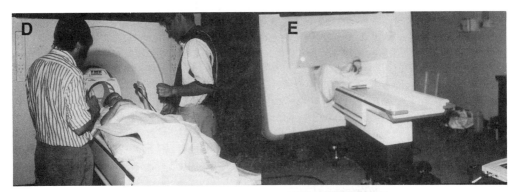

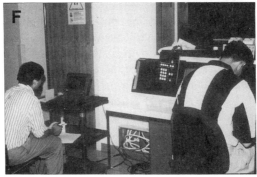

Figure 4.3.   This series of six pictures illustrates how fMRI is conducted at the Yale Center for the Study of Learning and Attention. The child is instructed about the tasks he will see (Panels A and B) and then lies in the magnet, a conventional 1.5-tesla unit (Panel C). He holds a response bulb (Panel D) and observes the tasks projected on a screen viewed through a periscope (Panel E). These images are generated by a microcomputer in the control room (Panel F).

Table 4.1.   Tasks and subtractions

Task	Stimuli	Processes engaged
Line	// \ / // \ /	Visuospatial
Case	BtBT BtBT	Visuospatial + Orthographic
Rhyme	LETE JEAT	Visuospatial + Orthographic + Phonological
Category	CORN RICE	Visuospatial + Orthographic + Phonological + Semantic

sense word strings rhyme. This task engages visuospatial, orthographic, and assembled phonological processing (subjects must map the letter strings onto the appropriate phonological representations). In a semantic category task, subjects determine whether two words belong to the same semantic category. This task engages visuospatial, orthographic, phonological, and semantic information processing.

By subtracting the line task from the case task, activation in regions associated with orthographic processing are isolated, because the two tasks both engage visuospatial processing, but only the case task engages letter processing (see Table 4.1). By subtracting the case task from the rhyme task, regions associated with assembled phonological processing (i.e., mapping from orthography to phonology) are isolated, because the tasks differ primarily on the phonological dimension. By subtracting the rhyme task from the semantic category task, regions associated with lexical semantic processing are isolated, because only the semantic category task engages this type of processing (i.e., by using nonsense word stimuli in the rhyme task, spurious activation of semantic sites should be minimized).

Of the tasks described, investigators focus on the rhyme judgment task, in particular, because it taps phonological processing, which, as indicated throughout this chapter, is the core deficit in reading disability. If scientists can determine the organization and localization of those neural systems that engage phonological processing, they will have taken a major step forward in understanding the neural basis of both reading and dyslexia. The isolation of the neural networks that underlie phonological processing is a necessary prerequisite to the study of dyslexia. The study of phonological processing and the identification of activation patterns associated with phonological processing in individuals with dyslexia would make it possible, for the first time, to have a biological signature of a specific learning disability—in this case, reading disability or dyslexia. With this goal in mind, the authors have undertaken a systematic series of experiments designed to determine the neural systems responsible for phonological processing and to determine how the functional organization of these systems differ in individuals with and without dyslexia.

A recent study examined nonimpaired, right-handed readers (19 men and 19 women) while they performed the above-described tasks (Shaywitz et al., 1995). The study focused on those brain regions that previous neuropsychological and neuroimaging investigations indicated were of relevance for language function (Demonet et al., 1994; Frackowiack, 1994; Petersen & Fiez, 1993). Behavioral research on word recognition has isolated two types of coding relevant to lexical identification: orthographic (i.e., pertaining to letter encoding) and phonological (i.e., pertaining to phoneme encoding) (Coltheart et al., 1993; Lukatela & Turvey, 1991; Pugh et al., 1994). Initial analyses identified one region uniquely associated with orthographic processing (i.e., the extrastriate). A second region, located within the superior aspect of the inferior frontal gyrus (IFG), roughly encompassing Brodmann's areas 44 and 45 (which we term IFG) and previously shown to be activated in speech tasks when phonetic decisions are required (Demonet et al., 1992; Demonet et al., 1994), was found to be uniquely associated with phonological processing on rhyme judgments. The rhyme judgment task was also associated with activation at sites in both the superior temporal gyrus and middle temporal gyrus, areas that fall within traditional language regions. The semantic task, however, activated both of these areas significantly more strongly than did the rhyme task, which suggests that these regions subserve both phonological and lexical semantic processing. The IFG, in contrast, was uniquely associated with phonological processing. Of particular interest were differences in brain activation during phonological processing in men compared with that during phonological processing in women. As shown in Figure 4.4 on page *xxxi*, activation during the performance of the rhyming task in men was lateralized to the left IFG. In contrast, activation during this same task in women was bilateral in the IFG. Error rates for both the semantic and rhyme tasks were extremely low (on average, one error per 20 trials) and did not vary systematically by task or by sex.

These findings provided the first clear evidence of sex differences in the functional organization of the brain for language and indicated that these differences exist in phonological processing. At one level, these findings support and extend a long-held hypothesis that suggests that language functions are more likely to be highly lateralized in males but represented in both cerebral hemispheres in females (Halpern, 1992; Hampson & Kimura, 1992; Harshman et al., 1983; Hellige, 1993; Hines, 1990; Iaccino, 1993; McClone, 1980; Witelson & Kigar, 1992). On another level, and of particular relevance to the scientific study of reading and reading disability, these data indicate that it is possible to isolate specific components of language and, at the same time, relate these language processes to distinct patterns of functional organization in the brain. It is possible, therefore, to conduct studies that link cognitive function and brain organization, not only in individuals without reading impairments, but also, potentially, in subjects with histories of dyslexia. These data suggest that the activation of the IFG region during the performance of a rhyming task may provide a neural signature for phonological processing, the core cognitive component in reading and dyslexia. This discovery of a biological marker for phonological processing in reading means that investigators can now approach the most basic cognitive deficit in reading disability from the perspective of brain organization. Neural systems relating to phonological processing can be investigated in both individuals without reading impairments and individuals with dyslexia.

FUTURE DIRECTIONS

The discovery of a biological signature for reading and, potentially, dyslexia has significant implications, not only for our understanding of the fundamental neural mechanisms underlying reading and reading disability, but also for the identification and diagnosis of dyslexia and for the assessment of the effects of interventions on dyslexia. For example, it has become possible to examine the development over time of the neural mechanisms serving reading in both individuals with dyslexia and individuals without reading impairments. In the above-described study, it was established that, for nonimpaired readers, the neural systems engaged by mature men and women during phonological processing differ significantly. It is not known, however, whether there are also differences in these neural systems in boys and girls or at what age these differences emerge. Studies designed to address this question, that is, how the neural locus of reading changes over the course of development in boys and girls individually, have been undertaken to determine, for the first time, what happens in the brain as children mature. These studies not only address this development in boys and girls without reading disorders, but also address the development of the functional organization of the brain for phonological processing in boys and girls with well-defined dyslexia.

The discovery of a biological signature or marker for reading (and potentially for dyslexia) offers a unique opportunity to identify and diagnose dyslexia in older individuals. Studies, therefore, have been undertaken to examine the functional organization of the brain for phonological processing in the following three groups of older individuals: individuals without reading impairments; individuals with dyslexia; and individuals who have compensated, either wholly or partially, for their reading impairment. The authors hypothesize that the functional organization of phonological processing will differ among all three groups. It is possible that the neural signature for phonological processing may provide the most sensitive index of dyslexia in individuals who appear to have compensated for their reading disability. Finally, the discovery of a biological signature for reading offers an unprecedented opportunity to assess the effects of interventions on reading in nonimpaired readers as well as in individuals with dyslexia. It is reasonable to suggest that brain activation patterns obtained while subjects engage in tasks that tap phonological processing represent the most precise measure of phonological processing. By using activation patterns obtained while individuals perform phonological tasks, it is possible to determine the functional organization in the brains of individuals with dyslexia, impose interventions, and measure the effects of those interventions on the brain. If measurable effects on brain organization are seen after the intervention, it is possible to repeat the fMRI to determine whether these differences persist after the intervention ends.

CONCLUSIONS

With these fMRI studies, the field of dyslexia research has taken a significant step forward in the quest to understand the underlying neural basis of reading and dyslexia. fMRI allows scientists to identify and isolate those brain regions activated while a child actually reads a word. The ability to pinpoint the specific neural network that serves reading has moved the field considerably closer to understanding, treating, and even preventing learning disabilities. Once the particular neural networks engaged by reading have been identified, these can be mapped and quantified. Researchers then can identify the specific locations of those networks within the brain, as well as their sizes, compositions, and the specific intensities of their activation when reading takes place and use these as potential biological markers for studying and better understanding why some children and adults cannot learn to read. In the 1990s, the field of dyslexia research is in the process of harnessing the extraordinary power of modern neurobiology to improve the lives of children and adults with learning disabilities. Society is on the cusp of a true revolution in its ability to use science to inform public policy—a revolution in which biological discoveries serve the health and education of our children.

Children and adults with learning disabilities no longer will be at the mercy of vague impressions or misguided notions of learning disability. We no longer have to grope in the dark, for scientific discoveries illuminate our paths.

REFERENCES

Baader, J. (1763). *Observationes medicae incisionibus cadaverum anatomicis illustratae*. Augsburg & Freiburg, Germany: Ignatius & Anton Wagner.

Bell, L.C., & Perfetti, C.A. (1994). Reading skill: Some adult comparisons. *Journal of Educational Psychology, 86*, 244–255.

Bruck, M. (1990). Word-recognition skills of adults with childhood diagnoses of dyslexia. *Developmental Psychology, 26*, 439–454.

Bruck, M. (1992). Persistence of dyslexics' phonological awareness deficits. *Developmental Psychology, 28*, 874–886.

Coltheart, M., Curtis, B., Atkins, P., & Haller, M. (1993). Models of reading aloud: Dual-route and parallel-distributed-processing approaches. *Psychology Review, 100*, 589–608.

Critchley, M. (1981). Dyslexia: An overview. In G.T. Pavlidis & T.R. Miles (Eds.), *Dyslexia research and its applications to education* (pp. 1–11). Chichester, England: John Wiley & Sons.

Damasio, A.R., & Damasio, H. (1992). Brain and language. *Scientific American, 267*, 89–95.

Demonet, J.F., Chollet, F., Ramsey, S., Cardebat, D., Nespoulous, J.-L., Wise, R., Rascol, A., & Frackowiak, R. (1992). The anatomy of phonological and semantic processing in normal subjects. *Brain, 115*, 1753–1768.

Demonet, J.F., Price, C., Wise, R., & Frackowiak, R.S.J. (1994). A PET study of cognitive strategies in normal subjects during language tasks: Influence of phonetic ambiguity and sequence processing on phoneme monitoring. *Brain, 117*, 671–682.

Ferrier, D. (Ed.). (1890). *The Croonian lectures on cerebral localisation*. London: Smith, Elder and Co.

Fletcher, J.M., Shaywitz, S.E., Shankweiler, D.P., Katz, L., Liberman, I.Y., Stuebing, K.K., Francis, D.J., Fowler, A., & Shaywitz, B.A. (1994). Cognitive profiles of reading disability: Comparisons of discrepancy and low achievement definitions. *Journal of Educational Psychology, 85*, 1–18.

Frackowiak, R.S.J. (1994). Functional mapping of verbal memory and language. *Trends in Neurosciences, 17*, 109–115.

Francis, D.J., Shaywitz, S.E., Stuebing, K.K., Shaywitz, B.A., & Fletcher, J.M. (1994). The measurement of change: Assessing behavior over time and within a developmental context. In G.R. Lyon (Ed.), *Frames of reference for the assessment of learning disabilities: New views on measurement issues* (pp. 29–58). Baltimore: Paul H. Brookes Publishing Co.

Friston, K.J., Frith, C.D., Liddle, P.F., & Frackowiak, R.S.J. (1993). Functional connectivity: The principal-component analysis of large (PET) data sets. *Journal of Cerebral Blood Flow and Metabolism, 13*, 5–14.

Goswami, U., & Bryant, P. (1992). Rhyme, analogy, and children's reading. In P.B. Gough, L.C. Ehri, & R. Treiman (Eds.), *Reading acquisition* (pp. 49–64). Hillsdale, NJ: Lawrence Erlbaum Associates.

Gough, P.B., Ehri, L.C., & Treiman, R. (Eds.). (1992). *Reading acquisition*. Hillsdale, NJ: Lawrence Erlbaum Associates.

Gough, P.B., & Tunmer, W.E. (1986). Decoding, reading, and reading disability. *Remedial and Special Education, 7*, 6–10.

Halpern, D. (1992). *Sex differences in cognitive abilities*. Hillsdale, N.J.: Lawrence Erlbaum Associates.

Hampson, E., & Kimura, D. (1992). Sex differences and hormonal influences on cognitive function in humans. In J.B. Becker, S.M. Breedlove, & D. Crews (Eds.), *Behavioral endocrinology* (pp. 357–398). Cambridge, MA: The MIT Press.

Harshman, R., Remington, R., & Krashen, S. (1983). *Sex, language and the brain. III. Evidence from dichotic listening for adult sex differences in verbal lateralization*. Unpublished manuscript, University of Western Ontario, Canada.

Hellige, J. (1993). *Hemispheric asymmetry: What's right and what's left*. Cambridge, MA: Harvard University Press.

Hines, M. (1990). Gonadal hormones and human cognitive development. In J. Balthazart (Ed.), *Hormones, brain and behavior in vertebrates: Sexual differentiation, neuroanatomical aspects, neurotransmitters and neuropeptides* (Vol. 1, pp. 51–63). Basel, Switzerland: Karger.

Iaccino, J. (1993). *Left brain–right brain differences.* Hillsdale, NJ: Lawrence Erlbaum Associates.

Kavale, K.A. (1987). Response to Lyon. In S. Vaughn & C.S. Bos (Eds.), *Research in learning disabilities: Issues and future directions* (pp. 80–82). Boston: Little, Brown.

Lefly, D.L., & Pennington, B.F. (1991). Spelling errors and reading fluency in compensated adult dyslexics. *Annals of Dyslexia, 41,* 143.

Liberman, I.Y. (1971). Basic research in speech and lateralization of language: Some implications for reading disability. *Bulletin of the Orton Society, 21,* 71–87.

Liberman, I.Y., & Shankweiler, D. (1991). Phonology and beginning to read: A tutorial. In L. Rieben & C.A. Perfetti (Eds.), *Learning to read: Basic research and its implications.* Hillsdale, NJ: Lawrence Erlbaum Associates, Inc.

Liberman, I.Y., Shankweiler, D., & Liberman, A.M. (1989). The alphabetic principle and learning to read. In D. Shankweiler & I.Y. Liberman (Eds.), *International Academy for Research in Learning Disabilities Monograph Series: Number 6. Phonology and reading disability: Solving the reading puzzle* (pp. 1–33). Ann Arbor: University of Michigan Press.

Lou, H.C., Henriksen, L., & Bruhn, P. (1984). Focal cerebral hypoperfusion in children with dysphasia and/or attention deficit disorder. *Archives of Neurology, 42,* 825–829.

Lou, H.C., Henriksen, L., & Bruhn, P. (1990). Focal cerebral dysfunction in developmental learning disabilities. *Lancet, 335,* 8–11.

Lukatela, G., & Turvey, M.T. (1991). Phonological access of the lexicon: Evidence from associative priming and pseudo homophones. *Journal of Experimental Psychology, 17,* 951–966.

Lyon, G.R. (1995). Toward a definition of dyslexia. *Annals of Dyslexia, 45,* 3–30.

Lyon, G.R. (1987). Learning disabilities research: False starts and broken promises. In S. Vaughn & C.S. Bos (Eds.), *Research in learning disabilities: Issues and future directions* (pp. 69–85). Boston: Little, Brown.

McClone, J. (1980). Sex differences in human brain asymmetry: A critical survey. *Behavioral and Brain Sciences, 3,* 215–227.

Morgan, W.P. (1896). A case of congenital word blindness. *British Medical Journal,* 1378.

Perfetti, C.A. (1985). *Reading ability.* New York: Oxford University Press.

Petersen, S.E., & Fiez, J.A. (1993). The processing of single words studied with positron emission tomography. *Annual Review of Neuroscience, 16,* 509–530.

Pugh, K., Rexer, K., & Katz, L. (1994). Evidence for flexible coding in visual word recognition. *Journal of Experimental Psychology, 20,* 807–825.

Sergent, J. (1994). Brain-imaging studies of cognitive function. *Trends in Neurosciences, 17,* 221–227.

Shankweiler, D., Crain, S., Katz, L., Fowler, A.E., Liberman, A.M., Brady, S.A., Thornton, R., Lundquist, E., Dreyer, L., Fletcher, J.M., Stuebing, K.K., Shaywitz, S.E., & Shaywitz, B.E. (1995). Cognitive profiles of reading-disabled children: Comparison of language skills in phonology, morphology, and syntax. *Psychological Science, 6,* 149–156.

Shaywitz, B.A., Shaywitz, S.E., Pugh, K.R., Constable, R. Todd, Skudlarski, P., Fulbright, R.K., Bronen, R.A., Fletcher, J.M., Shankweiler, D.P., Katz, L., & Gore, J.C. (1995). Sex differences in the functional organization of the brain for language. *Nature, 373,* 607–609.

Shaywitz, S.E., Escobar, M.D., Shaywitz, B.A., Fletcher, J.M., & Makuch, R. (1992). Evidence that dyslexia may represent the lower tail of a normal distribution of reading ability. *New England Journal of Medicine, 326,* 145–150.

Shaywitz, S.E., & Shaywitz, B.A. (1994). Learning disabilities and attention disorder. In K.F. Swaiman (Ed.), *Pediatric neurology: Principles and practice* (Vol. 2, pp. 1119–1151). St. Louis, MO: C.V. Mosby.

Shaywitz, S.E., & Shaywitz, B.A. (1996). Unlocking learning disabilities: The neurological basis. In S. Cramer & B. Ellis (Eds.), *Learning disabilities: Lifelong issues* (pp. 255–260). Baltimore: Paul H. Brookes Publishing Co.

Stanovich, K.E. (1988). Explaining the differences between the dyslexic and the garden-variety poor reader: The phonological-core variable-difference model. *Journal of Learning Disabilities, 21,* 590–604.

Stanovich, K.E., & Siegel, L.S. (1994). Phenotypic performance profile of children with reading disabilities: A regression-based test of the phonological-core variable-difference model. *Journal of Educational Psychology, 86,* 24–53.

Torgesen, J.K., Wagner, R.K., Bryant, B.R., & Pearson, N. (1992). Toward development of a kindergarten group test for phonological awareness. *Journal of Research and Development in Education, 25,* 13–21.

Wagner, R.K., & Torgesen, J.K. (1987). The nature of phonological processing and its causal role in the acquisition of reading skills. *Psychological Bulletin, 101,* 192–212.

Witelson, S.F., & Kigar, D.L. (1992). Sylvian fissure morphology and asymmetry in men and women: Bilateral differences in relation to handedness in men. *Journal of Comparative Neurology, 323,* 323–326.

Young, R. (1990). *Mind, brain and adaptation in the nineteenth century.* Oxford, England: Oxford University Press.

5

Neuroimaging in Attention-Deficit/Hyperactivity Disorder

Monique Ernst

Brain imaging in individuals with attention-deficit/hyperactivity disorder (ADHD) has been limited to research applications. At present, neither structural nor functional brain imaging can be used clinically as a diagnostic or prognostic tool for ADHD. Nonetheless, the scientific value of brain imaging as a tool to bring new insights to the underlying neural substrates of the symptoms of ADHD is unique. This chapter shows, through a review of the literature, how the findings derived from brain imaging studies of individuals with ADHD contribute to our understanding of the disorder. Before the results of brain imaging research are presented, a number of caveats relevant to their interpretation are addressed.

FACTORS THAT AFFECT
THE INTERPRETATION OF BRAIN IMAGING DATA

ADHD Samples

ADHD is defined by the *Diagnostic and Statistical Manual of Mental Disorders* (4th ed.) (American Psychiatric Association, 1994; see Table 5.1) as a disorder characterized by persistent inattention and/or hyperactivity-impulsivity starting before 7 years of age and leading to impaired functioning in at least two settings (i.e., school, home). Three subtypes—a predominantly inattentive type, a predominantly hyperactive/impulsive type, and a combined inattentive/hyperactive type—are described.

ADHD affects 3%–5% of school-age children and is 4–9 times more common in boys than in girls, depending on the setting (community versus clinic populations) (American Psychiatric Association, 1994; Barkley et al., 1990; Ross & Ross, 1982; Szatmari et al., 1989). A significant number of children with ADHD will continue to exhibit ADHD symptoms into adulthood (Gittelman et al., 1985; Hechtman, 1992; Klein & Mannuzza, 1991; Loney et al., 1981; Weiss, 1985).

The definition of ADHD has changed over time (see Table 5.2). This change has contributed to the selection of research samples with differing clinical characteristics, making comparisons among studies difficult. For instance, samples of children with ADHD who were diagnosed according to DSM-III-R (American Psychiatric Association, 1987) criteria include children who do not meet DSM-III (American Psychiatric Association, 1980) criteria (Newcorn et al., 1989). According to the DSM-IV field trial (Lahey et al., 1994), DSM-IV criteria identified more girls and preschool children with ADHD than did DSM-III-R criteria. Table 5.2 summarizes the various terms used to label ADHD and the characteristics of each. Those labels reflect the currents of thoughts about ADHD and their evolution over time.

The understanding of children presenting characteristics of restlessness, inattention, and impulsivity first focused on brain damage as an etiology, as evidenced by the

Table 5.1.   DSM-IV diagnostic criteria for ADHD

A.   The diagnosis of ADHD should be made when the following criteria of either inattention or hyperactivity-impulsivity are met:

1.   A child shows six (or more) of the following symptoms of inattention that have persisted for at least 6 months to a degree that is maladaptive and inconsistent with developmental level:
   a.   Often fails to give close attention to details or makes careless mistakes in schoolwork, work, or other activities
   b.   Often has difficulty sustaining attention in tasks or play activities
   c.   Often does not seem to listen when spoken to directly
   d.   Often does not follow through on instructions and fails to finish schoolwork, chores, or duties in the workplace (not caused by oppositional behavior or failure to understand instructions)
   e.   Often has difficulty organizing tasks and activities
   f.   Often avoids, dislikes, or is reluctant to engage in tasks that require sustained mental effort (e.g., schoolwork, homework)
   g.   Often loses things necessary for tasks or activities (e.g., toys, school assignments, pencils, books, tools)
   h.   Often is easily distracted by extraneous stimuli
   i.   Often is forgetful in daily activities

2.   A child shows six (or more) of the following symptoms of hyperactivity-impulsivity that have persisted for at least 6 months to a degree that is maladaptive and inconsistent with developmental level:

   Hyperactivity
   a.   Often fidgets with hands or feet or squirms in seat
   b.   Often leaves seat in classroom or in other situations in which remaining seated is expected
   c.   Often runs about or climbs excessively in situations in which it is inappropriate (in adolescents or adults, this symptom may be limited to subjective feelings of restlessness)
   d.   Often has difficulty playing or engaging in leisure activities quietly
   e.   Often is "on the go" or acts as if "driven by a motor"
   f.   Often talks excessively

   Impulsivity
   g.   Often blurts out answers before questions have been completed
   h.   Often has difficulty awaiting turn
   i.   Often interrupts or intrudes on others (e.g., butts into conversations or games)

The diagnosis of ADHD also should be made when the following criteria are met:

B.   Some hyperactive-impulsive or inattentive symptoms that cause impairment were present before age 7 years.
C.   Some impairment from the symptoms is present in two or more settings (e.g., at school [or work] and at home).
D.   There is clear evidence of clinically significant impairment in social, academic, or occupational functioning.
E.   The symptoms do not occur exclusively during the course of a pervasive developmental disorder, schizophrenia, or other psychotic disorder and are not better accounted for by another mental disorder (e.g., mood disorder, anxiety disorder, dissociative disorder, personality disorder).

Note: Adapted by permission of the American Psychiatric Association (1994).

ADHD, combined type, should be diagnosed when both criteria A1 and A2 are met for at least 6 months; ADHD, predominantly inattentive type, should be diagnosed when Criterion A1 has been met but Criterion A2 has not been met for at least 6 months; and ADHD, predominantly hyperactive-impulsive type, should be diagnosed when Criterion A2 has been met but Criterion A1 has not been met for at least 6 months.

Table 5.2.   Labels used for ADHD throughout history

Label	Date of use	Characteristics
Organic drivenness (Kahn & Cohen, 1934) Restlessness syndrome (Childers, 1935) Brain-injured child (Strauss & Lehtinen, 1947) Minimal brain damage Minimal brain dysfunction (MBD)	1930s–1960s	Severe restlessness, poor ability to sustain interest in activities, and impaired impulse control Believed to be caused by central nervous system damage, even when such neurological evidence was lacking; defects of forebrain structures held responsible for the disorder Characterized children without mental retardation who exhibited behavioral or perceptual disturbances and features such as motor clumsiness, cognitive impairments, and even parent–child conflict; hyperactivity not required for the diagnosis
Hyperkinetic impulsive disorder (Laufer et al., 1957) Hyperactive child syndrome Hyperkinetic reaction of childhood disorder (DSM-II, American Psychiatric Association, 1968)	Late 1960s–1970	Excessive activity level compared to normal children Concept of hyperactivity syndrome separated from that of brain damage syndrome (Chess, 1960; Werry & Sprague, 1970) Thalamic dysfunction leading to poor filtering of stimuli and cortical overstimulation; more generally, dissociation between cortical and subcortical regions responsible for sensory gating and resulting in cortical overloading (Knobel et al., 1959) Believed to be resolved by puberty
Attention deficit disorder and hyperactivity (ADD/+H) (DSM-III, American Psychiatric Association, 1980)	1980–1987	Inattention, impulsivity, and hyperactivity Impairments in sustained attention and impulse control held greater weight in the diagnosis than did hyperactivity Hyperactivity symptoms believed to be situational and usually decreased by adolescence, whereas attention and poor impulse control persisted Brain damage minor in the etiology of this disorder
ADHD (DSM-III-R, American Psychiatric Association, 1987)	1987–1994	Defined ADHD with a single item list of symptoms and a single cutoff score rather than using the previous three lists of inattention, impulsivity, and hyperactivity Considered a chronic disabling condition, with strong biological or hereditary predisposition Consideration of familial and environmental influences

(continued)

Table 5.2.   (continued)

Label	Date of use	Characteristics
ADHD (DSM-III-R, American Psychiatric Association, 1987) (continued)	1987–1994	Believed to result from insensitivity to consequences, such as reinforcement, punishment, or both Motivational factors, as opposed to attention deficits, the central role in the disorder
ADHD (DSM-IV, American Psychiatric Association, 1994)	1994–1996	Persistent pattern of inattention and/or hyperactivity-impulsivity present before 7 years of age and producing impairment in at least two social settings; two lists of symptoms—one for the inattention domain and one for the hyperactivity-impulsivity domain

label "minimal brain dysfunction" (MBD). Later, an organic basis for the behavioral symptoms lost its prominence, and interest turned toward psychophysiological conceptual models to explain the above-mentioned maladaptive behaviors. Hyperactivity was considered the primary symptom leading to inattention and impulsivity. Later still, inattention was thought to be the primary symptom. Working from the premise that ADHD is a primary impairment in attention, neuroanatomical and neurofunctional studies of ADHD can be interpreted in light of the various neurophysiological models of attention (Lyon & Krasnegor, 1996). For convenience, ADHD is used in this chapter as a generic term for the syndromes of hyperactivity and inattention cited in the literature, which do not necessarily conform fully to the DSM-IV definition of ADHD.

Another issue relating to sample homogeneity concerns the inclusion of children with comorbid disorders. Significant comorbidity of ADHD with disruptive disorders, mood disorders, anxiety disorders, and substance abuse have been reported (for a review, see Biederman et al., 1991). In addition, ADHD frequently is associated with learning disabilites. A large number of children with mental retardation present symptoms of inattention, hyperactivity, and impulsivity beyond what would be expected for a given mental age. It is important to note that hyperactivity and attention problems often are expressed as part of psychiatric disorders. For example, anxiety is associated with restlessness, depression with trouble concentrating, and psychosis with distractibility. This overlap of symptoms may complicate the diagnosis of comorbid ADHD. The hallmark of ADHD, however, is that symptoms start before 7 years of age and do not remit during childhood. The inclusion of children with ADHD and comorbid psychiatric disorders is of concern in brain imaging studies because findings may reflect abnormalities related to comorbidity rather than to ADHD.

Other important factors to consider in the interpretation of brain imaging studies are the effects of age and gender. Most research on ADHD has involved males because of its predominance in males and the desirability of homogeneous samples. Findings in females with ADHD, however, may differ in important ways from those in males.

LIMITATIONS OF BRAIN IMAGING STUDIES

The disparity among brain imaging techniques (i.e., magnetic resonance imaging [MRI] equipment and procedures; positron emission tomography [PET], single photon emission computed tomography [SPECT] equipment and radioactive tracers) and among experimental conditions (i.e., resting states, performing a cognitive task during functional imaging) introduces variance that impedes attempts to synthesize the literature. Another significant obstacle in the interpretation of brain imaging studies is the difficulty in collecting large subject samples, mostly because of financial restrictions. The reliability of conclusions primarily depends on replications of findings rather than large sample sizes; as a result, normative data are lacking in brain imaging. Most results, therefore, are considered indicative rather than definite. In addition, the radiation exposure that is associated with PET and SPECT has posed special ethical considerations for the studies of minors. This fact is reflected in the paucity of studies of children, in particular, control children.

In this regard, various strategies have been used to include control children. Some researchers have used medical controls, that is, patients who underwent brain imaging studies that were indicated for medical reasons (usually to rule out structural brain damage) and were read as normal clinically. The use of such control patients eliminates normal extremes or outliers and introduces bias because it artificially reduces normal variability. Other researchers have used control patients who have abnormalities restricted to one side of the brain. The healthy side of the brain was used for comparison with the data from patients with ADHD. Obviously, this is a less-than-optimal strategy, because it is not known whether the healthy brain regions have been modified to compensate for the impairments related to the brain abnormalities. The final strategy was to use the unaffected siblings of children from the patient groups. From an ethical point of view, siblings could benefit from participating in studies aimed at clarifying disorders that affect their family lives and that could eventually be passed onto their own offspring. Two opposing outcomes may be anticipated with this strategy. First, the use of siblings may decrease interindividual variability because of the presence of common genes and, thereby, increase the power to detect differences between affected and unaffected siblings. Second, the degree of genetic penetrance (i.e., the likelihood that a mutant gene will be expressed phenotypically) may mask differences between affected and unaffected family members. A control sibling may carry a genetic mutation associated with ADHD and not express the phenotype because of environmental, biochemical, or genetic protective factors.

HYPOTHESES THAT GUIDE NEUROIMAGING RESEARCH IN ADHD

Although it is exploratory, brain imaging research in ADHD is driven by neurophysiological hypotheses drawn from neuropsychology, psycopharmacology, neuroelectrophysiology, and animal models that have identified putative neural substrates of attention and motor activity. Neuropsychologists have identified various components of attention thought to be subserved by different underlying neural pathways. Cooley and Morris (1990) and Mirsky et al. (1991) described four main elements of attention—focus (or selective), sustained, shift, and divided attention—which can be tested behaviorally with neuropsychological tests (see Table 5.3). Posner and Petersen (1990) divided attention into three subsystems including "(a) orienting to sensory events, (b) detecting signals for focal (conscious) processing, and (c) maintaining a vigilant or alert state" (p. 26) and related these subsystems to neural circuits of the ventral occipital lobe, an anterior attention system, and arousal systems, respectively. Posner and Petersen (1990) and Posner et al. (1988) used brain imaging studies to investigate these

Table 5.3. Components of attention

Components of attention	Description	Neuropsychological tests	Brain regions/ neural networks[a]
Focused or selective attention	Ability to select target information and ignore irrelevant information	Stroop Color-Word Interference Test (Stroop, 1935) Talland Letter Cancellation Test (Talland, 1965) Trail Making Test (Reitan & Davidson, 1974) Digit Symbol Substitution, Arithmetic Test, and Digit Span Test (Wechsler, 1974)	Spatial selective attention (neglect symptom): right posterior and parietal cortical regions and cingulate gyrus, thalamus, and corpus striatum
Sustained attention	Ability to maintain focus and alertness over time	Continuous Performance Test (Rosvold et al., 1956) Span of Apprehension Test (Neale et al., 1969)	Anterior frontal lobe
Shifted attention	Ability to change focus of attention in a flexible and adaptive manner	Wisconsin Card Sorting Test (Grant & Berg, 1948) Reciprocal Motor Programs Test (Jones et al., 1988)	Posterior parietal lobe, thalamus, and midbrain
Attention for action	Ability to connect visuosensory input with relevant output systems	Wisconsin Card Sorting Test (Grant & Berg, 1948)	Frontal lobe
Divided attention	Ability to attend to two or more stimuli simultaneously	Dual-task interference paradigm	No hypothesis reported

Note: For review, see Cooley and Morris (1990), Mirsky et al. (1991), and Posner et al. (1988).
[a]Mainly identified through brain lesions.

hypotheses. A review of findings of the performance of children with ADHD on neuropsychological tests supports the notion that sustained attention is impaired predominantly (Barkley et al., 1992; Hooks et al., 1994). Performance on continuous performance tests (CPTs), posited to measure sustained attention, probably is most consistently deviant in children with ADHD compared with performances on other tests of attention. CPT tasks involve the presentation of stimuli that include a set number of predetermined targets to which subjects respond. CPTs vary in duration (a few minutes to a half hour), sensory modality (visual or auditory), stimuli (numbers, letters, drawings, and colors), and nature of the task (single target, double target, or sequential recognition). The differences among CPTs are factors to consider when comparing CPT performances. Most common measures assess omission errors, or misses, and commission errors, or false alarms. The use of CPTs in functional brain imaging is particularly relevant for the study of subjects with ADHD. It is conceivable that brain activity deviance in ADHD may be detected only during performance of a task that activates defective neural networks involved in ADHD attentional impairments.

Table 5.4 lists conceptual behavioral models used to understand the clinical presentation of ADHD. Each of these models carries its own clinical assumptions and implicates a given neural network. For example, the capacity to sustain attention has been associated with an optimal level of cortical arousal. This model implies that the structures that control arousal are dysfunctional. These structures include the reticular activating system, which mediates tonic arousal (Moruzzi & Magoun, 1949); the thala-

Table 5.4.   Conceptual models of ADHD

Theory	Characteristics	Studies using conceptual model
Defective moral control	Believed to be a chronic behavior impairment in children who were aggressive, defiant, and resistant to discipline and who showed spitefulness, cruelty, and dishonesty	Still (1902)
Hypoarousal	Problems with alertness, arousal, selectivity, sustained attention, distractibility, and span of apprehension Most apparent when children are required to engage in dull, boring, repetitive tasks (e.g., schoolwork, homework, chores)	Satterfield and Dawson (1971) Ullman et al. (1978) Milich et al. (1982) Zentall (1985) Luk (1985)
Defective inhibitory processes	Inability to inhibit internal (i.e., thoughts, emotions) or external (i.e., motor activity) responses to internal or external stimuli	Douglas (1972)
Motivation deficit disorder and impaired rule-governed behavior	Corresponds to impairments in reward systems, reflected by reduced activation of the brain reward structures and dysfunction of cortical-limbic pathways Failure to respond to rules and instructions, especially when they are not repeated or reinforced Lack of correspondence between behavior and previously stated rules	Rosenthal and Allen (1978); Sroufe (1975) Douglas (1983) Zettle and Hayes (1983) Draeger et al. (1986)
Impaired delayed response	Inability to delay responses to stimuli, internal or external, which leads to hyperactivity, as well as difficulty in concentrating	Barkley (1990)
Disorder in sensory gating	Sensory inputs incorrectly gated into motor systems—"relevant" stimuli do not lead to action, and irrelevant stimuli do lead to action (function is assumed to be performed by the basal ganglia)	Heilman et al. (1991)

Note: For review, see Barkley (1990).

mus, which mediates phasic arousal (Sharpless & Jasper, 1956); and, possibly, the limbic system, particularly the hippocampus (Thompson & Bettinger, 1970). It also is possible, however, that defective inhibitory processes could result from frontal lobe dysfunction, analogous to the disinhibition syndrome produced by frontal lesions.

As synthesized by Heilman et al. (1991), the neurological and neuropsychological literature pertaining to ADHD behavior offers the following pathophysiological substrates to the various symptoms of ADHD: ADHD, itself, may be a variant of the neglect syndrome, which implicates the dorsolateral and medial frontal lobe, cingulate and parietal cortices, striatum, and reticular formation, particularly in the right hemisphere. Motor impersistence, the inability to sustain a given motor activity, has been associated with right frontal cortical dysfunction in patients with acquired lesions. Failure of response inhibition, the inability to inhibit responses to irrelevant stimuli, is associated with dysfunction of the orbital, inferior lateral, and medial (including the supplementary motor area and cingulate) frontal cortical regions. Impairments in frontal-striatal gating of behavior involve a large neural network, composed of prefrontal cortex (in particular, the dorsolateral and frontal eye fields regions), caudate, pars reticulata of the substantia nigra, ventral anterior nucleus of the thalamus, anterior cingulate gyrus, and limbic system. In addition, the supplementary motor area may play a critical role in the adaptation of motor activity to internal and external contexts. Motor restlessness is somewhat similar to akathisia (side effect of neuroleptic agents that is characterized by motor restlessness, leading to an inability to sit still or lie quietly) and may reflect dopamine hypoactivity in the prefrontal mesocortex. Motor restlessness also implicates the ventral tegmental region, in which lesions result in marked motor restlessness in rats.

Among the various theoretical models proposed as a basis for ADHD, there is agreement as to the role of the frontal, parietal, and cingulate cortices in attention processing, particularly regions on the right side of the brain (Heilman et al., 1991; Mennemeier et al., 1994; Morecraft et al., 1993; Voeller, 1986). Most evidence stems from cortical lesions, which produce a syndrome of neglect characterized by loss of attention to stimuli originating from a given spatial area, usually contralateral to the site of the lesion. This syndrome occurs most consistently when the right side of the brain is damaged and has been seen in patients with lesions of the frontal and parietal cortices and subcortical regions, such as the thalamus and striatum. Functional brain imaging studies support the critical role of the frontal cortex (Cohen et al., 1988; Deutsch et al., 1987), parietal cortex (Heinze et al., 1994), and cingulate (Pardo et al., 1990) in attention processing.

Of all of the above-mentioned brain regions, it is the frontal lobe to which the most prominent role in attention has been attributed (Luria, 1973; Mesulam, 1986; Stuss & Benson, 1984). Frontal lesions in humans and animals produce behaviors that mimic the hyperactivity, inattention, and impulsivity symptoms of ADHD (Benson, 1991; Heilman et al., 1991; Mattes, 1980). Barkley et al. (1992) reviewed 22 neuropsychological studies of children with ADHD. Tests of response inhibition were the most sensitive in discriminating children with ADHD from children without ADHD. Impairments in response inhibition have been associated with frontal lobe lesions in humans (Drewe, 1975; Leimkuhler & Mesulam, 1985), particularly when medial frontal lesions occurred on the right side (Verfaellie & Heilman, 1987); in addition, impairments in response inhibition were produced by medial frontal lesions in dogs (Dabrowska, 1972) and by orbital or inferior lateral frontal lesions in monkeys (Iversen & Mishkin, 1970).

Stimulants, such as methylphenidate, dextroamphetamine, and pemoline, are effective pharmacological treatments of ADHD symptoms. Their therapeutic effects are mediated by the activation of the dopaminergic and noradrenergic systems. Although the exact mechanism of action of stimulants remains unclear, stimulant efficacy supports the role of frontal-striatal structures in ADHD. Noradrenergic structures, in particular, the locus ceruleus, also may contribute to ADHD pathophysiology.

In conclusion, the various behavioral and neuropathophysiological models of ADHD proposed in the literature suggest that the brain areas important for the expression of ADHD symptoms may be located principally in the frontal, cingulate, and parietal cortices and the striatum. The neurotransmitter systems proposed as major contributors to ADHD behavior are the dopaminergic and noradrenergic systems. It is clear that attentional processes are subserved by a large and complex interconnected neural network. Functional brain imaging can be used to clarify the neuropathophysiological basis of ADHD.

NEUROIMAGING RESEARCH IN ADHD

Structural Studies

Computed Tomography

It is difficult to make comparisons among computed tomography (CT) studies of ADHD (Bergström & Bille, 1978; Nasrallah et al., 1986; Shaywitz et al., 1983) because of the use of different diagnostic definitions of ADHD, different designs (e.g., open or blind, with or without a control group), and different methods of analysis (i.e., qualitative, quantitative). In one study, Bergström and Bille (1978) studied 46 children with MBD. MBD was defined by the presence of incoordination and impairment in sensory–motor integration. Of the 46 children, 15 (32.6%) presented gross CT abnormalities of cerebral atrophy, ventricular asymmetry, or ventriculomegaly. The clinical presentations of three of these children were described carefully and resembled cerebral palsy more than ADHD. In addition, the analysis was qualitative, and the design did not involve a control group.

By using a quantitative measurement, control group, and blind analysis, Shaywitz et al. (1983) studied 35 children and adolescents diagnosed with ADHD according to DSM-III criteria (29 boys and 6 girls; age range, 4–18 years; mean, 11.0 ± 3.5 years). The control subjects had normal IQs and no histories of seizures or ADHD. Shaywitz et al. (1983) did not specify the clinical indications for performing a CT scan in the control group, and comorbid psychiatric disorders in the ADHD group were not mentioned. The results revealed no significant differences between the two groups in any of the measurements obtained for biventricular width, widths of the left and right anterior horns of the lateral ventricles, width of the brain plus ventricle, widths of the right and left hemispheres, and two derived measures—the cerebroventricular index (Evan's index = biventricular width / width of brain + ventricle) and the asymmetry index (BL − BR / BL + BR, where BL and BR are the widths of the left and right hemispheres at the bifrontal line measured from the internal table to the septum pellucidum). Moreover, no sex differences were found in any of the measurements, and none of the brain measurements correlated significantly with IQ or handedness. Shaywitz et al. (1983) did not provide results pertaining to the effects of age.

Nasrallah et al. (1986) studied 24 men with hyperactivity, 22 of whom had documented histories of childhood ADHD treated with stimulants (mean age, 23.2 ± 1.9 years), and 27 control males (mean age, 28.7 ± 8.3 years). The hyperactive group had been part of a cohort of boys who were diagnosed at the age of 8.7 ± 1.9 years with hyperkinesis/MBD and who presented symptoms of hyperactivity, fidgetiness, inattention, and motor incoordination. No information was provided regarding the status of these symptoms at the time of the CT scan. Of the 24 men with hyperactivity, 7 had histories of alcohol abuse. The control subjects were individuals who had been in vehicle accidents and who had normal neurological examinations and CT scans, part of the routine medical workup. Brain measurements consisted of lateral ventricular size expressed as the ventricle-to-brain ratio, third ventricular size, sulcal widening visually rated by a neuroradiologist blind to diagnosis on a 4-point rating scale, and cerebellar atrophy. The men with hyperactivity showed greater sulcal widening, suggesting mild cerebral atrophy, and cerebellar atrophy than did control subjects. Unfortunately, the relatively high proportion of individuals with histories of alcohol abuse (30% of the hyperactive group) clouded the interpretation of the results, because findings of CT studies have reported an association between alcoholism and cerebral atrophy (Epstein et al., 1977).

In summary, one of the three above-mentioned studies had negative findings. Of the two studies with positive findings of either gross abnormalities or mild cerebral atrophy, one used children with neurological impairments, and the other used adults with histories of ADHD (30% of whom also abused alcohol) and without clinical assessment concurrent to the CT study. In addition, left-to-right ratios (Shaywitz et al., 1983) and sizes of frontal cortices were not reported to be deviant. CT findings, therefore, did not provide convincing findings specific to ADHD.

Magnetic Resonance Imaging

The first MRI studies of ADHD were conducted by Hynd et al. (1990), Hynd et al. (1991), Hynd et al. (1993), and Semrud-Clikeman et al. (1993). In a first report, Hynd et al. (1990) compared three groups: 10 children with ADHD, as defined by DSM-III and DSM-III-R (8 boys and 2 girls; mean age, 120.6 ± 40.4 months); 10 children with developmental reading disorder (8 boys and 2 girls; mean age, 118.90 ± 24.55 months); and 10 control children (8 boys and 2 girls; mean age, 141.20 ± 24.07 months). All 30 children had IQs within the normal range. Comorbidity was diagnosed in seven children with ADHD (five with conduct disorder/oppositional defiant disorder and two with anxiety disorder). Sizes and areas of the left and right anterior (from a line drawn horizontally across the tip of the genu) and posterior (from a line drawn horizontally across the posterior tip of the splenium) regions, lengths of the right and left insular regions, and total brain areas were measured on a single axial slice at the level of the region of planum temporale. Children in the ADHD group had bilaterally smaller anterior cortices, especially on the right, than did those in the control group. In addition, the frontal lobe asymmetry (left smaller than right) that is present in normal children was not observed in children with ADHD. No other measures differentiated children with ADHD from normal children.

These findings led to an examination of the corpus callosum. The corpus callosum, composed of connective interhemispheric fibers (Innocenti, 1981; Pandya et al., 1971), subserves bihemispheric connection and lateralization of function. The anterior corpus callosum contains fibers that connect the premotor, orbitofrontal, and prefrontal right and left cortices (Pandya et al., 1971; Pandya & Seltzer, 1986), whereas the posterior corpus callosum contains fibers that connect the peristriatal, properistriatal, and juxtastriatal right and left regions (visual association cortical areas) (Alexander & Warren, 1988; Pandya et al., 1971). Hynd et al. (1991) hypothesized that the anterior corpus callosum would be smaller in individuals with ADHD than in normal subjects, because it connects the right and left frontal lobes. Both the anterior (genu) and posterior (splenium) regions of the corpus callosum were significantly smaller in children with ADHD ($n = 7$; 5 boys and 2 girls; mean age, 109.0 ± 61.07 months) than in normal children ($n = 10$; 8 boys and 2 girls; mean age, 141.50 ± 24.36 months) (Hynd et al., 1991).

The reduction in the size of the splenium, but not of the anterior part of the corpus callosum, was replicated in a subsequent study (Semrud-Clikeman et al., 1993) in which a group of males with "pure" ADHD ($n = 15$; mean age, 155.6 ± 47.5 months), in contrast with the above-described study in which the ADHD sample included comorbid diagnoses (mainly disruptive behavior disorders), was used. All children with ADHD received medication for at least 6 months before the study. The children who did not respond to stimulant medication ($n = 5$) tended to have smaller corpora callosa than those who did respond ($n = 10$). No significant correlation was noted between size of corpus callosum regions and age.

In contrast with these findings, Giedd et al. (1994) reported that only the anterior regions of the corpus callosum (rostrum and rostral body) were smaller in boys with ADHD ($n = 18$; mean age, 11.9 ± 2.5 years) than in normal boys ($n = 18$; mean age, 10.5 ± 2.3 years), who were matched for age, weight, height, Tanner stage, and handedness. Giedd et al. (1994) did not mention drug treatment or drug response.

Additional work was undertaken to assess other brain structures, such as the basal ganglia, hypothesized to play a significant role in attention processes and motor activity. In an MRI study, Hynd et al. (1993) reported that the heads of the left caudate nuclei were significantly smaller in subjects with ADHD ($n = 11$; 8 males and 3 females; ages not reported) than in normal subjects ($n = 11$; 6 males and 5 females; ages not reported). Castellanos et al. (1994) reported smaller total brain volumes and losses of normal caudate volume asymmetry (right greater than left) in a large group of 50 males with ADHD (age range, 6–19 years) compared with 48 well-matched control males (age range, 6–18 years). The loss of caudate asymmetry in the ADHD group reflected the decrease of right caudate volume compared with the control group. Total brain volume, IQ, and comorbid disorders did not influence this finding. All patients had been exposed to stimulant treatment before the MRI study. Comorbid disorders included conduct disorder ($n = 8$), oppositional defiant disorder ($n = 21$), and learning disorder ($n = 13$).

In summary, the right frontal cortices, corpora callosa (posterior area in one study and anterior in two studies), and the heads of the caudate nuclei (left in one study and right in one study) were found to be smaller in subjects with ADHD than in control subjects. Discrepancies in the results must be examined in light of the differences in sample characteristics and methodologies used in these MRI studies. However, the direction of the results, in general, is in accordance with above-mentioned pathophysiological models of ADHD, which propose the frontal cortex and striatum, particularly on the right side, as the brain regions most likely to be involved in ADHD symptoms. The functional significance and the clinical relevance of these structural brain abnormalities in subjects with ADHD could be further clarified by using functional brain imaging, as illustrated below.

Functional Brain Imaging

Cerebral Blood Flow

Lou et al. (1984, 1990) and Lou et al. (1989) conducted three [133]xenon-inhalation and SPECT studies of cerebral blood flow in children with ADHD. Data were collected when children were at rest with their eyes open. SPECT primarily yields a three-dimensional qualitative measure of cerebral blood flow, which is believed to reflect metabolic and functional activity of the brain: The greater the cerebral blood flow, the more active the brain. Resolution of the images in these three studies was 17 mm, and only one axial slice through the striatum and thalamus was examined.

The first study (Lou et al., 1984) examined a heterogeneous sample of 11 children who were clinically diagnosed with attention deficit disorder (ADD) (10 boys and 1 girl; age range, 6.5–15 years) and had varying degrees of congenital and neonatal complications (4 of 11 children), dysphasia (6 of 11 children), mild mental retardation (2 of 11 children), and other neuropsychological impairments (7 of 11 children). Of the 11 children, 6 received methylphenidate until 1 week before the study. The ADD group was compared with nine control children (six boys and three girls; age range, 7–15 years), all of whom were siblings of the children with ADD. The use of siblings as controls was directed by convenience rather than a scientific hypothesis. Lou et al. (1984) reported hypoperfusion of the frontal lobes of all 11 children with ADD compared with the control children. In addition, the caudate nuclei of 7 of the 11 children with ADD had decreased cerebral blood flow; in contrast, the occipital lobes of those seven children were relatively hyperperfused. Six of the children with ADD underwent SPECT scans twice—once before and once 30 min after oral administration of their treatment dose of methylphenidate (10 mg–30 mg). All six children showed increased perfusion in the frontal and caudate regions after treatment. The findings are difficult to interpret given the heterogeneity of the patient group, lack of criteria for the diagnosis of ADD, and absence of information regarding comorbid psychiatric disorders.

Extending the 1984 study, in the second study, Lou et al. (1989) enlarged the patient group from 11 children with ADD to 19 children and subdivided it into children with pure ADHD ($n = 6$) and children with ADHD and comorbid neurological or neuropsychiatric symptoms ($n = 13$). The control group was the same as that studied by Lou et al. (1984) ($n = 9$; 6 boys and 3 girls; age range, 7–15 years; siblings of ADD patients). Five of six children with pure ADHD had histories of neonatal complications. Consistent with results of the first study, the right striatal region (10.6% decrease) was hypoperfused, whereas the occipital lobe (13.7% increase) and left sensorimotor and primary auditory region (9.6% increase) were hyperperfused. Approximately 30–60 min after methylphenidate had been administered (10 mg–30 mg) to four children with pure ADHD and 9 with ADHD and comorbidities, cerebral blood flow increased significantly (by 7%) in the left striatal region and left and right posterior periventricular regions. The results of this second study cannot be regarded as an independent replication of those of the first study because of the overlap of samples.

In the third study, Lou et al. (1990) studied a new control group of 15 normal children (8 boys and 7 girls; median age, 11 years; age range, 6–17 years), 4 of whom were siblings of children with ADHD. The patient group was enlarged by the addition of children with dysphasia. The extent of overlap of patients between this study and the two preceding ones remains unclear. Of the children with pure ADHD, nine (seven boys and two girls) showed a 10.7% decrease in blood flow in the striatal regions (without mention of laterality), a 6.8% decrease in the posterior periventricular region (6.8%), and an increase in occipital regions compared with the control group.

The consistency of the results among these three studies may be ascribed to the large overlap among samples, and the results cannot be interpreted as replications. The patient samples were heterogeneous and included patients with histories of perinatal brain insults. It is difficult to conclude whether the reported abnormalities are related to ADHD or associated pathology. No standardized instruments were used to make the diagnosis of ADHD. The results, however, are in keeping with the theoretical framework of the pathogenesis of ADHD, which implicates abnormalities in the frontal cortex and striatum (more so on the right side than on the left side).

Brain Glucose Metabolic Rates

Zametkin et al. (1993) and Zametkin et al. (1990) studied adults and adolescents with ADHD by using PET and [^{18}F]fluorodeoxyglucose (FDG) to measure cerebral glucose utilization (see Chapter 2). The following section presents three groups of PET and FDG studies: studies of adults, studies of adolescents, and studies in which stimulants were used.

Studies of Adults Before studying children with ADHD, Zametkin et al. (1990) investigated ADHD in adults. The decision to do so was guided by the difficulty in performing functional neuroimaging research in minors and by the observation that many parents of children with ADHD had clear symptoms of ADHD themselves. This study proved to be seminal, because it showed, for the first time, definite and quantifiable central neurophysiological differences between carefully screened adults with ADHD and normal adults.

All 25 adults with ADHD (18 men and 7 women; mean age 37.4±6.9 years) had childhood histories of ADHD, met Utah criteria for ADHD in adults (Wender et al., 1981; Wender et al., 1985), and had children who were diagnosed as having ADHD. This group of 25 patients was compared with a group of 50 normal adults (28 men and 22 women; mean age, 36.3±11.7 years). No subjects had ever been treated with stimulants. PET scans were acquired during the performance of an auditory CPT while subjects' eyes were covered.

The global glucose metabolism (mean of regional glucose metabolic rates for all gray matter–rich areas examined in this study) was 8.1% lower in adults with ADHD than in normal adults ($p = 0.03$). Of the brain regions sampled, 50% (30 of 60) of those in adults with ADHD had significantly reduced glucose metabolic rates compared with rates in control subjects. These brain regions were four subcortical areas—the right thalamus, right caudate, right hippocampus, and cingulate. Those cortical regions that significantly differentiated adults with ADHD from control adults were located bilaterally and predominantly in the superior cortical regions. When normalized (individual regional values divided by global metabolic values), the regional metabolic rates of the four regions in the left premotor and left somatosensory areas were decreased significantly, thereby indicating that the greatest reductions were in these regions. The reductions in brain metabolism were greater in women than in men; the difference, however, was not statistically significant.

In conclusion, although the decreases seen in frontal and striatal brain glucose metabolism in studies by Zametkin et al. (1990) are consistent with Lou et al.'s (1990) findings, the decreases seen in somatosensory and occipital areas contradict the increased blood flow in these regions reported by Lou et al. (1990). When comparing these studies, it is important to consider the differences in sample characteristics (children versus adults), experimental conditions (resting state with eyes open versus during CPT with eyes covered), physical measures (cerebral blood flow versus glucose metabolism), techniques (PET versus SPECT), and analysis of the results (single-plane versus five-plane analysis, 17-mm versus 6-mm image resolution, and normalized data versus absolute and normalized values). Despite these discrepancies among study samples and methods, however, the findings that these studies share support the involvement of the brain regions already hypothesized to mediate symptoms of ADHD. The direction of

changes (i.e., hypoactivity) must be investigated further to understand the role of neurotransmitters and neural circuits, particularly the corticostriatal-cortical loops.

   Studies of Adolescents   Given the positive results of Zametkin et al.'s 1990 study,
Zametkin et al. (1993) initiated an FDG PET study in adolescents. Indeed, the interpretation of data collected in adults with childhood disorders is difficult, because the primary effects of the disorder cannot be isolated from secondary or long-lasting environmental influences. To minimize radioactivity exposure, the radiation dose was reduced
to one fifth of that used in adults.

   In this study, 20 adolescents (15 boys and 5 girls; mean age, 14.7 ± 1.7 years) who
fulfilled DSM-III-R ADHD criteria were compared with 19 control adolescents (13 boys
and 6 girls; mean age, 14.4 ± 1.4 years) (Ernst, Liebenauer, Jons, et al., 1994; Ernst, Liebenauer, King, et al., 1994). Subjects received no medication for 2 weeks before undergoing PET scans. A preliminary report originating from scans of the first half of the
ADHD and control samples found few differences between groups (Zametkin et al.,
1993). When the sample size was increased (Ernst, Liebenauer, Jons, et al., 1994; Ernst,
Liebenauer, King, et al., 1994), no significant differences were seen in either global or regional glucose metabolic rates between adolescents with ADHD and normal adolescents. Similar to the findings in adults, however, girls showed greater deviance in metabolic rates than did boys. In contrast with boys with ADHD, girls with ADHD ($n = 5$)
showed a significant (15%) global brain metabolism reduction compared with girls
without ADHD ($n = 6$).

   In conclusion, the following two issues emerged from the findings in adults and adolescents: The decreased brain glucose metabolism found in adults with ADHD was not
found in adolescents with ADHD, which suggests an age effect; and females with
ADHD, both adults and adolescents, showed more metabolic deviance than did males
with ADHD, which suggests a gender effect. Regarding the age effect, several factors
may account for the lack of metabolic differences between adolescents with ADHD and
normal adolescents. First, the adolescent control group was not as pure as the control
group in the adult study, because 63% (12 of 19) of the normal adolescents had first-
degree relatives with ADHD, whereas none of the normal adults had family histories of
ADHD pathology. Second, 75% adolescents with ADHD previously had been exposed
to treatment with stimulants, whereas none of the adults with ADHD had been exposed to stimulants. Third, it is conceivable that the adults with ADHD were more severely impaired than were the adolescents with ADHD, because the adults were part of
the only 40%–60% of patients with childhood ADHD who retain symptoms of ADHD
in adulthood; alternatively, positive findings in adults with ADHD may reflect secondary effects of ADHD, such as daily enhanced mental effort to perform routine tasks,
mood changes, or behavioral strategies to compensate for their impairments. Finally,
because adolescence is an important physiological and psychological transition period,
brain glucose metabolism in adolescents may be subject to greater interindividual and,
possibly, intraindividual variations than that in adults, which would decrease the statistical power to find differences among adolescent groups. Larger sample sizes may be
needed to reach enough statistical power to elicit differences between groups.

   Regarding the gender effect, greater deviance of brain glucose metabolism in females than in males may reflect sex-related clinical differences in ADHD. For example,
more cognitive and language impairments have been reported in females (Ackerman et
al., 1983; Berry et al., 1985; Brown et al., 1991; James & Taylor, 1990; Shaywitz & Shaywitz, 1987) and more hyperactivity and conduct problems have been reported in males
(Barkley, 1989; Befera & Barkley, 1985; Breen, 1989). The greater effect of ADHD on brain

metabolism in females also may result from an interaction between sex steroids and neural substrates that underlie ADHD on brain activity.

Influence of Sexual Maturation on Cerebral Glucose Metabolism in Girls Because of the more pronounced findings in cerebral glucose metabolism rate in females, an additional sample of eight girls with ADHD (mean age, 14.5±1.9 years) and eight control girls (mean age, 14.8±1.6 years) was examined (Ernst, Liebenauer, Jons, et al., 1994). Contrary to expectations, no differences in global and regional glucose brain metabolism were found between the girls with ADHD and the control girls. The only difference, across all demographic and behavioral variables, between the new sample of 16 girls and the previous sample of 11 girls was that the 8 girls with ADHD in the new sample were significantly less sexually mature (mean Tanner stage, 3.7±1.0) than were the 5 girls with ADHD in the previous sample (mean Tanner stage, 5.0±0.0). Within each group separately, Tanner stage was correlated negatively with brain glucose metabolism (i.e., the more sexually mature the girl, the lower the brain glucose utilization). The correlation was statistically significant in the control girls ($r = -0.85$; $p = 0.01$) but did not reach significance in the girls with ADHD ($r = -0.44$; $p = 0.28$). Because girls with ADHD were at a lower average Tanner stage, it is possible that the decreased brain glucose metabolism observed in women with ADHD and more sexually mature girls with ADHD was masked by the influence of sexual maturation on cerebral glucose metabolism.

It is clear that more studies on the influence of sex hormones and of sex chromosomes on brain glucose metabolism and, more generally, on brain development are needed to better understand findings of functional brain imaging studies in adolescents. That sex hormones do affect brain development is, however, well documented in animals. For example, the size of the corpus callosum was found to be reduced significantly in female rats compared with male rats, and this decrease was, in part, produced by estrogen exposure (Mack et al., 1993). In humans, the size of the splenium, as well as the sizes of the sylvian fissure and the anterior commissure, were found to be influenced by handedness in males but not in females (Witelson, 1989, 1993). In rats, lateralization was shown to be influenced by gender, and stronger left hemisphere specialization was seen in males than in females (Fitch et al., 1993). Estrogen was reported to increase dendritic spine formation and synaptic density in the ventromedial hypothalamic nucleus in the rat. In addition, the administration of estradiol to castrated male rats did not induce synaptic formation, probably because males may have a permanently higher density of neural wiring (Frankfurt & McEwen, 1991). Studies on brain maturation have shown earlier myelination, neuronal connections, and lateralization in females than in males, which result in greater maturity at birth for females than for males (Seeman & Lang, 1990). In humans, MRI studies of normal women and women with Turner syndrome (45,X karyotype) showed bilateral cerebral abnormalities, particularly on the right side, and this abnormality was more severe in patients with X monosomy than in those with mosaicism (see Chapter 7) (Murphy et al., 1993). Activation studies in which PET and [15]O were used to measure blood flow during memory tasks showed that differential regional activation occurred as a function of gender, thereby suggesting the use of either gender-specific cognitive strategies or gender-specific neural circuitry involved in cognitive tasks (Andreasen et al., 1993). Finally, with regard to neurotransmitter systems, the role of estrogen as a dopamine antagonist has potentially strong implications in the expression of ADHD symptoms, which are closely related to dopamine activity (Di Paolo et al., 1982; Fields & Gordon, 1982; Van Hartesveldt & Joyce, 1986).

Effects of Stimulants on Cerebral Glucose Metabolism   Zametkin et al. (1990) have examined the effects of stimulants on cerebral glucose metabolism in adults with ADHD. On the basis of animal studies that showed increased brain glucose metabolism after the stimulant injection (Bell et al., 1983; Eison et al., 1981; Porrinio et al., 1984; Wechsler et al., 1979), it was hypothesized that the reduction of brain glucose metabolism observed in adults with ADHD could be reversed by stimulants (DuPaul & Barkley, 1990). Zametkin et al. (1990) expected to observe increased brain glucose metabolism, especially in the striatal and frontal regions, after the administration of a stimulant.

Matochik et al. (1994) and Matochik et al. (1993) reported two studies—one of acute and one of chronic stimulant treatment—of adults with ADHD using [18F]FDG PET. In the acute study, 27 adult outpatients with ADHD underwent scans once while they were not receiving medication and once after receiving a single oral dose of either dextroamphetamine (0.25 mg/kg; $n = 13$) or methylphenidate hydrochloride (0.35 mg/kg; $n = 14$). The repeated scans were completed 1–4 months apart in counterbalanced order. The PET procedure was identical to that used in the adult study by Zametkin et al. (1990), in which subjects were studied while performing auditory CPT with their eyes covered. The acute administration of dextroamphetamine or methylphenidate had only a minimal effect on global glucose metabolic rates. When the data were normalized (regional/global), the regional metabolic rates of 7 of 60 regions changed significantly after dextroamphetamine administration. These seven regions were predominantly on the right side of the brain (five right and two left) and comprised four regions with increased metabolism (anterior medial frontal, right posterior temporal, right thalamus, and right caudate) and three regions with decreased metabolism (right rolandic, left anterior frontal, and right anterior frontal). Of interest is the increased metabolism in the right caudate nucleus. After methylphenidate administration, the normalized regional metabolism of five regions, all on the left side, were significantly changed; two increased (left posterior frontal and left parietal) and three decreased (anterior medial frontal, left parietal, and left parieto-occipital).

The chronic administration of stimulants (Matochik et al., 1994) also resulted in minimal changes in brain metabolism. A sample of 37 adults with ADHD was studied twice, not receiving treatment and then receiving treatment, at the end of 6–15 weeks of dextroamphetamine ($n = 18$; mean dose, $19 \pm$ mg/day) or methylphenidate ($n = 19$; mean dose, 29 ± 10 mg/day) administration. Subjects were randomly assigned to receive either dextroamphetamine or methylphenidate, and dosages were titrated individually to achieve optimal therapeutic efficacy. Global and absolute regional brain metabolic rates were unchanged after the administration of stimulants. Normalized metabolic rates changed in only 2 of the 60 regions studied and only after methylphenidate treatment (decreased metabolism was seen in the right anterior putamen and increased metabolism was seen in the right posterior orbitofrontal region). The lack of effect of either of the stimulants on brain metabolism stood in sharp contrast with the 68% clinical response rate (positive clinical response was defined as an 8-point decrease on a modified self-rated Conners scale [Conners, 1969]).

The results of these two studies were unexpected. It is possible that the FDG PET technique was not sensitive enough to detect the effects of stimulants. For instance, PET spatial resolution limits the structures that can be studied. In addition, the nucleus accumbens, which is one of the brain structure activities most consistently altered by stimulants in animal studies (Porrino & Lucignani, 1987; Porrino et al., 1984), cannot reliably be examined with PET because of its small size. Porrino et al. (1984) reported that the nucleus accumbens was the only structure in rats to have an increased metabolic rate after injections of 0.2 mg/kg and 0.5 mg/kg of amphetamine. It is of interest that no metabolic rate change in the nucleus accumbens was found after caffeine administration, which has no reported beneficial effect on ADHD symptoms. The nucleus accumbens receives input from the limbic system, the ventral tegmental (dopaminergic), and the prefrontal association cortex (glutaminergic) and projects to the basal ganglia (γ-aminobutyric acidergic) and substantia nigra. Its role is central to the gating of cognitive and motivational input onto motor systems, which have been proposed to be defective in ADHD (Heilman et al., 1991).

Another reason to expect stimulants to increase brain glucose metabolism stemmed from findings in animal studies (Bell et al., 1983; Eison et al., 1981; Porrino et al., 1984; Wechsler et al., 1979) that reported increased brain glucose utilization after stimulant injection. To more closely approximate the conditions in animal experiments (Ernst, Zametkin, et al., 1994), brain glucose metabolism was measured before and after a 0.15 mg/kg intravenous injection of dextroamphetamine in adults with ADHD. Preliminary results in eight adults with ADHD failed to disclose any significant changes in global or absolute regional glucose metabolic rates. Only 3 of 60 regional normalized metabolic rates differed between conditions. Glucose metabolism was decreased in two regions (right temporal cortex and right hippocampus) and increased in one (right parietal cortex). Again, the minimal changes in brain glucose metabolism were in contrast with the striking changes in affective (more energetic, increased concentration) and physiological states (significant increases in diastolic and systolic blood pressure) induced by the intravenous injection of dextroamphetamine. Discrepant results between studies of animals and humans also have been reported in studies of cocaine effects on brain metabolism. Studies of animals showed increased brain metabolism (London et al., 1986), whereas studies of humans reported decreases in brain metabolism globally and in 26 of 29 regions examined in individuals who abused multiple substances (London et al., 1990). Many variables may account for the differing results in humans and animals; the most important of these are the effects of species and of experimental conditions.

The results of the four above-described PET studies, which assessed brain metabolism in adolescents with ADHD and after stimulant administration in adults with ADHD, have been somewhat disappointing. These studies, however, illustrate clearly the difficulty of using and interpreting data from functional brain imaging studies. It is possible that FDG may not be the appropriate tracer for use in functional brain imaging studies of ADHD in functional brain imaging. The use of behavioral activation tasks that tap specific cognitive impairments and neurotransmitter-dependent tracers may improve the results of PET studies. In ADHD, activation tasks should target sustained attention and impulsivity. Hyperactivity is now thought to be part of the domain of impulsivity, which is conceptualized as a motor disinhibition disorder (see DSM-IV). The neurotransmitter system most relevant to ADHD pathology seems to be the dopaminergic system. PET studies of ADHD subjects using [18F]fluorodopa to quantify presynaptic dopamine accumulation have been undertaken at the National Institute of Mental Health, National Institutes of Health, Bethesda, Maryland. Finally, females with ADHD may exhibit greater deviance in brain metabolism and may be more sensitive to the influence of sexual maturation on brain activity than males with ADHD.

CONCLUSIONS AND FUTURE DIRECTIONS

It is likely that the slow progress made in the understanding of the neurochemistry of ADHD stems, in part, from the difficulty in isolating and studying patient samples that are demographically and clinically homogenous. In this respect, future advances in brain imaging research may help refine the selection of uniform groups by clarifying the neuropathophysiology that underlies ADHD. The further development of fMRI, therefore, may play a significant role, because of its exquisite spatial resolution and because the absence of radiation exposure will make it easier to enroll normal children. It is clear, however, that any significant gain in knowledge about ADHD, one of the most prevalent psychiatric disorders in childhood, which has both genetic and environmental determinants, will require the integration of findings from multiple scientific fields such as brain imaging, neuropsychology, genetics, and neurochemistry.

REFERENCES

Ackerman, P.T., Dykman, R.A., & Oglesby, D.M. (1983). Sex and group differences in reading and attention disordered children with and without hyperkinesis. *Journal of Learning Disabilities, 16*, 407–414.

Alexander, M.P., & Warren, R.L. (1988). Localization of callosal auditory pathways: A CT case study. *Neurology, 38*, 802–804.

American Psychiatric Association. (1968). *Diagnostic and statistical manual of mental disorders* (2nd ed.). Washington, DC: Author.

American Psychiatric Association. (1980). *Diagnostic and statistical manual of mental disorders* (3rd ed.). Washington, DC: Author.

American Psychiatric Association. (1987). *Diagnostic and statistical manual of mental disorders* (3rd ed., Rev.). Washington, DC: Author.

American Psychiatric Association. (1994). *Diagnostic and statistical manual of mental disorders* (4th ed.). Washington, DC: Author.

Andreasen, N.C., McEwen, B.S., Gorski, R.A., Witelson, S., & Frank, E. (1993). Gender differences and the brain. *Society for Neuroscience Abstracts, 19*, NR3.4.

Barkley, R.A. (1989). Hyperactive girls and boys: Stimulant drug effects on mother–child interactions. *Journal of Child Psychology and Psychiatry and Allied Disciplines, 30*, 379–390.

Barkley, R.A. (1990). *Attention deficit hyperactivity disorder: A handbook for diagnosis and treatment.* New York: Guilford Press.

Barkley, R.A., Anastopoulos, A.D., Guevremont, D.C., & Fletcher, K.E. (1990). Adolescents with ADHD: Patterns of behavioral adjustment, academic functioning, and treatment utilization. *Journal of the American Academy of Child and Adolescent Psychiatry, 30*, 752–761.

Barkley, R.A., Grodzinsky, G., & DuPaul, G.J. (1992). Frontal lobe functions in attention deficit disorder with and without hyperactivity: A review and research report. *Journal of Abnormal Child Psychology, 20*, 163–188.

Befera, M.S., & Barkley, R.A. (1985). Hyperactive and normal girls and boys: Mother–child interaction, parent psychiatric status and child psychopathology. *Journal of Child Psychology and Psychiatry and Allied Disciplines, 26*, 439–452.

Bell, R.D., Alexander, G.M., & Schwartzman, R.J. (1983). Methylphenidate decreases local glucose metabolism in the motor cortex. *Pharmacology, Biochemistry, and Behavior, 18*, 1–5.

Benson, D.F. (1991). The role of frontal dysfunction in attention deficit hyperactivity disorder. *Journal of Child Neurology, 6*, 9–12.

Bergström, K., & Bille, B. (1978). Computed tomography of the brain in children with minimal brain damage: A preliminary study of 46 children. *Neuropädiatrie, 9*, 378–384.

Berry, C.A., Shaywitz, S.E., & Shaywitz, B.A. (1985). Girls with attention deficit disorder: A silent minority? A report on behavioral and cognitive characteristics. *Pediatrics, 76*, 801–809.

Biederman, J., Newcorn, J., & Sprich, B.A. (1991). Comorbidity of attention deficit hyperactivity disorder with conduct, depressive, anxiety and other disorders. *American Journal of Psychiatry, 148*, 564–577.

Breen, M.J. (1989). Cognitive and behavioral differences in ADHD boys and girls. *Journal of Child Psychology and Psychiatry and Allied Disciplines, 30*, 711–716.

Brown, R.T., Madan-Swain, A., & Baldwin, K. (1991). Gender differences in a clinic-referred sample of attention-deficit-disordered children. *Child Psychiatry and Human Development, 22*, 111–128.

Castellanos, F.X., Giedd, J.N., Eckburg, P., Marsh, W.L., Vaituzis, C., Kaysen, D., Hamburger, S.D., & Rapoport, J.L. (1994). Quantitative morphology of the caudate nucleus in attention-deficit hyperactivity disorder. *American Journal of Psychiatry, 151*, 1791–1796.

Chess, S. (1960). Diagnosis and treatment of the hyperactive child. *New York State Journal of Medicine, 60*, 2379–2385.

Childers, A.T. (1935). Hyperactivity in children having behavior disorders. *American Journal of Orthopsychiatry, 5*, 227–243.

Cohen, R.M., Semple, W.E., Gross, M., Holcomb, H.H., Dowling, M.S., & Nordahl, T.E. (1988). Functional localization of sustained attention: Comparison to sensory stimulation in the absence of instruction. *Neuropsychiatry, Neuropsychology, and Behavioral Neurology, 1*(1), 3–20.

Conners, C.K. (1969). A teacher rating scale for use in drug studies with children. *American Journal of Psychiatry, 126*, 152–156.

Cooley, E.L., & Morris, R.D. (1990). Attention in children: A neuropsychologically based model for assessment. *Developmental Neuropsychology, 6*, 239–274.

Dabrowska, J. (1972). On the mechanisms of go–no go symmetrically reinforced tasks in dogs. *Acta Neurobiologia Experimentals (Warszawa), 32*, 345–359.

Deutsch, G., Papanicolaou, A.C., Bourbon, W.T., & Eisenberg, H.M. (1987). Cerebral blood flow evidence of right frontal activation in attention demanding tasks. *International Journal of Neuroscience, 36*, 23–28.

Di Paolo, T., Poyet, P., & Labrie, F. (1982). Effect of prolactin and estradiol on rat striatal dopamine receptors. *Life Sciences, 31*, 2921–2929.

Douglas, V.I. (1972). Stop, look, and listen: The problem of sustained attention and impulse control in hyperactive and normal children. *Canadian Journal of Behavioral Science, 4*, 259–282.

Douglas, V.I. (1983). Attention and cognitive problems. In M. Rutter (Ed.), *Developmental neuropsychiatry* (pp. 280–329). New York: Guilford Press.

Draeger, S., Prior, M., & Sanson, A. (1986). Visual and auditory attention performance in hyperactive children: Competence or compliance. *Journal of Abnormal Child Psychology, 14*, 411–424.

Drewe, E.A. (1975). Go–no go learning after frontal lobe lesions in humans. *Cortex, 11*, 8–16.

DuPaul, G.J., & Barkley, R.A. (1990). Medication therapy. In R.A. Barkley (Ed.), *Attention-deficit hyperactivity disorder: A handbook for diagnosis and treatment* (pp. 573–612). New York: Guilford Press.

Eison, M.S., Eison, A.S., & Ellison, G. (1981). The regional distribution of D-amphetamine and local glucose utilization in rat brain during continuous amphetamine administration. *Experimental Brain Research, 43*, 281–288.

Epstein, P., Pisani, V., & Fawcett, J. (1977). Alcoholism and cerebral atrophy. *Alcoholism: Clinical and Experimental Research, 1*, 61–65.

Ernst, M., Liebenauer, L.L., Jons, P.H., King, A.C., Cohen, R.M., & Zametkin, A.J. (1994). Sexual maturation and brain metabolism in ADHD and normal girls [Abstract]. *Scientific Proceedings of the 41st Annual Meeting of the American Academy of Child and Adolescent Psychiatry, X*, NR-9.

Ernst, M., Liebenauer, L.L., King, A.C., Fitzgerald, G.A., Cohen, R.M., & Zametkin, A.J. (1994). Reduced brain metabolism in hyperactive girls. *Journal of the American Academy of Child and Adolescent Psychiatry, 33*(6), 858–868.

Ernst, M., Zametkin, A.J., Matochik, J.A., Liebenauer, L.L., Fitzgerald, G.L., & Cohen, R.M. (1994). Effects of intravenous dextroamphetamine on brain metabolism in adults with attention deficit hyperactivity disorder (ADHD): Preliminary findings. *Psychopharmacology Bulletin, 30*, 219–225.

Fields, J.Z., & Gordon, J.H. (1982). Estrogen inhibits the dopaminergic supersensitivity induced by neuroleptics. *Life Sciences, 30*, 229–234.

Fitch, R.H., Brown, C.P., O'Connor, K., & Tallal, P. (1993). Functional lateralization for auditory temporal processing in male and female rats. *Behavioral Neuroscience, 107*(5), 844–850.

Frankfurt, M., & McEwen, B.S. (1991). 5,7-Dihydroxytryptamine and gonadal steroid manipulation alter spine density in ventromedial hypothalamic neurons. *Neuroendocrinology, 54*(6), 653–657.

Giedd, J.N., Castellanos, X., Casey, B.J., Kozuch, P., King, A.C., Hamburger, S.D., & Rapoport, J.L. (1994). Quantitative morphology of the corpus callosum in attention deficit hyperactivity disorder. *American Journal of Psychiatry, 151*, 665–669.

Gittelman, R., Mannuzza, S., Shenker, R., & Bonagura, N. (1985). Hyperactive boys almost grown up. *Archives of General Psychiatry, 42*, 937–947.

Grant, D.A., & Berg, E.A. (1948). A behavioral analysis of degree of reinforcement and ease of shifting two new responses in a Weigl-type card sorting problem. *Journal of Experimental Psychology, 38*, 404–411.

Hechtman, L. (1992). Long-term outcome in attention-deficit hyperactivity disorder. *Psychiatric Clinics of North America, 1*, 553–565.

Heilman, K.M., Voeller, K.K.S., & Nadeau, S.E. (1991). A possible pathophysiologic substrate of attention deficit hyperactivity disorder. *Journal of Child Neurology, 6*, S76–S81.

Heinze, H.J., Mangun, G.R., Burchert, W., Hinrichs, H., Scholz, M., Munte, T.F., Gos, A., Scherg, M., Johannes, S., Hundeshagen, H., Gazzaniga, M.S., & Hillyard, S.A. (1994). Combined spatial and temporal imaging of brain activity during visual selective attention in humans. *Nature, 372*, 543–546.

Hooks, K., Milich, R., & Lorch, E.P. (1994). Sustained and selective attention in boys with attention deficit hyperactivity disorder. *Journal of Clinical Child Psychology, 23*, 69–77.

Hynd, G.W., Marshall, R., & Gonzalez, J.J. (1993). *Asymmetry of the caudate nucleus in ADHD: An exploratory study of gender and handedness effects.* Paper presented at the annual meeting of the Society for Research in Child and Adolescent Psychopathology, Santa Fe, New Mexico.

Hynd, G.W., Semrud-Clikeman, M., Lorys, A.R., Novey, E.S., & Eliopulos, D. (1990). Brain morphology in developmental dyslexia and attention deficit disorder/hyperactivity. *Archives of Neurology, 47*, 919–926.

Hynd, G.W., Semrud-Clikeman, M., Lorys, A.R., Novey, E.S., Eliopulos, D., & Lyytinen, H. (1991). Corpus callosum morphology in attention deficit hyperactivity disorder: Morphometric analysis of MRI. *Journal of Learning Disabilities, 24*, 141–146.

Innocenti, G.M. (1981). Development of interhemispheric cortical connections. *Neuroscience Research Program Bulletin, 20*, 532–540.

Iversen, S.D., & Mishkin, M. (1970). Perseverative interference in monkeys following selective lesions of the inferior prefrontal convexity. *Experimental Brain Research, 11*, 376–386.

James, A., & Taylor, E. (1990). Sex differences in the hyperkinetic syndrome of childhood. *Journal of Child Psychology and Psychiatry and Allied Disciplines, 31*, 437–446.

Jones, B.P., Henderson, M., & Welch, C.A. (1988). Executive functions in unipolar depression before and after electroconvulsive therapy. *International Journal of Neuroscience, 38*, 287–297.

Kahn, E., & Cohen, L.H. (1934). Organic driveness: A brain stem syndrome and an experience. *New England Journal of Medicine, 210*, 748–756.

Klein, R.G., & Mannuzza, S. (1991). Long-term outcome of hyperactive children: A review. *Journal of the American Academy of Child and Adolescent Psychiatry, 30*, 383–387.

Knobel, M., Wolman, M.B., & Mason, E. (1959). Hyperkinesis and organicity in children. *Archives of General Psychiatry, 1*, 310–321.

Lahey, B.B., Applegate, B., McBurnett, K., Greenhill, L., Hynd, G.W., Barkley, R.A., Newcorn, J., Jensen, P., & Richters, J. (1994). DSM-IV field trials for attention deficit hyperactivity disorder in children and adolescents. *American Journal of Psychiatry, 151*, 1673–1685.

Laufer, M., Denhoff, E., & Solomons, G. (1957). Hyperkinetic impulse disorder in children's behavior problems. *Psychosomatic Medicine, 19*, 38–49.

Leimkuhler, M.E., & Mesulam, M.M. (1985). Reversible go–no go deficits in a case of frontal lobe tumor. *Annals of Neurology, 18*, 617–619.

London, E.D., Cascella, N.G., Wong, D.F., Phillips, R.L., Dannals, R.F., Links, J.M., Herning, R., Grayson, R., Jaffe, J.H., & Wagner, H.N. (1990). Cocaine-induced reduction of glucose utilization in human brain. *Archives of General Psychiatry, 47*, 567–574.

London, E.D., Wilkerson, G., Goldberg, S.R., & Risner, M.E. (1986). Effects of L-cocaine on local cerebral glucose utilization in the rat. *Neuroscience Letters, 68*, 73–78.

Loney, J., Kramer, J., & Milich, R. (1981). The hyperactive child grows up: Predictors of symptoms, delinquency, and achievement at follow-up. In K.D. Gadow & J. Loney (Eds.), *Psychosocial aspects of drug treatment for hyperactivity* (pp. 381–415). Boulder, CO: Westview Press.

Lou, H.C., Henriksen, L., & Bruhn, P. (1984). Focal cerebral hypoperfusion in children with dysphasia and/or attention deficit disorder. *Archives of Neurology, 41*, 825–829.

Lou, H.C., Henriksen, L., & Bruhn, P. (1990). Focal cerebral dysfunction in developmental learning disabilities. *Lancet, 335*, 8–11.

Lou, H.C., Henriksen, L., Bruhn, P., Borner, H., & Nielsen, J.B. (1989). Striatal dysfunction in attention deficit and hyperkinetic disorder. *Archives of Neurology, 46*, 48–52.

Luk, S. (1985). Direct observations studies of hyperactive behaviors. *Journal of the American Academy of Child Psychiatry, 24*, 338–344.

Luria, A.R. (1973). The frontal lobes and the regulation of behavior. In K.H. Prihbram & A.R. Luria (Eds.), *Psychophysiology of the frontal lobes* (pp. 3–26). Orlando, FL: Academic Press.

Lyon, G.R., & Krasnegor, N.A. (Eds.). (1996). *Attention, memory, and executive function.* Baltimore: Paul H. Brookes Publishing Co.

Mack, C.M., Fitch, R.H., Cowell, P.E., Schrott, L.M., & Denenberg, V.H. (1993). Ovarian estrogen acts to feminize the female rat's corpus callosum. *Brain Research: Developmental Brain Research, 15,* 115–119.

Matochik, J.A., Liebenauer, L.L., King, A.C., Szymanski, H.V., Cohen, R.M., & Zametkin, A.J. (1994). Cerebral glucose metabolism in adults with attention-deficit hyperactivity disorder after chronic stimulant treatment. *American Journal of Psychiatry, 151,* 658–664.

Matochik, J.A., Nordahl, T.E., Gross, M., Semple, W.E., King, A.C., Cohen, R.M., & Zametkin, A.J. (1993). Effects of acute stimulant medication on cerebral metabolism in adults with hyperactivity. *Neuropsychopharmacology, 8,* 377–386.

Mattes, J.A. (1980). The role of frontal lobe dysfunction in childhood hyperkinesis. *Comprehensive Psychiatry, 21,* 358–369.

Mennemeier, M.S., Chatterjee, A., Watson, R.T., Wertman, E., Carter, L.P., & Heilman, M. (1994). Contributions of the parietal and frontal lobes to sustained attention and habituation. *Neuropsychologia, 32*(6), 703–716.

Mesulam, M.M. (1986). Editorial: Frontal cortex and behavior. *Annals of Neurology, 19,* 320–325.

Milich, R., Loney, J., & Landau, S. (1982). The independent dimensions of hyperactivity and aggression: A validation with playroom observation data. *Journal of Abnormal Psychology, 91,* 183–198.

Mirsky, A.F., Anthony, B.J., Duncan, A.C., Ahearn, M.B., & Kellam, S.G. (1991). Analysis of the elements of attention: A neurological approach. *Neuropsychological Reviews, 2*(2), 109–145.

Morecraft, R.J., Geula, C., & Mesulam, M.M. (1993). Architecture of connectivity within a cingulo-fronto-parietal neurocognitive network for directed attention. *Archives of Neurology, 50,* 279–284.

Moruzzi, G., & Magoun, H.W. (1949). Brain stem reticular formation and activation of the EEG. *Electroencephalography and Clinical Neurophysiology, 1,* 455–473.

Murphy, D.G., DeCarli, C., Daly, E., Haxby, J.V., Allen, G., White, B.J., McIntosh, A.R., Powell, C.M., Horwitz, B., Rapoport, S.I., & Shapiro, M.B. (1993). X-chromosome effects on female brain: A magnetic resonance imaging study of Turner's syndrome. *Lancet, 13,* 1197–2000.

Nasrallah, H.A., Loney, J., Olsen, S.C., McCalley-Whitters, M., Kramer, J., & Jacoby, C.G. (1986). Cortical atrophy in young adults with a history of hyperactivity in childhood. *Psychiatry Research, 17,* 241–246.

Neale, T.M., McIntyre, C.W., Fox, R., & Cromwell, R.L. (1969). Span of apprehension in acute schizophrenics. *Journal of Abnormal Psychology, 74,* 593–596.

Newcorn, J.H., Halperin, J.M., Healey, J.M., O'Brien, J.D., Pascualvaca, D.M., Wolf, L.E., Morganstein, A., Sharma, V., & Young, J.G. (1989). Are ADDH and ADHD the same or different? *Journal of the American Academy of Child and Adolescent Psychiatry, 285,* 734–738.

Pandya, D.N., Karol, E.A., & Heilbronn, D. (1971). The topographical distribution of interhemispheric projections in the corpus callosum of the rhesus monkey. *Brain Research, 32,* 31–43.

Pandya, D.N., & Seltzer, B. (1986). The topography of commissural fibers. In F. Lepore, M. Ptito, & H.H. Jasper (Eds.), *Two hemispheres — one brain* (pp. 47–73). New York: Alan R. Liss.

Pardo, J.V., Pardo, P.J., Janer, K.W., & Raichle, M.E. (1990). The anterior cingulate cortex mediates processing selection in the Stroop attentional conflict paradigm. *Proceedings of the National Academy of Sciences of the United States of America, 87,* 256–259.

Porrino, L.J., & Lucignani, G. (1987). Different patterns of local brain energy metabolism associated with high and low doses of methylphenidate: Relevance to its action in hyperactive children. *Biological Psychiatry, 22,* 126–138.

Porrino, L.J., Lucignani, G., Dow-Edwards, D., & Sokoloff, L. (1984). Correlation of dose-dependent effects of acute amphetamine administration on behavior and local cerebral metabolism in rats. *Brain Research, 307,* 311–320.

Posner, M.I., & Petersen, S.E. (1990). The attention system of the human brain. *Annual Review of Neuroscience, 13,* 25–42.

Posner, M.I., Petersen, S.E., Fox, P.T., & Raichle, M.E. (1988). Localization of cognitive operations in the human brain. *Science, 240,* 1627–1631.

Reitan, R.M., & Davidson, L.A. (Eds.). (1974). *Clinical neuropsychology: Current status and applications.* Washington, DC: V.H. Winston and Sons.

Ross, D.M., & Ross, S.A. (1982). *Hyperactivity: Current issues, research, and theory.* New York: John Wiley & Sons.

Rosvold, H.E., Mirsky, A.F., Sarason, I., Bransome, E.D., & Beck, L.H. (1956). A continuous performance test of brain damage. *Journal of Consulting and Clinical Psychology, 20*, 343–350.

Satterfield, J.H., & Dawson, M.E. (1971). Electrodermal correlates of hyperactivity in children. *Psychophysiology, 8*, 191–197.

Seeman, M.V., & Lang, M. (1990). The role of estrogens in schizophrenia gender differences. *Schizophrenia Bulletin, 16*, 185–194.

Semrud-Clikeman, M., Filipek, P.A., Biederman, J., Steingard, R., Kennedy, D., Renshaw, P., & Bekken, K. (1993). *Attention deficit disorder: Differences in the corpus callosum by MRI morphometric analysis*. Paper presented at the annual meeting of the Society for Research in Child and Adolescent Psychopathology, Santa Fe, New Mexico.

Sharpless, S., & Jasper, H. (1956). Habituation of the arousal reaction. *Brain, 79*, 655–680.

Shaywitz, B.A., Shaywitz, S.E., Byrne, T., Cohen, D.J., & Rothman, S. (1983). Attention deficit disorder: Quantitative analysis of CT. *Neurology, 33*, 1500–1503.

Shaywitz, S.E., & Shaywitz, B.A. (1987). Attention deficit disorder: Current perspectives. *Pediatric Neurology, 3*, 129–135.

Still, G.F. (1902). Some abnormal psychical conditions in children. *Lancet, i*, 1008–1012, 1077–1082, 1163–1168.

Strauss, A.A., & Lehtinen, L.E. (1947). *Psychopathology and education of the brain-injured child*. New York: Grune & Stratton.

Stroop, J.R. (1935). Studies of interference in serial verbal reactions. *Journal of Experimental Psychology, 18*, 643–662.

Stuss, D.T., & Benson, D.F. (1984). Neuropsychological studies of the frontal lobes. *Psychological Bulletin, 95*, 3–28.

Szatmari, P., Offord, D.R., & Boyle, M. (1989). Ontario Child Health Study: Prevalence of attention deficit disorder with hyperactivity. *Journal of Child Psychology and Psychiatry and Allied Disciplines, 30*, 219–230.

Talland, G.A. (1965). *Deranged memory*. New York: Academic Press.

Thompson, R.F., & Bettinger, L.A. (1970). Neural substrates of attention. In D.I. Mostofsky (Ed.), *Attention: Contemporary theory and analysis* (pp. 367–401). New York: Appleton-Century-Crofts.

Ullman, D.G., Barkley, R.A., & Brown, H.W. (1978). The behavioral symptoms of hyperkinetic children who successfully responded to stimulant drug treatment. *American Journal of Orthopsychiatry, 48*, 425–437.

Van Hartesveldt, C., & Joyce, J.N. (1986). Effects of estrogen on the basal ganglia. *Neuroscience and Biobehavioral Reviews, 10*, 1–14.

Verfaellie, M., & Heilman, K.M. (1987). Response preparation and response inhibition after lesions of the medial frontal lobe. *Archives of Neurology, 44*, 1265–1271.

Voeller, K.K.S. (1986). Right hemisphere deficit syndrome in children. *American Journal of Psychiatry, 143*, 1004–1009.

Wechsler, D. (1974). *Wechsler Intelligence Scale for Children–Revised*. New York: Psychological Corporation.

Wechsler, L.R., Savaki, H., & Sokoloff, L. (1979). Effects of D- and L-amphetamine on local cerebral glucose utilization in the conscious rat. *Journal of Neurochemistry, 32*, 15–22.

Weiss, G. (1985). Follow up studies on outcome of hyperactive children. *Psychopharmacology Bulletin, 21*, 169–177.

Wender, P.H., Reimberr, F.W., & Wood, D.R. (1981). Attention deficit disorder ("minimal brain dysfunction") in adults. *Archives of General Psychiatry, 38*, 449–456.

Wender, P.H., Wood, D.R., & Reimberr, F.W. (1985). Pharmacological treatment of attention deficit disorder, residual type (ADD, RT, "minimal brain dysfunction," "hyperactivity") in adults. *Psychopharmacology Bulletin, 21*, 222–231.

Werry, J.S., & Sprague, R.L. (1970). Hyperactivity. In G.C. Costello (Ed.), *Symptoms of psychopathology* (pp. 397–417). New York: John Wiley & Sons.

Witelson, S.F. (1989). Hand and sex differences in the isthmus and genu of the human corpus callosum: A postmortem morphological study. *Brain, 112*, 799–835.

Witelson, S.F. (1993). Anterior commissure in relation to corpus callosum anatomy: Hand preference and sex. *Society for Neuroscience Abstracts, 19*, NR232–236.

Zametkin, A.J., Liebenauer, L.L., Fitzgerald, G.A., King, A.C., Minkunas, D.V., Herscovitch, P., Yamada, E.M., & Cohen, R.M. (1993). Brain metabolism in teenagers with attention deficit hyperactivity disorder. *Archives of General Psychiatry, 50*, 333–340.

Zametkin, A.J., Nordahl, T.E., Gross, M., King, A.C., Semple, W.E., Rumsey, J., Hamburger, S., & Cohen, R.M. (1990). Cerebral glucose metabolism in adults with hyperactivity of childhood onset. *New England Journal of Medicine, 323,* 1361–1366.

Zentall, S.S. (1985). A context for hyperactivity. In K.D. Gadow & I. Bialer (Eds.), *Advances in learning and behavioral disabilities* (Vol. 4, pp. 273–343). Greenwich, CT: JAI Press.

Zettle, R.D., & Hayes, S.C. (1983). Rule-governed behavior: A potential theoretical framework for cognitive-behavioral therapy. In P.C. Kendall (Ed.), *Advances in cognitive–behavioral research* (Vol. 1, pp. 73–118). New York: Academic Press.

6

Neuroimaging Studies of Autism
—————— Judith M. Rumsey ——————

DEFINITIONS AND DIAGNOSIS

Autism is a rare behavioral syndrome rather than a disease. It is defined by a cluster of associated symptoms and a characteristic early age of onset and chronic course rather than by an underlying etiology. The core symptoms are impairments of reciprocal social interaction, impairments of verbal and nonverbal communication, and a markedly restricted repertoire of activities and interests (*Diagnostic and Statistical Manual of Mental Disorders* [4th ed.], American Psychiatric Association, 1994). Prevalence is estimated to be 2–5 cases per 10,000 individuals (American Psychiatric Association, 1994). Although patients' conditions improve with maturation, autism nearly always is a life-long disorder.

First identified by Kanner in 1943, autism has come to be regarded as one of the best-validated diagnoses in child psychiatry. In his historic paper, Kanner (1943) described a group of children who showed severe impairments in their attachment and social interactions with others, including their parents; restricted, bizarre interests and preoccupations; and language and communication abnormalities. Yet, in some cases, islets of normal or even exceptional functioning, for example, impressive rote memory and visuoperceptual skills (e.g., ability to complete form boards and puzzles) were noted.

In 1944 in Vienna, Asperger (1991) described a similar group of children with "autistic psychopathy." Impressed with behavioral similarities between some of these children and their parents, Asperger speculated about possible genetic factors. Even earlier, Heller (1908), a Viennese educator, had described a small group of children with an insidious loss of language and mental abilities between the ages of 3 and 4 years, which left them severely impaired with autistic symptoms.

The *Diagnostic and Statistical Manual of Mental Disorders* (3rd ed.) (DSM-III) (American Psychiatric Association, 1980) introduced the term *pervasive developmental disorder* (PDD) for children meeting the descriptions noted above. The term *infantile autism* was restricted to those children who had a pervasive lack of responsiveness to others with an onset before 30 months of age. The revision of this edition of the diagnostic manual (DSM-III-R) (American Psychiatric Association, 1987) broadened the definition of autism by eliminating the age of onset criteria and relaxing the criteria for social abnormality. Impaired social interaction and communication and restricted activities and interests were required for a DSM-III-R diagnosis of autistic disorder. In addition, the operationalization of each criterion with lists of symptoms characteristic of individuals at different ages and developmental levels rendered the diagnosis of older patients somewhat less problematic.

As a result of these relaxed criteria, DSM-III-R identified many more children as having autism than did the more restrictive DSM-III criteria (Volkmar et al., 1994). Studies in which DSM-III-R criteria were used, therefore, may well include many less classic cases of autism than may those in which DSM-III criteria were used. The evolving diagnostic criteria for autism are listed in Table 6.1.

DSM-IV retained the three major criteria contained in DSM-III-R but separated the two subgroups previously described by Asperger (1991) and Heller (1908). In DSM-IV, Asperger's disorder was differentiated from autistic disorder by a lack of developmental language delay. Asperger's disorder is thought to have a somewhat later onset than autistic disorder as well as motor delays or clumsiness not typically seen in autism. Childhood disintegrative disorder (Heller's syndrome) is differentiated from autism by a loss of previously acquired skills after a period of normal development. Whether these disorders are variants of autism or reflect distinct etiologies is unclear. These diagnostic distinctions will allow future research to clarify this issue. Because the few neuroimaging studies of Asperger's syndrome in the literature were completed prior to the adoption of differential criteria for Asperger's disorder by the American Psychiatric Association, these studies are included in this chapter.

Methods for applying diagnostic criteria primarily involved clinical judgments until the development of the Autism Diagnostic Interview (LeCouteur et al., 1989) and its revision, the Autism Diagnostic Interview–Revised (Lord et al., 1994). This standardized interview is designed for use with a patient's primary caregiver; it provides a lifetime assessment of the range of behaviors relevant to the diagnosis of PDDs in individuals from preschool age through adulthood and applies an algorithm for distinguishing PDDs by using DSM criteria from nonautistic mentally disabled individuals. The revision of this interview was linked to DSM-IV criteria for the diagnosis of autism. Although this instrument has not yet been validated for discriminating among PDDs, new data along these lines appear promising (Lord, unpublished data, 1995).

Table 6.1.   Diagnostic criteria for autism

DSM-III (American Psychiatric Association, 1980):   Infantile autism
A.   Onset before 30 months of age
B.   Pervasive lack of responsiveness to other people (autism)
C.   Gross deficits in language development
D.   When speech is present, peculiar speech patterns such as immediate and delayed echolalia, metaphorical language, and pronomial reversal
E.   Bizarre responses to various aspects of the environment (e.g., resistance to change, peculiar interest in or attachments to animate or inanimate objects)
F.   Absence of delusions, hallucinations, loosening of associations, and incoherence, as in schizophrenia
DSM-III-R (American Psychiatric Association, 1987):   Autistic disorder
A.   Qualitative impairment in reciprocal social interaction
B.   Qualitative impairment in verbal and nonverbal communication and in imaginative activity
C.   Markedly restricted repertoire of activities and interests
D.   Onset during infancy or childhood
DSM-IV (American Psychiatric Association, 1994):   Autistic disorder[a]
A.   1.   Qualitative impairment in social interaction
     2.   Qualitative impairments in communication
     3.   Restricted, repetitive, and stereotyped patterns of behavior, interests, and activities
B.   Delays or abnormal functioning, before 3 years of age, in social interaction, language as used in social communication, or symbolic or imaginative play
C.   Not better accounted for by Rett's disorder or childhood disintegrative disorder

[a]Separate diagnostic categories exist for Asperger's disorder, childhood disintegrative disorder, and Rett's disorder (the latter has a highly distinctive course and is diagnosed only in females).

ETIOLOGY AND COMORBIDITY

Decades of research have drastically altered early beliefs about the syndrome of autism. Psychogenic theories concerning etiology (i.e., the idea that emotionally cold parents caused social withdrawal in their children) have given way to neurogenic theories and hypotheses, although the biology of the disorder remains poorly understood. Early beliefs that emotional disturbance interfered with or masked normal intellectual functioning, which led to psychoanalytic attempts to break through a glass shell, have been replaced by a realization that cognitive impairments in autism are a real and permanent part of the disorder (Rutter, 1983). Approximately 75% of patients with autism also have mental retardation with IQs below 70 (American Psychiatric Association, 1994), and even patients with autism without mental retardation demonstrate cognitive impairments (Rumsey, 1992; Rumsey & Hamburger, 1988). Although many earlier researchers considered autism to be a precocious form of schizophrenia or a psychosis (Bender, 1955; Goldfarb, 1964; Reiser, 1963), autism has been found to be distinct from schizophrenia in its age of onset, developmental course, and pattern of family history (DeMyer et al., 1973; Green et al., 1984; Kolvin, 1971; Kolvin et al., 1971; Rutter, 1970).

Many patients with autism (approximately one fifth to one third) develop epileptic seizures (Deykin & MacMahon, 1979; Volkmar & Nelson, 1990). Most (although not all) seizures occur in lower-functioning patients, and the risk for developing seizures is greatest in early childhood and adolescence.

Rubella (Chess et al., 1971), neurofibromatosis, tuberous sclerosis, and fragile X syndrome, a genetic disorder that accounts for a high percentage of mental retardation in males (see Chapter 7), place children at risk for developing autism (Folstein & Piven, 1991). The majority of cases of autism, however, are idiopathic (i.e., they have no known etiology).

Autism is thought to have multiple etiologies that likely affect widely distributed brain systems. Distinct etiologies may not produce distinct behavioral syndromes in a simple one-to-one fashion when there is variability in the brain regions and circuits affected. The link between etiology (e.g., the disease process) and behavioral manifestations, therefore, is thought to depend more on the particular brain regions and circuits affected.

VARIABILITY IN CLINICAL PRESENTATION

The behavioral presentation of autism is highly heterogeneous. Autism may be diagnosed in individuals at almost any level of intelligence—from severe levels of mental retardation to above-average IQ levels. As mentioned above, however, most children with autism (approximately 75%) have mental retardation with IQs below 70. Uneven cognitive profiles, such as those demonstrated on the widely used Wechsler intelligence tests (e.g., high digit span and block design scores, low comprehension and picture arrangement scores), frequently are seen in these patients (Rumsey, 1992). Even those patients with high IQs share the core social disabilities and may display cognitive deficits (Rumsey, 1992). The subgroup of patients with IQs above 70 is most likely to be subdivided between those with autistic disorder and Asperger's disorder when DSM-IV criteria are applied.

Delayed language development frequently brings these children with autism to professional attention. Language disabilities in autism range from mutism to dysphasia to eventual development of good basic language skill with impaired pragmatics (i.e., the social use of language) and/or dysprosodies (i.e., abnormalities of speech rate, rhythm, and intonation) (Tager-Flusberg, 1981). The style of social interaction also varies, particularly in older patients. Some patients remain aloof and/or passive; others display odd or stilted approaches to others or intrusive personality styles (Wing, 1992). Attentional disturbances include abnormally prolonged attention to certain repetitive activities, distractibility, and inability or unwillingness to focus attention (e.g., on faces, books). Other variable symptoms include abnormalities of posture and motor behavior, such as toe walking and stereotypies, hypo- or hyperresponsivity to sensory stimuli (e.g., sounds, spinning objects, touch, pain stimuli), lability of mood, and self-injurious behavior (e.g., wrist biting).

IMPLICATIONS FOR NEUROIMAGING STUDIES AND METHODOLOGICAL CONSIDERATIONS

Several of the above-discussed factors may affect neuroimaging studies. The fact that autism is believed to be heterogeneous in etiology and is associated with several co-morbid conditions, including epilepsy, neurofibromatosis, tuberous sclerosis, fragile X syndrome, mental retardation, and developmental language disorder, likely influences neuroimaging findings. The variation in clinical presentation, such as the prominence and type of communication disorder (e.g., mutism, good language with striking dys-prosodic speech), well may have different neuroanatomical and neuropsysiological correlates.

Neuroimaging findings may be more highly associated with these comorbid factors than with autism, per se. For example, some abnormalities seen in patients with autism and epilepsy or mental retardation may be caused by the comorbid seizure disorder or the mental retardation independent of autism. Medications used to treat seizures or behavioral symptoms seen in patients with autism also may affect neurophysiology and neuroanatomy, thereby presenting another potential confounding factor for imaging studies. For example, anticonvulsants can decrease cerebral blood flow and metabolism (Gaillard et al., 1996; Theodore et al., 1989).

Patient cooperation also presents difficulties for such studies. In some studies, investigators have sedated difficult patients before performing scans. Although this practice should only improve the quality of anatomical scans, medications may influence brain physiology, thereby presenting a confounding factor for functional neuroimaging studies. Even when patient cooperation is sufficient for scanning without medication, the subjective anxiety and stress experienced by patients with autism may exceed the anxiety and stress experienced by the control subjects with whom they are compared and may, as a result, influence results on physiological scans. Many patients with autism cannot accurately or adequately self-report on their anxiety levels. Some patients have too-severe language impairments, whereas others lack adequate self-awareness and reflection; as a result, external observers must judge the anxiety levels of such patients. Objective physiological measures of arousal and anxiety might be useful, although the additional equipment such measures require could potentially exacerbate anxiety levels in patients.

Given the nature of autism as an early onset disorder, it seems best to study young patients to diminish the effects of interventions, aging, and the like. The diagnosis of children younger than 3 years of age, however, may be less certain than later diagnosis. Few children younger than 6 years of age, even healthy children, are able to voluntarily (i.e., without sedation) remain still long enough for anatomical magnetic resonance imaging (MRI) scanning. Given the rarity of the disorder, investigators frequently must include a wide age range of patients with autism, which increases age-related variability.

Functional neuroimaging studies require even greater cooperation than do anatomical studies and, until the emergence of functional MRI (fMRI), required exposure to radiation. Because children are more sensitive to the effects of radiation than are adults, safety factors have severely limited the use of these techniques in children. Most previous functional imaging studies of autism have, therefore, involved adult subjects. The study of adults can present more difficult diagnostic issues, because standard diagnostic criteria were adopted by the medical profession only as recently as 1980. Thus, their childhood diagnoses may be less reliable or valid than those of younger patients.

The few functional imaging studies of children with autism that have been completed to date have been unable, for ethical/safety reasons, to include normal children as control subjects. Instead, investigators usually have selected as controls other patients, who may themselves have abnormal brain function, or have compared children to normal adults, in whom brain metabolism is known to differ from that in children (Chugani et al., 1987).

Control subjects should match patients in age and gender, because both variables are associated with anatomical and physiological differences. Brain metabolism shows age-related differences both globally and regionally (Chugani et al., 1987). Females tend to have smaller brains (Giedd et al., 1996) and higher rates of brain metabolism and blood flow (Baxter et al., 1987; Gur et al., 1982; Rodrigues et al., 1988; Yoshii et al., 1988). Although the relative sizes of many individual structures (compared with the whole brain) are not thought to differ by gender or age, some structures do show such differences (Cowell et al., 1992; Giedd et al., 1996; Pujol et al., 1993).

In functional imaging studies, the state under which subjects are studied is important. The first functional imaging studies in autism were completed while subjects were in a resting state, perhaps the most neutral state with which to begin. In addition, when tasks are involved, performance may vary widely given the heterogeneity seen within autism. Differences in brain physiology may correlate with poor performance, thereby raising a chicken-and-egg question when causal interpretations are sought. Other methodological considerations include various technical limitations, which are beyond the scope of this chapter. The reader is referred to Chapter 2 for a discussion of these factors.

AUTOPSY STUDIES

Because the brains of individuals who have developmental disorders seldom are autopsied, only a small number of neuropathological studies have been completed. The major work in this area is that of Bauman and Kemper (Bauman, 1991; Bauman & Kemper, 1985), who have reported on five well-documented cases of patients with autism, several of whom experienced seizures. In all cases, the brains were well developed and were without gross lesions, abnormalities of gyral configuration, myelination, or obvious gliosis. Microscopic examination of the cerebral cortex failed to disclose abnormalities of cellular lamination, structure, or number. Abnormalities, in all cases, were limited to limbic and cerebellar circuits.

Relative to the brains of control subjects, the brains of individuals with autism showed increased cell-packing density (increased numbers of neurons per unit volume) and reduced nerve cell size bilaterally in the hippocampal complex, subiculum, entorhinal cortex, portions of the amygdala, mamillary body, and medial septal nucleus. Several brains of individuals with autism showed similar abnormalities in the anterior cingulate. Cerebellar findings have included a variable loss of Purkinje cells and, to a lesser extent, granule cells, primarily in the neocerebellar cortex, with some involvement of the anterior cerebellum and vermis. These defects are thought to have been acquired early in development.

All abnormalities reported in the forebrain involve structures known to be connected through closely interrelated circuits, which comprise a portion of the limbic system. These abnormalities, therefore, have implications for motivation, emotion, learning, and memory. The significance of the cerebellar findings is unclear, but recent research suggests that the cerebellum may play some role in the modulation of emotion and higher cortical functions (Leiner et al., 1986; Watson, 1978). Consistent with these findings, Coleman et al. (1985) reported normal cell counts in the primary auditory cortex, auditory association cortex, and Broca's speech area of a woman with autism, and Ritvo et al. (1986) reported decreased Purkinje cell counts in the cerebella of four patients with autism.

Because these findings are microscopic in nature, in vivo structural imaging studies are not expected to show gross abnormalities when evaluated clinically in many, perhaps most, cases. Nonetheless, it is possible that quantitative studies may be sensitive to subtle differences in the sizes or shapes of affected brain structures.

FUNCTIONAL NEUROIMAGING STUDIES

Functional neuroimaging studies of autism published before 1995 include seven positron emission tomography (PET) studies, three single photon emission computed tomography (SPECT) studies, and one spectroscopy study. The first of these was a PET study published by Rumsey et al. (1985), who studied a group of 10 healthy men with clear childhood diagnoses of autism that met restrictive DSM-III criteria. All 10 men had good childhood diagnostic records (several had been diagnosed by Professor Leo Kanner), and most of the men were unusually high functioning with little or no history of neuroleptic use. Patients and age- and gender-matched normal control subjects were studied in a resting, sensory-restricted state with their eyes closed and ears plugged.

The group of men with autism showed diffusely elevated glucose metabolism, although there was substantial overlap of individual values between autistic and control subjects (4.87 mg/100 g/min versus 5.84 mg/100 g/min; $p < 0.05$). Regional values reflected this global hypermetabolism but failed to suggest additional focal or localized abnormalities; that is, specific brain regions did not show particularly high or low values relative to global brain metabolism. The anxiety ratings of the patients completed by external observers did not differ from those of the control subjects and did not correlate with global metabolic rates in this small sample.

After increasing the patient sample to 14, Horwitz et al. (1988) explored metabolic patterns thought to reflect functional relationships among brain regions with a correlational analysis. The rationale for examining correlations between brain regions was as follows: If two brain regions are coupled functionally, a change in one will effect a change in another, resulting in significant correlations between these regions. Regions that are intercorrelated, therefore, were hypothesized to be functionally related; and differences between groups in the strength or direction of these correlations were hypothesized to reflect differences in these functional relationships.

Relative to control subjects, men with autism showed reduced intercorrelations within and between the frontal and parietal lobes and, most strikingly, between the frontal and parietal neocortex and subcortical regions (Horwitz et al., 1988). Normal male control subjects showed many large positive correlations within and between the frontal and parietal lobes and fewer, but generally positive, correlations between the frontal and parietal cortex and subcortical regions and between different subcortical regions. Men with autism showed lower correlations within and between the frontal and parietal lobes and large negative correlations with subcortical regions, including those in the striatum and thalamus, in contrast with the positive correlations seen in control subjects. These differences were hypothesized to reflect dysfunction in the neural systems associated with directed attention, such as the reciprocal frontal–parietal interactions that mediate approach–avoidance equilibrium with the external environment (Mesulam, 1986). The differences in neocortical–subcortical relationships well may reflect dysfunction in neural systems that subserve affective and motivational aspects of attention (Mesulam, 1985).

Buchsbaum and colleagues (Buchsbaum et al., 1992; Heh et al., 1989; Siegel et al., 1992) studied glucose metabolism in high-functioning adults with autism during the performance of a visual vigilance task, thought to measure the ability to sustain attention, on which patients performed as well as control subjects. In contrast with the hypermetabolism reported by Rumsey et al. (1985), normal levels of global brain glucose metabolism were seen. Regional differences were few but included relative decreases in the right posterior thalamus and right putamen in the 7 patients reported by Buchsbaum et al. (1992) and relative decreases in the left putamen and high metabolism in the posterior calcarine cortex in the 16 patients reported by Siegel et al. (1992). The increased variability seen in patients compared with that seen in control subjects attested to the considerable heterogeneity seen in autism.

Stimulated by autopsy (Bauman & Kemper, 1985) and anatomical MRI (Courchesne et al., 1988) findings in the cerebellum, Heh et al. (1989) sampled glucose metabolism in 10 regions of the cerebellar hemispheres and vermis, as well as in the pons, on a single PET slice through the cerebellum at the level of the superior posterior vermis, superior cerebellar peduncles, and pons. No significant differences between patients and control subjects were seen, raising the possibility that glucose metabolism may be relatively insensitive to the sort of neuropathological changes reported in the cerebellum in autism.

DeVolder et al. (1987) in Belgium studied glucose metabolism in 18 children with autism, ages 2–18 years—many of whom were sedated for scanning. Control subjects were adults (known to show lower brain metabolic rates than children) (Chugani et al., 1987) and a small group of children with varied brain pathologies. Although the children with autism showed more variable metabolic rates, no significant differences were seen overall in group means.

Herold et al. (1988) in England examined brain metabolism and blood flow on a single PET slice through the basal ganglia and temporal gray matter in eight young men with autism and IQs in the range of mild mental retardation to average intelligence, while the subjects listened to the music of their choice. One subject had a history of epilepsy; one, cortical atrophy, as determined by clinical computed tomography (CT), and three, enlarged ventricles, as determined by quantitative study. Glucose and oxygen metabolism and cerebral blood flow all were normal.

One other study, which used SPECT with a good sample size ($n = 21$), reported normal global and regional cerebral blood flow (Zilbovicius et al., 1992). Two smaller studies (George et al., 1992; Ozbayrak et al., 1991) have reported hypoperfusion (i.e., decreased blood flow). One of these, a clinical case study (Ozbayrak et al., 1991), reported left posterior (primarily occipital) hypoperfusion in a patient with Asperger's syndrome and complicating conditions. The other, a study of four men with autism (George et al., 1992), reported global and regional hypoperfusion. Failure to control for gender and the presence of seizures and anticonvulsant use on the part of three of four subjects with autism may have been responsible for the finding of hypoperfusion. Taken as a whole, the research literature has failed to demonstrate consistently and convincingly abnormal brain metabolism or blood flow in autism.

Efforts to label various classes of receptors in the brain with the use of PET were begun only in the 1990s. This application of neuroimaging should enable investigators to determine whether various chemical receptors are distributed normally in location and number. Appendix A at the end of this chapter lists functional neuroimaging studies.

SPECTROSCOPY

Magnetic resonance spectroscopy (MRS) is a newly evolving technique for studying brain chemistry in vivo. Using ^{31}P MRS to assay brain energy metabolism in the dorsal prefrontal cortex of 11 high-functioning adolescents and adults with autism studied in a resting state, Minshew et al. (1993) found decreased levels of phosphocreatine (PCr) and decreased levels of esterified ends on α-adenosine triphosphate (α-ATP). Levels of phosphomonoester (PME), inorganic phosphate (Pi), phosphodiester (PDE), ionized ends (α-ATP and β-adenosine diphosphate ([β-ADP]), middles (β-ATP), and intracellular pH were found to be normal in relationship to those of a well-matched control group. The decrease in PCr in the absence of changes in intracellular pH suggested increased utilization of PCr to maintain ATP levels, or a hypermetabolic state. The decrease in esterified ends could be of multiple origins. One possibility is that it signals an undersynthesis and enhanced degradation of cell membranes, which may provide a molecular metabolic basis for histoanatomical findings of a truncation in the development of the dendritic tree (Raymond et al., 1989).

The ^{31}P MRS metabolite levels were correlated with performance on a number of neuropsychological tests. Specifically, as neuropsychological test performance declined in the subjects with autism, levels of the most labile high-energy phosphate compound and of membrane building blocks decreased, and levels of membrane breakdown products increased. This pattern was consistent across neuropsychological tests in the group with autism and was not present in the control group. The findings of this study provided preliminary evidence of alterations in brain energy metabolism and phospholipid metabolism that may relate to the neurophysiological and neuropathological abnormalities that have been reported in autism (Minshew & Dombrowski, 1994; Minshew et al., 1993).

ANATOMICAL NEUROIMAGING

Anatomical neuroimaging studies in autism began with the introduction of X-ray CT scanning in the early 1970s. Given the limitations of CT, these early studies examined cerebral asymmetries, ventricular size, and the sizes of the basal ganglia and thalamus. Taken as a whole, those studies that included patients with associated infectious, metabolic, or genetic disorders reported abnormalities more often than did those that excluded such cases of autism and failed to yield consistent findings. Because many studies that have used the superior technology offered by MRI have been reported, the early CT studies are not reviewed here (for such a review, see Minshew & Dombrowski, 1994).

MRI has been used to examine a variety of brain structures in autism. For review purposes, these studies are categorized in Appendix B (at the end of this chapter) in three groups—those that focused primarily on forebrain structures, those that focused on posterior fossa structures, and those that included both groups of structures.

With respect to forebrain structures, Piven et al. (1990) reported developmental anomalies of the cerebral cortex in 7 of 13 physically healthy, well-diagnosed, relatively high-functioning men with autism. Scans of patients and control subjects were rated for the presence or absence of cortical anomalies by two neurologists experienced in MRI interpretation, who were unaware of subjects' diagnoses (control or patient). Five patients showed polymicrogyria (i.e., numerous small convolutions or microgyria), one had schizencephaly (i.e., abnormal clefts in brain substance) and macrogyria (i.e., large gyri), and one had macrogyria; in contrast, no control subjects were rated as having any abnormality. These anomalies found in the patients develop during the first 6 months of gestation, when neurons normally migrate to take their proper positions in the layered cortex. Figure 6.1 illustrates these findings.

Because the above-described malformations were not confined to any particular lobe and were detected with similar frequency in both the right and left hemispheres, they are unlikely to cause autistic behavior directly. Rather, by their common timing in development, they may be linked to an underlying mechanism etiologically related to autism. Piven et al. (1990) suggested that fetal anoxia, maternal cytomegalovirus infection, single gene defects, and other extrinsic and intrinsic factors may play a role in these anomalies.

Similar cortical anomalies were reported in two patients with Asperger's syndrome studied by Berthier et al. (1990). Both patients had histories of motor clumsiness; social isolation and peculiarities, including excessive shyness and obsessive or idiosyncratic interests; and average verbal IQs. One had aprosodic, monotonous speech. One patient showed a left middle frontal macrogyria and right temporo-occipital polymicrogyria; and one showed bilateral inferior frontal polymicrogyria with greater involvement on the left side.

Decreases in parietal lobe volume were reported in a sample of 21 patients with idiopathic autism, 6–32 years of age, by Courchesne et al. (1993). A neuroradiologist who was blind to diagnoses systematically evaluated a long list of brain structures on the scans of patients and control subjects. Of 21 patients, 9 (43%) were identified as having abnormal findings; no control subjects were so identified. All nine affected patients showed parietal lobes that were abnormal in appearance. Of these, seven patients had bilateral superior parietal cortical volume loss, as manifested in sulcal widening in seven patients, and this loss extended into adjacent superior frontal or occipital regions in four of the seven. Three patients showed white matter volume loss and thinning of the corpus callosum, especially along the posterior body. Possible origins for these findings include early disrupted development and late-onset progressive atrophy.

One behavioral correlate was impairment in the ability to shift attention. Although they were able to focus attention normally, patients with autism and parietal lobe abnormalities detected on MRIs showed significant deficits in their ability to shift attention accurately and rapidly, similar to those deficits seen in patients with acquired parietal lesions (Courchesne, Townsend, et al., 1994). Such a deficit may underlie the

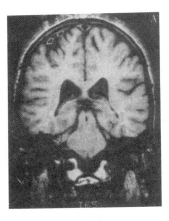
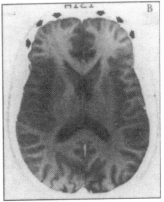
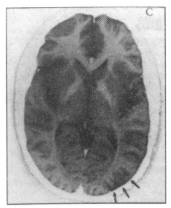
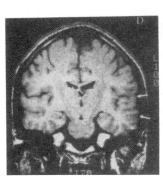
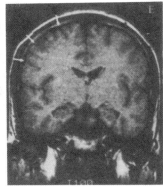
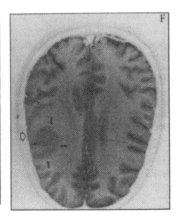
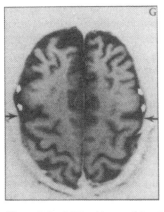

A. 19-year-old male; nonverbal IQ=116. T_1-weighted coronal image showing a right su-
    perior parietal polymicrogyria (open arrows).

B. 27-year-old male; nonverbal IQ=107. Inverted T_2-weighted axial image showing a
    bilateral frontopolar polymicrogyria (black arrows).

C. 35-year-old male; nonverbal IQ=67. Inverted T_2-weighted axial image showing a left
    parieto-occipital polymicrogyria (black arrows).

D. 22-year-old male; nonverbal IQ=95. T_1-weighted coronal image showing a left tem-
    poral polymicrogyria (white arrows). This subject also had left temporal-occipital and
    left-middle frontal polymicrogyria.

E. 21-year-old male; nonverbal IQ=65. T_1-weighted coronal image showing a right su-
    perior parietal polymicrogyria (white arrows).

F. 30-year-old male; nonverbal IQ$\leq$130. Inverted T_2-weighted axial image showing a left
    precentral macrogyria (open arrows) and a focal region of thickened cortex (black
    arrows).

G. 53-year-old male; nonverbal IQ$\leq$130. Inverted T_2-weighted axial image showing bi-
    lateral central parietal clefts (schizencephaly) (black arrows) and a wide postcentral
    gyrus (macrogyria) (open arrows).

Figure 6.1.   MRI evidence of developmental cortical malformations in seven patients with autism. (From Piven,
J., Berthier, M.L., Starkstein, S.E., Nehme, E., Pearlson, G., & Folstein, S. [1990]. Magnetic resonance imaging
evidence for a defect of cerebral cortical development in autism. *American Journal of Psychiatry, 147*, p. 737;
reprinted by permission.)

preference for repetitive, predictable, or invariant stimulation and activities seen in autism. Deficits in such a critical cognitive operation in infancy also might compromise
social, affective, and cognitive development through their adverse effects on joint social attention, that is, the coordination of attention between two individuals, such as a
mother and her child.

Heterotopic gray matter, along with other varied findings, also has been reported by Gaffney and Tsai (1987) in a clinical, qualitative study of 14 patients with autism. Other findings, which are in need of replication, include altered asymmetries of the volumes of the frontal lobes (Hashimoto et al., 1989) and small right lenticular nuclei relative to those of medical (rather than healthy) control subjects (Gaffney et al., 1989). The latter study involved some patients who experienced seizures or neurofibromatosis.

The investigation of posterior fossa structures in autism was prompted by Courchesne et al.'s (1988) report of cerebellar abnormalities in autism. After a case study revealed hypoplasia (i.e., incomplete development) of the neocerebellar portion of the vermis in a young man with autism (Courchesne et al., 1987), scans of 18 patients with idiopathic autism were compared with scans of 12 medical control subjects whose scans had been judged by two neuroradiologists to be normal. Lobules I–V, composing the anterior vermis, and lobules VI and VII, composing the neocerebellar, superior posterior vermis were measured. The result was the identification of a developmental hypoplasia of the neocerebellar portion of the vermis, lobules VI and VII, as illustrated in Figure 6.2.

Although previously the cerebellum was afforded a role only in motor function, recent work suggests a possible role for the cerebellum in learning and cognition (Leiner et al., 1986; Watson, 1978), which raises the possibility that neocerebellar maldevelopment may affect cognition negatively and directly (Courchesne et al., 1988). Alternatively, through its extensive connections with other brain regions, the maldevelopment of the neocerebellum may have an indirect impact on attention, cortical modulation, sensory modulation, autonomic regulation, and motor and behavioral initiation.

Cerebellar activity (especially that of vermian lobules VI and VII) modulates brain stem, thalamic, hippocampal, and cerebral cortical responses to visual, auditory, and somatosensory stimulation and may play a role in attention control analogous to the one it plays in motor control; that is, it may subserve effortless, accurate, and timely shifts in attention (Courchesne, Townsend, et al., 1994).

Courchesne et al. (1993) speculated that cerebellar abnormalities may even play a causal role in the development of parietal abnormalities. Citing Killackey's (1990) characterization of the cerebellum as a constituent of the "labeled line system" that is involved in the functional and structural development of the cerebral cortex, Courchesne et al. (1993) have hypothesized that a patchy loss of Purkinje cells in the cerebellar cortex and posterior vermian lobules may result in aberrant excitatory input to corresponding patches of cerebral cortex. Such abnormal input then may affect aberrant cortical specialization and development.

Despite these intriguing hypotheses, a number of nonreplicative studies of the above-described findings, which report normal midsagittal areas of the vermian lobules, including lobules VI–VII, have appeared in the literature (Ekman et al., 1991; Garber & Ritvo, 1992; Garber et al., 1989; Hashimoto, Murakawa, et al., 1992; Hashimoto, Tayama, Miyazaki, Murakawa, & Kuroda, 1992; Hashimoto et al., 1993; Holttum et al., 1992; Kleinman et al., 1992; Nowell et al., 1990). Because the fourth ventricle lies in front of the vermis, several investigators have measured this structure as well, and, in general, it has been normal in size (see Appendix B).

Piven et al. (1992) reported smaller cerebellar lobules VI–VII when they compared 15 high-functioning males with idiopathic autism with control subjects who were matched for age and parental socioeconomic status (SES) but not when they compared

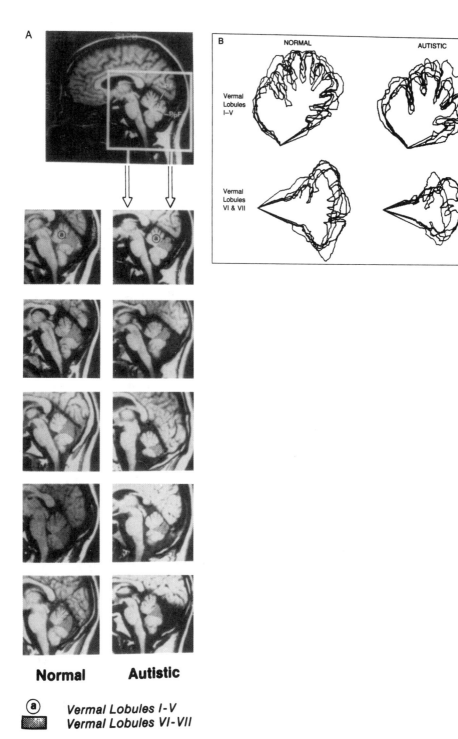

Normal **Autistic**

(a) *Vermal Lobules I-V*
/// *Vermal Lobules VI-VII*

Figure 6.2.   Magnetic resonance scans (A) and tracings (B) of the vermal lobules of five patients with autism who have vermal hypoplasia and of five control subjects. A) Midline sagittal views of the vermis. The patients have vermal hypoplasia, in that lobules VI and VII are smaller than those of control subjects; lobules I–V and lobule VIII are normal, except for a hypoplastic lobule VIII in the third scan from the bottom. PF = primary fissure; PpF = prepyramidal fissure. B) Superimposed outlines of the lobules of five patients and those of five control subjects (the same 10 subjects represented in A). Lobules VI and VII of the patients are appreciably smaller than are those of the control subjects; lobules I–V of both groups are similar in area. (From Courchesne, E., Yeung-Courchesne, R., Press, G.A., Hesselink, J.R., & Jernigan, T.L. [1988]. Hypoplasia of cerebellar vermal lobules VI and VII in autism. *New England Journal of Medicine, 318*, p. 1351; reprinted by permission.)

patients with autism with a contrast group matched for age and nonverbal IQ, which included four patients with mental retardation. The area of lobules I–V was larger in the patients with autism than in the age- and IQ-matched control subjects, but did not differ from that in the SES-matched control subjects. The midsagittal brain area in subjects with autism was larger than that in either control group, and this was found to have a significant effect on the area of the cerebellar lobules and fourth ventricle. To adjust for differences in brain size, the ratio of cerebellar lobules VI–VII to lobules I–V was examined and found to be significantly smaller in patients with autism relative to the SES-matched control subjects but not relative to the IQ-matched control group. It is significant that there was no a priori exclusion criterion for control subjects who had unusual or abnormal scan results, because that practice may artificially reduce normal variability. As a result, control group bias was avoided.

Patients with other developmental disorders, including fragile X syndrome, which has some association with autistic behavior (Reiss, Aylward, et al., 1991; Reiss, Freund, et al., 1991), also have been reported to show neocerebellar hypoplasia on midsagittal MRIs. This finding raises the possibility that neocerebellar hypoplasia may not be specific to autism and may be seen in a variety of developmental disorders, although the underlying etiologies and pathologies still may differ among these disorders.

Courchesne and colleagues (Courchesne, Saitoh, et al., 1994) enlarged their samples from 18 to 50 patients and from 12 to 53 control subjects. When the distributions of values for vermian lobules VI–VII were examined in these enlarged samples, values in the control subjects were distributed normally, whereas those in the patients with autism were not. Although the bulk of the distribution of patient values was shifted downward, some patients had unusually high values, indicating large lobules VI–VII. Courchesne, Saitoh, et al. (1994), therefore, reported two distinct subgroups of patients with autism — one contained 86% of the patients who had vermian hypoplasia, and the other contained 12% of the patients who had vermian hyperplasia. The subgroup with hypoplasia consisted of 43 patients with a mean midsagittal area for lobules VI–VII that was 16% smaller than was the mean in the control subjects. The subgroup with hyperplasia's mean midsagittal area for lobules VI–VII was 34% larger than was that of the control group.

No differences were seen among the two subgroups with autism and the control group in the size of the ventral pons, a brain stem structure and relay for the cerebrocerebellar pathway. The corpus callosum, a major cerebrocerebral pathway, however, was smaller than normal in the subgroup with hyperplasia. The wide age range studied (2–40 years of age) may complicate the latter finding, however, because age-related changes in the corpus callosum have been measured with MRI (Cowell et al., 1992; Pujol et al., 1993).

Although the etiological mechanisms that underlie hyperplasia are unclear, one possibility is a failure of regressive mechanisms. Normal development involves an initial phase of overgrowth and overproduction of neurons followed by subsequent cell death and synaptic pruning to eliminate excess neurons and neural connections (Cowan et al., 1984). Such events are thought to be regulated genetically. Thus, genetic defects that affect regressive events conceivably may result in hyperplasia. An excess of neurons or connections might interfere with normal brain function.

Extending findings of earlier studies on the cerebellum, Murakami et al. (1989) reported smaller cerebellar hemispheres in a subsample of the group studied by Courchesne et al. (1988), thereby indicating more widespread involvement of the cerebellum, which is compatible with autopsy findings of reduced Purkinje cell counts in both the hemispheres and vermis of the cerebellum (Bauman & Kemper, 1985; Ritvo et al., 1986). Murakami et al. (1989) also reported a moderate correlation between the area measurement of vermian lobules VI–VII and the cumulative slice measurement of the cerebellar hemispheres in the patient group in contrast with a low correlation in control subjects. The latter finding must be interpreted cautiously given the small sample sizes and the tendency for correlations to be unreliable in small samples.

Some investigators have reported smaller brain stems in individuals with autism (Hashimoto, Murakawa, et al., 1992; Hashimoto, Tayama, Miyazaki, Murakawa, & Kuroda, 1992; Hashimoto et al., 1993; Hashimoto, Tayama, Miyazaki, Sakurama, et al., 1992), whereas others have found that brain stem structures (i.e., pons, midbrain) are of normal size (Courchesne, Saitoh, et al., 1994; Ekman et al., 1991; Hsu et al., 1991; Piven et al., 1992).

In summary, a good number of anatomical MRI studies of autism, most involving small samples and limited statistical power, have been published. Relatively few studies have the strength of comparing patients to truly normal control subjects (i.e., control subjects diagnosed as normal on the basis of some a priori evaluation). Given the number of cerebellar studies published, it is surprising that so little attention has been given to the cerebellar hemispheres, particularly in light of autopsy findings that implicate the hemispheres. Quantitative findings with respect to the cerebellum seem to be influenced significantly by the nature of the control groups.

The cerebral cortical findings, which are more qualitative in nature, are intriguing, albeit heterogeneous. This heterogeneity is consistent with the view that autism is a syndrome with multiple etiologies and diverse behavioral symptoms. It may be that separate syndromes, such as those included in DSM-IV or other, as of yet unidentified, syndromes, may be found to be associated with diverse findings in the future.

CONCLUSIONS AND FUTURE DIRECTIONS

PET and SPECT studies of glucose metabolism and blood flow have failed to reveal consistent global or regional abnormalities in autism, although correlational approaches and activation studies appear to hold promise. New work in labeling brain receptors with the use of these techniques also is of great interest. Anatomical MRI studies suggest some intriguing findings, for example, increased brain size (i.e., macrocephaly), cortical anomalies (not seen in the few cases autopsied), and alterations of cerebellar size (still in need of independent replication when this book went to press). The low consistency of the findings likely reflects heterogeneity in the patient samples studied, the presence of comorbid disorders, important differences in control groups, the subtlety of brain-related abnormalities in autism, and numerous methodological differences.

Despite autopsy studies that suggested limbic pathology, neuroimaging studies have left limbic structures and circuits relatively unexplored. It is hoped that future studies will examine these structures carefully in autism.

The heterogeneity seen in clinical courses and symptoms may contribute to inconsistent findings. New diagnostic criteria designed to subdivide the pervasive developmental disorders may reduce some of the heterogeneity seen in neuroimaging studies.

The heterogeneity seen across levels of analysis—behavioral, neuropsychological, anatomical, and physiological—suggests that attempts to link these different levels of analysis may prove to be a fruitful strategy. Although the core behavioral impairments are thought to be social in nature, additional refinement and reduction of this construct is needed to attempt to relate it to underlying biology. The core neuropsychological deficits that underlie the social behavioral impairments remain poorly understood and require definition and refinement. Promising candidates for core deficits include the ability to disengage and shift attention, which may underlie deficits in joint social attention, thereby linking attentional and social dysfunctions. It is encouraging to see attempts to link such deficits to anatomical and physiological findings (Courchesne, Townsend, et al., 1994; Minshew et al., 1993). Functional neuroimaging studies could further explore the anatomical localization of circuits involved in such operations.

Neuroimaging technologies, both anatomical and physiological, continue to advance at a truly remarkable pace and hold promise for advancing our understanding of autism. Attempts to link biology and behavior in autism will require sophistication both in the application of evolving imaging modalities and in the refinement of behavioral constructs—diagnostic, social-behavioral, and neuropsychological.

REFERENCES

American Psychiatric Association. (1980). *Diagnostic and statistical manual of mental disorders* (3rd ed.). Washington, DC: Author.

American Psychiatric Association. (1987). *Diagnostic and statistical manual of mental disorders* (3rd ed., Rev.). Washington, DC: Author.

American Psychiatric Association. (1994). *Diagnostic and statistical manual of mental disorders* (4th ed.). Washington, DC: Author.

Asperger, H. (1991). "Autistic psychopathy" in childhood. In U. Frith (Ed. and Trans.), *Autism and Asperger syndrome* (pp. 37–92). Cambridge, England: Cambridge University Press.

Bauman, M.L. (1991). Microscopic neuroanatomic abnormalities in autism. *Pediatrics, 87*(Suppl.), 791–796.

Bauman, M.L., & Kemper, T.L. (1985). Histoanatomic observations of the brain in early infantile autism. *Neurology, 35,* 866–874.

Baxter, L.R., Mazziotta, J.C., Phelps, M.E., Selin, C.J., Guze, B.H., & Fairbanks, L. (1987). Cerebral glucose metabolic rates in normal human females versus normal males. *Psychiatry Research, 21,* 237–245.

Bender, L. (1955). Twenty years of clinical research on schizophrenic children, with special reference to those under six years of age. In G. Caplan (Ed.), *Emotional problems of early childhood* (pp. 503–515). New York: Basic Books.

Berthier, M.L., Starkstein, S.E., & Leiguarda, R. (1990). Developmental cortical anomalies in Asperger's syndrome: Neuroradiological findings in two patients. *Journal of Neuropsychiatry, 2,* 197–201.

Buchsbaum, M.S., Siegel, B.V., Jr., Wu, J.C., Hazlett, E., Sicotte, N., & Haier, R. (1992). Brief report: Attention performance in autism and regional brain metabolic rate assessed by positron emission tomography. *Journal of Autism and Developmental Disorders, 22,* 115–125.

Chess, S., Korn, S.J., & Fernandez, P.B. (1971). *Psychiatric disorders of children with congenital rubella.* New York: Brunner/Mazel.

Chugani, H.T., Phelps, M.E., & Mazziotta, J.C. (1987). Positron emission tomography study of human brain functional development. *Annals of Neurology, 22,* 487–497.

Coleman, P.D., Romano, J., Lapham, L., & Simon, W. (1985). Cell counts in the cerebral cortex of an autistic patient. *Journal of Autism and Developmental Disorders, 15,* 245–255.

Courchesne, E., Hesselink, J.R., Jernigan, T.L., & Yeung-Courchesne, R. (1987). Abnormal neuroanatomy in a nonretarded person with autism: Unusual findings with magnetic resonance imaging. *Archives of Neurology, 44,* 335–341.

Courchesne, E., Press, G.A., & Yeung-Courchesne, R. (1993). Parietal lobe abnormalities detected with MR in patients with infantile autism. *American Journal of Roentgenology, 160,* 387–393.

Courchesne, E., Saitoh, O., Yeung-Courchesne, R., Press, G.A., Lincoln, A.J., Haas, R.H., & Schreibman, L. (1994). Abnormality of cerebellar vermian lobules VI and VII in patients with infantile autism: Identification of hypoplastic and hyperplastic subgroups with MR imaging. *American Journal of Roentgenology, 162*, 123–130.

Courchesne, E., Townsend, J.P., Akshoomoff, N.A., Yeung-Courchesne, R., Press, G.A., Murakami, J.W., Lincoln, A.J., James, H.E., Saitoh, O., Egaas, B., Haas, R.H., & Schreibman, L. (1994). A new finding: Impairment in shifting attention in autistic and cerebellar patients. In S.H. Broman & J. Grafman (Eds.), *Atypical cognitive deficits in developmental disorders: Implications for brain function* (pp. 101–137). Hillsdale, NJ: Lawrence Erlbaum Associates.

Courchesne, E., Yeung-Courchesne, R., Press, G.A., Hesselink, J.R., & Jernigan, T.L. (1988). Hypoplasia of cerebellar vermal lobules VI and VII in autism. *New England Journal of Medicine, 318*, 1349–1354.

Cowan, W.M., Fawcett, J.W., O'Leary, D.D.M., & Stanfield, B.B. (1984). Regressive events in neurogenesis. *Science, 225*, 1258–1265.

Cowell, P.E., Allen, L.S., Zalatimo, N.S., & Denenberg, V.H. (1992). A developmental study of sex and age interactions in the human corpus callosum. *Developmental Brain Research, 66*, 187–192.

DeMyer, M.K., Barton, S., DeMyer, W.E., Norton, J.A., Allen, J., & Steele, R. (1973). Prognosis in autism: A follow-up study. *Journal of Autism and Developmental Disorders, 3*, 199–246.

DeVolder, A., Bol, A., Michel, C., Congneau, M., & Goffinet, A.M. (1987). Brain glucose metabolism in children with the autistic syndrome: Positron tomography analysis. *Brain Development, 9*, 581–587.

Deykin, E.Y., & MacMahon, B. (1979). The incidence of seizures among children with autistic symptoms. *American Journal of Psychiatry, 136*, 1310–1312.

Ekman, G., DeChateau, P., Marions, O., Sellden, H., Wahlung, L.O., & Wetterberg, L. (1991). Low field magnetic resonance imaging of the central nervous system in 15 children with autistic disorder. *Acta Paediatrica Scandinavica, 80*, 243–247.

Folstein, S.E., & Piven, J. (1991). Etiology of autism: Genetic influences. *Pediatrics, 87*(Suppl.), 767–773.

Gaffney, G.R., Kuperman, S., Tsai, L.Y., & Minchin, S. (1989). Forebrain structure in infantile autism. *Journal of the American Academy of Child and Adolescent Psychiatry, 28*, 534–537.

Gaffney, G.R., Kuperman, S., Tsai, L.Y., Minchin, S., & Hassanein, K.M. (1987). Midsagittal magnetic resonance imaging of autism. *British Journal of Psychiatry, 151*, 831–833.

Gaffney, G.R., & Tsai, L.Y. (1987). Brief report: Magnetic resonance imaging of high level autism. *Journal of Autism and Developmental Disorders, 17*, 433–438.

Gaillard, W.D., Zeffiro, T., Fazilat, S., Reeves, P., & Theodore, W.H. (1996). Valproate's effect on cerebral metabolism and blood flow: An [18]FDG and [15]O water PET study. *Epilepsia*.

Garber, H.J., & Ritvo, E.R. (1992). Magnetic resonance imaging of the posterior fossa in autistic adults. *American Journal of Psychiatry, 149*, 245–247.

Garber, H.J., Ritvo, E.R., Chiu, L.C., Griswold, V.J., Kashanian, A., Freeman, B.J., & Oldendorf, W.H. (1989). A magnetic resonance imaging study of autism: Normal fourth ventricle size and absence of pathology. *American Journal of Psychiatry, 146*, 532–534.

George, M., Costa, D., Kouris, K., Ring, H., & Ell, R. (1992). Cerebral blood flow abnormalities in adults with infantile autism. *Journal of Nervous and Mental Disease, 180*, 413–417.

Giedd, J.N., Snell, J.W., Lange, N., Rajapakse, J.C., Kaysen, D., Vaituzis, C., Vauss, Y.C., Hamburger, S.D., Kozuch, P., & Rapoport, J.L. (1996). Quantitative magnetic resonance imaging of human brain development: Ages 4–18. *Cerebral Cortex*.

Goldfarb, W. (1964). An investigation of childhood schizophrenia. *Archives of General Psychiatry, 11*, 620–634.

Green, W.H., Campbell, M., Hardesty, A.S., Grega, D.M., Padron-Gayol, M., Shell, J., & Erlenmeyer-Kimling, L. (1984). A comparison of schizophrenic and autistic children. *Journal of the American Academy of Child Psychiatry, 23*, 399–409.

Gur, R.C., Gur, R.E., Obrist, W.D., Hungerbuhler, J.P., Younkin, D., Rosen, A.D., Skolnick B.E., & Reivich, M. (1982). Sex and handedness differences in cerebral blood flow during rest and cognitive activity. *Science, 217*, 659–661.

Hashimoto, T., Murakawa, K., Miyazaki, M., Tayama, M., & Kuroda, Y. (1992). Magnetic resonance imaging of the brain structures in the posterior fossa in retarded autistic children. *Acta Paediatrica, 81*, 1030–1034.

Hashimoto, T., Tayama, M., Miyazaki, M., Murakawa, K., & Kuroda, Y. (1992). Brainstem and cerebellar vermis involvement in autistic children. *Journal of Child Neurology, 7*, 149–153.

Hashimoto, T., Tayama, M., Miyazaki, M., Murakawa, K., Shimakawa, S., Yoneda, Y., & Kuroda, Y.Y. (1993). Brainstem involvement in high functioning autistic children. *Acta Neurologica Scandinavica, 88*, 123–128.

Hashimoto, T., Tayama, M., Miyazaki, M., Sakurama, N., Yoshimoto, T., Murakawa, K., & Kuroda, Y. (1992). Reduced brainstem size in children with autism. *Brain Development, 14*, 94–97.

Hashimoto, T., Tayama, M., Mori, K., Fujino, K., Miyazaki, M., & Kuroda, Y. (1989). Magnetic resonance imaging in autism: Preliminary report. *Neuropediatrics, 20*, 142–146.

Heh, C., Smith, R., Wu, J., Hazlett, E., Russell, A., Asarnow, R., Tanguay, P., & Buchsbaum, M. (1989). Positron emission tomography of the cerebellum in autism. *American Journal of Psychiatry, 146*, 242–245.

Heller, T. (1908). Uber dementia infantilis: Verblodungsprozess im kindesalter. *Zeitschrift fur die Erforschung und Behandlung jugendlichen Schwachsinns, 2*, 17–28.

Herold, S., Frackowiak, R.S.J., LeCouteau, A., Rutter, M., & Howlin, P. (1988). Cerebral blood flow and metabolism of oxygen and glucose in young autistic adults. *Psychological Medicine, 18*, 823–831.

Holttum, J.R., Minshew, N.J., Sanders, R.S., & Phillips, N.E. (1992). Magnetic resonance imaging of the posterior fossa in autism. *Biological Psychiatry, 32*, 1091–1101.

Horwitz, B., Rumsey, J., Grady, C., & Rapoport, S.I. (1988). The cerebral metabolic landscape in autism: Intercorrelations of regional glucose utilization. *Archives of Neurology, 45*, 749–755.

Hsu, M., Yeung-Courchesne, R., Courchesne, E., & Press, G.A. (1991). Absence of magnetic resonance imaging evidence of pontine abnormality in infantile autism. *Archives of Neurology, 48*, 1160–1163.

Kanner, L. (1943). Autistic disturbances of affective contact. *Nervous Child, 2*, 217–250.

Killackey, H.P. (1990). Neocortical expansion: An attempt toward relating phylogeny and ontogeny. *Journal of Cognitive Neuroscience, 2*, 1–17.

Kleinman, M.D., Neff, S., & Rosman, N.P. (1992). The brain in infantile autism: Are posterior fossa structures abnormal? *Neurology, 42*, 753–760.

Kolvin, I. (1971). Studies in the childhood psychoses. I. Diagnostic criteria and classification. *British Journal of Psychiatry, 118*, 381–384.

Kolvin, I., Ounsted, C., Humphrey, M., & McNay, A. (1971). Studies in the childhood psychoses. II. The phenomenology of childhood psychoses. *British Journal of Psychiatry, 118*, 385–395.

LeCouteur, A., Rutter, M., Lord, C., Rios, P., Robertson, S., Holdgrafer, M., & McLennan, J. (1989). Autism Diagnostic Interview: A standardized investigator-based instrument. *Journal of Autism and Developmental Disorders, 19*, 363–387.

Leiner, H.C., Leiner, A.L., & Dow, R.S. (1986). Does the cerebellum contribute to mental skills? *Behavioral Neuroscience, 100*, 443–454.

Lord, C., Rutter, M., & LeCouteur, A. (1994). Autism Diagnostic Interview–Revised: A revised version of a diagnostic interview for caregivers of individuals with possible pervasive developmental disorders. *Journal of Autism and Developmental Disorders, 24*, 659–685.

Lord, C., Pickles, A., McLennan, J., Rutter, M., Bregman, J., Folstein, S., Fombonne, E., Leboyer, S., & Minshew, N. (1995). Diagnosing autism: Analysis of data from the Autism Diagnostic Interview. Unpublished data.

Mesulam, M.M. (1985). Attention, confusional states, and neglect. In M.M. Mesulam (Ed.), *Principles of behavioral neurology* (pp. 125–168). Philadelphia: F.A. Davis Company.

Mesulam, M.M. (1986). Frontal cortex and behavior. *Annals of Neurology, 19*, 320–325.

Minshew, N.J., & Dombrowski, B.S. (1994). In vivo neuroanatomy of autism: Neuroimaging studies. In M. Bauman & T. Kemper (Eds.), *The neurobiology of autism*. Baltimore: The Johns Hopkins University Press.

Minshew, N.J., Goldstein, G., Dombrowski, S.M., Panchalingam, K., & Pettegrew, J.W. (1993). A preliminary ^{31}P MRS study of autism: Evidence for undersynthesis and increased degradation of brain membranes. *Biological Psychiatry, 33*, 762–773.

Murakami, J.W., Courchesne, E., Press, G.A., Yeung-Courchesne, R., & Hesselink, J.R. (1989). Reduced cerebellar hemisphere size and its relationship to vermal hypoplasia in autism. *Archives of Neurology, 46*, 689–694.

Nowell, M.A., Hackney, D.B., Muraki, A.S., & Coleman, M. (1990). Varied MR appearance of autism: Fifty-three pediatric patients having the full autistic syndrome. *Magnetic Resonance Imaging, 8*, 811–816.

Ozbayrak, K., Kapucu, O., Erdem, E., & Aras, T. (1991). Left occipital hypoperfusion in a case with the Asperger syndrome. *Brain Development, 13*, 454–456.

Piven, J., Berthier, M.L., Starkstein, S.E., Nehme, E., Pearlson, G., & Folstein, S. (1990). Magnetic resonance imaging evidence for a defect of cerebral cortical development in autism. *American Journal of Psychiatry, 147*, 734–739.

Piven, J., Nehme, E., Simon, J., Barta, P., Pearlson, G., & Folstein, S. (1992). Magnetic resonance imaging in autism: Measurement of the cerebellum, pons, and fourth ventricle. *Biological Psychiatry, 31*, 491–504.

Pujol, J., Vendrell, P., Junqué, C., Martí-Vilalta, J.L., & Capdevila, A. (1993). When does human brain development end?: Evidence of corpus callosum growth up to adulthood. *Annals of Neurology, 34*, 71–75.

Raymond, G., Bauman, M., & Kemper, T. (1989). The hippocampus in autism: Golgi analysis. *Annals of Neurology, 26*, 483–484.

Reiser, D.E. (1963). Psychosis of infancy and early childhood, as manifested by children with atypical development. *New England Journal of Medicine, 269*, 790–798, 844–850.

Reiss, A.L., Aylward, E., Freund, L.S., Bujan, N., & Joshi, P. (1991). Neuroanatomy of fragile X syndrome: The posterior fossa. *Annals of Neurology, 29*, 26–32.

Reiss, A.L., Freund, L., Tseng, J.E., & Joshi, P. (1991). Neuroanatomy in fragile X females: The posterior fossa. *American Journal of Human Genetics, 49*, 279–288.

Ritvo, E.R., Freeman, B.J., Scheibel, A.B., Duong, P.T., Robinson, H., Guthrie, D., & Ritvo, A. (1986). Lower Purkinje cell counts in the cerebella of four autistic subjects: Initial findings of the UCLA–NSAC autopsy research project. *American Journal of Psychiatry, 13*, 862–866.

Rodrigues, G., Warkentin, S., Risberg, J., & Rosadini, G. (1988). Sex differences in regional cerebral blood flow. *Journal of Cerebral Blood Flow and Metabolism, 8*, 783–789.

Rumsey, J.M. (1992). Neuropsychological studies of high-level autism. In E. Schopler & G. Mesibov (Eds.), *High-functioning individuals with autism* (pp. 41–64). New York: Plenum Press.

Rumsey, J.M., Duara, R., Grady, C., Rapoport, J.L., Margolin, R.A., Rapoport, S.I., & Cutler, N.R. (1985). Brain metabolism in autism: Resting cerebral glucose utilization rates as measured with positron emission tomography. *Archives of General Psychiatry, 42*, 448–455.

Rumsey, J.M., & Hamburger, S. (1988). Neuropsychological findings in high-functioning men with infantile autism, residual state. *Journal of Clinical and Experimental Neuropsychology, 10*, 201–221.

Rutter, M. (1970). Autistic children: Infancy to adulthood. *Seminars in Psychiatry, 2*, 435–450.

Rutter, M. (1983). Cognitive deficits in the pathogenesis of autism. *Journal of Child Psychology and Psychiatry, 24*, 513–531.

Siegel, B.V., Jr., Asarnow, R., Tanguay, P., Call, J.D., Abel, L., Ho, A., Lott, I., & Buchsbaum, M.S. (1992). Regional cerebral glucose metabolism and attention in adults with a history of childhood autism. *The Journal of Neuropsychiatry and Clinical Neurosciences, 4*, 406–414.

Tager-Flusberg, H.B. (1981). On the nature of linguistic functioning in early infantile autism. *Journal of Autism and Developmental Disorders, 11*, 45–56.

Theodore, W.H., Bairamian, D., Newmark, M.E., Fishbein, D., Porter, R.J., DiChiro, G., Deitz, M., Baldwin, P., Margolin, R., Brooks, R., & Jacobs, G. (1989). The effect of antiepileptic drugs on cerebral glucose metabolism. *Advances in Epileptology, 17*, 139–141.

Volkmar, F., Klin, A., Siegel, B., Szatmari, P., Lord, C., Campbell, M., Freeman, B.J., Cicchetti, D.V., Rutter, M., Kline, W., Buitelaar, J., Hattab, Y., Fombonne, E., Fuentes, J., Werry, J., Stone, W., Kerbeshian, J., Hoshino, Y., Bregman, J., Loveland, K., Szymanski, L., & Towbin, K. (1994). Field trial for autistic disorder in DSM-IV. *American Journal of Psychiatry, 151*, 1361–1367.

Volkmar, F.R., & Nelson, D.S. (1990). Seizure disorders in autism. *Journal of the American Academy of Child and Adolescent Psychiatry, 29*, 127–129.

Watson, P.J. (1978). Nonmotor functions of the cerebellum. *Psychological Bulletin, 85*, 944–967.

Wing, L. (1992). Manifestations of social problems in high-functioning autistic people. In E. Schopler & G. Mesibov (Eds.), *High-functioning individuals with autism* (pp. 129–142). New York: Plenum Press.

Yoshii, F., Barker, W.W., Chang, J.Y., Loewenstein, D., Apicella, A., Smith, D., Boothe, T., Ginsberg, M.D., Pascal, S., & Duara, R. (1988). Sensitivity of cerebral glucose metabolism to age, gender, brain volume, brain atrophy and cerebral risk factors. *Journal of Cerebral Blood Flow and Metabolism, 8*, 654–661.

Zilbovicius, M., Garreau, B., Tzourio, N., Mazoyer, B., Bruck, B., Martinot, J., Raynaud, C., Samson, Y., Syrota, A., & Lelord, G. (1992). Regional cerebral blood flow in childhood autism: A SPECT study. *American Journal of Psychiatry, 149*, 924–930.

A

Functional Neuroimaging Studies

Functional neuroimaging studies

Investigators	Autistic patients (number, gender, criteria, ages, etc.)	Control subjects	Findings
PET studies			
Buchsbaum et al. (1992)	Seven patients (five males, two females); Semistructured Interview for Childhood Disorders and Schizophrenia; range, 19–36 years (mean, 23 years); full scale IQ of at least 70 (same subjects as Heh et al., 1989)	Thirteen males (mean age, 24 years)	Few differences in glucose metabolism during a visual vigilance task Less glucose metabolism asymmetry in patients than in control subjects Decreased metabolism in right putamen and right thalamus in patients
DeVolder et al. (1987)	Eighteen patients; DSM-III; range, 2–18 years	Fifteen adults, six children; three with unilateral brain pathology	More variable glucose metabolic rates and regional patterns (posterior to prefrontal ratio) in patients but no mean differences at rest
Heh et al. (1989)	Seven patients (five males, two females); Semistructured Interview for Childhood Disorders and Schizophrenia; range, 19–36 years (mean, 23 years)	Eight age-matched control subjects (seven males, one female), age range, 30–35 years (mean age, 24 years)	Normal glucose metabolism on a single slice through the cerebellum during a visual vigilance task
Herold et al. (1988)	Eight males; DSM-III-R; range, 21–25 years (mean, 22 years); mild retardation to normal intelligence; one patient with epilepsy; one patient with cortical atrophy on CT	Eight healthy normal control subjects (six males, two females), age range, 22–53 years (mean age, 33 years)	Normal glucose and oxygen metabolism and normal blow flow on a single slice through the basal ganglia and temporal gray matter while listening to music of choice

(*continued*)

Investigators	Autistic patients (number, gender, criteria, ages, etc.)	Control subjects	Findings
PET studies (*continued*)			
Horwitz et al. (1988)	Fourteen males; DSM-III; range, 18–39 years (mean, 27 years); most with verbal and performance IQs of greater than 80 (10 subjects from study by Rumsey et al., 1985)	Fourteen healthy, age- and gender-matched, normal control subjects	Correlations of glucose metabolic rates within and between frontal and parietal lobes and between these regions and subcortical regions were reduced in patients relative to control subjects
Rumsey et al. (1985)	Ten males; DSM-III; range, 18–36 years (mean, 26 years); seven with verbal and performance IQs of 82–126; all with normal CTs	Fifteen healthy, age- and gender-matched, normal control subjects	Diffusely elevated glucose metabolism in a resting, sensory-restricted state
Siegel et al. (1992)	Sixteen patients (12 males, four females); DSM-III; range, 18–38 years (mean, 23 years); full-scale IQs of 74–135 (mean, 90); two with comorbid schizophrenia	Twenty-six normal healthy control subjects (19 males, seven females), mean age, 27 years	Few differences in glucose metabolism during visual vigilance task Normal global metabolism Reversed asymmetry (left greater than right) in anterior rectal gyrus Low metabolism in the left putamen and high metabolism in the posterior calcarine cortex
SPECT studies			
George et al. (1992)	Four males; DSM-III; range, 22–34 years (mean, 28 years); three patients receiving anticonvulsant medication; all patients with normal CTs and minimal verbal skills	Four healthy, age-matched control subjects (two males, two females)	Global hypoperfusion with the greatest local hypoperfusion in the right lateral temporal and right, left, and midfrontal lobes during rest with eyes open in a quiet, darkened room
Ozbayrak et al. (1991)	One 22-year-old male; Asperger's syndrome, cyanotic at birth; paranoid psychotic episode at	None (clinical case study)	Left occipital hypoperfusion, including parts of the parietal and superior temporal regions

(continued)

Investigators	Autistic patients (number, gender, criteria, ages, etc.)	Control subjects	Findings
SPECT studies (*continued*)			
Ozbayrak et al. (1991) (*continued*)	age 15; receiving electroconvulsive therapy and neuroleptics; tardive dyskinesia; verbal IQ of 90 and performance IQ of 61; normal CT and MRI		
Zilbovicius et al. (1992)	Twenty-one patients (12 males, nine females); DSM-III-R; range, 5–11 years (mean, 7.5 years); nonverbal IQs of 10–75 (mean, 36); patients studied after premedication	Fourteen control subjects (10 males, four females) with developmental language disorder, mean age, 8.7 years, nonverbal IQs of 80–125 (mean, 96), patients studied at rest without premedication	Normal global and regional cortical blood flow at rest
MRS studies			
Minshew et al. (1993)	Eleven males; DSM-III-R and Autism Diagnostic Interview; range, 12–36 years; high-functioning (IQs of greater than 70) adolescents and adults	Eleven age-, gender-, IQ-, race-, and SES-matched, normal healthy control subjects	In the dorsal prefrontal cortex, decreased levels of phosphocreatinine and esterified ends of α-ATP with normal levels of phosphomonoester and phosphodiester and normal intracellular pH levels, suggesting increased use of phosphocreatinine to maintain ATP levels (hypermetabolic state) Abnormalities correlated with perseveration on the Wisconsin Card Sorting Test and with scores on language tests

B

MRI Neuroanatomical Studies

MRI studies

Investigators	Autistic patients (number, gender, criteria, ages, etc.)	Control subjects	Findings
Forebrain			
Berthier et al. (1990)	Two patients with Asperger's syndrome; may not meet DSM-IV criteria; 17 years; both with delayed language development	None (clinical case studies)	Left frontal macrogyria and right temporoparietal polymicrogyria in one patient Bilateral frontal opercular polymicrogyria in one patient
Courchesne et al. (1993)	Twenty-one patients; DSM-III; range, 6–32 years; 18 patients from previous study of the cerebellar vermis	Twelve medical control subjects with normal scans; 23 nonautistic patients with varied brain abnormalities; 17 nonautistic patients with nonspecific MRI finding	Nine patients (43%) with abnormal parietal lobe findings Seven patients with parietal volume loss, extending to the adjacent superior or occipital lobes in four of the seven Two patients with thinning of the corpus callosum Normal frontal and temporal lobes; limbic structures; basal ganglia; diencephalons and brain stems; and lateral, third, and fourth ventricles
Gaffney et al. (1989)	Thirteen patients (10 males, three females); DSM-III; range, 4–19 years; IQs of 65–139 (mean, 85); two patients with seizures; one patient with neurofibromatosis	Thirty-three age-matched medical control subjects (18 males, 15 females) with normal scans (two subjects with seizures, one subject with neurofibromatosis	Smaller right lenticular nuclei Enlarged frontal horns and body of lateral ventricles Normal basal ganglia, thalami, and cortices

(continued)

Investigators	Autistic patients (number, gender, criteria, ages, etc.)	Control subjects	Findings
Forebrain *(continued)*			
Hashimoto et al. (1989)	Eighteen patients (15 males, three females); DSM-III; range, 2–9 years (mean, 3.8 years); IQs of 38–121 (mean, 66)	Eleven subjects with mental retardation, age range, 2–4 years (mean age, 2.8 years); 18 medical control subjects (7 males, 11 females), age range, 2–11 years (mean age, 7.1 years)	Altered symmetry of frontal lobe volume in both patients with autism and those with mental retardation (more severe in autism)
Piven et al. (1990)	Thirteen males; DSM-III-R and Autism Diagnostic Interview; range, 19–53 years; nonverbal IQs of 65–130	Thirteen age- and IQ-matched control subjects (10 employees, three psychiatric patients)	Seven patients (54%) with developmental cortical anomalies; five with polymicrogyria, one with schizencephaly, and one with macrogyria
Posterior fossa			
Courchesne et al. (1987)	One male; DSM-III; 21 years; nonverbal IQ of 112; healthy; dysprosodic speech	None	Hypoplasia of declive, folium, and tuber in the posterior vermis, and hypoplasia of only medial aspect of each cerebellar hemisphere Pathological changes in the right posterior cerebral hemisphere: enlarged right posterior horn of the lateral ventricle, right posterior cerebral hemisphere larger than left, and slight increase in sulcal width in right parieto-occipital cortex
Courchesne et al. (1988)	Eighteen patients (16 males, two females); DSM-III; range, 6-30 years; verbal IQs of 45–111 (mean, 77) and performance IQs of 70–112 (mean, 88)	Twelve medical control subjects (nine males, three females) with normal scans, age range, 9–37 years (mean age, 24 years)	Hypoplasia of neocerebellar lobules VI and VII

(continued)

Investigators	Autistic patients (number, gender, criteria, ages, etc.)	Control subjects	Findings
Posterior fossa (_continued_)			
Courchesne, Saitoh, et al. (1994)	Fifty patients (41 males, nine females); DSM-III; range, 2–40 years (18 patients from previous study, 32 new patients)	Fifty-three control subjects (43 males, four females), age range, 3–37 years, 41 new subjects	New sample replicated difference in vermal lobules VI–VII but not lobules I–V Two subgroups: 43 individuals (86%) with hypoplasia of vermian lobules VI–VII; 12% with hyperplasia of lobules VI–VII and I–V Both subgroups with normal midsagittal area of the pons Only hyperplasia subgroup with smaller corpora callosa
Garber et al. (1989)	Twelve patients (nine males, three females); DSM-III; range, 18–38 years (mean, 27 years)	Twelve age-matched control subjects (eight males, four females)	Normal midsagittal areas of the cerebrum, pons, fourth ventricle, cerebellar vermis, and lobules I–V and VI–VII and normal ratio
Garber and Ritvo (1992)	Twelve patients (nine males, three females); DSM-III; range, 18–38 years	Twelve age-matched control subjects (eight males, four females)	Normal midsagittal areas of the pons, fourth ventricle, cerebellar vermis, and lobules I–V and VI–VII and normal ratio
Hashimoto, Murakawa, et al. (1992)	Twelve patients (eight males, four females); DSM-III-R and Kanner's criteria; range, 5–10 years (mean, 6.6 years); IQs of 33–73 (mean, 49)	Fifteen control subjects with idiopathic mental retardation, age range, 5–10 years (mean age, 7.7 years), IQs of 42–78 (mean IQ, 60). Medical control subjects	Smaller brain stems (midbrain, medulla) in both those with autism and those with mental retardation Normal midsagittal areas for cerebellar vermian lobules I–V, VI–VII, and VIII–X in both those with autism and those with mental retardation

(_continued_)

Investigators	Autistic patients (number, gender, criteria, ages, etc.)	Control subjects	Findings

Posterior fossa
(*continued*)

Hashimoto, Tayama, Miyazaki, Murakawa, and Kuroda (1992)	Twenty-one patients (15 males, six females); DSM-III-R and Kanner's criteria; range, 2–7 years (mean, 4.3 years); developmental quotients or IQs of 20–129 (mean, 64)	Twenty-one medical control subjects, age range, 2–7 years (mean age, 3.9 years), IQs of 94–123 (mean IQ, 108)	Smaller brain stems (midbrain, pons, medulla) Smaller cerebellar vermian lobules VIII–X Normal cerebellar lobules I–V and VI–VII
Hashimoto, Tayama, Miyazaki, Sakurama, et al. (1992)	Twenty-nine patients (27 males, two females); DSM-III-R and Kanner's criteria; range, 2–7 years (mean, 4.9 years); 10 with developmental quotients or IQs of 80–129; 10 with developmental quotients or IQs of 21–76	Fifteen age- and gender-matched medical control subjects	Smaller brain stem width, especially in the low developmental quotient/IQ group
Hashimoto et al. (1993)	Twelve patients (11 males, one female); DSM-III-R and Kanner's criteria; range, 2–12 years (mean, 6 years); developmental quotients or IQs of greater than 80	Twenty-four age- and gender-matched medical control subjects (21 males, three females)	Smaller midbrain and medulla Normal pons and vermian lobules I–V, VI–VII, and VIII–X Positive correlation between age and vermian size in autistic patients but not in control subjects
Holttum et al. (1992)	Eighteen males; DSM-III-R and Autism Diagnostic Interview; range, 12–41 years (mean, 20 years); full scale and verbal IQs of greater than 70	Eighteen normal, age-, gender-, IQ-, race-, and SES-matched control subjects (mean age, 20 years)	Normal midsagittal areas of the cerebellar vermis and vermian lobules I–V, VI–VII, and VIII–X Normal fourth ventricle area
Hsu et al. (1991)	Thirty-four patients (27 males, 7 females); range, 2–39 years (mean, 18.9 years); 11 with mental retardation	Forty-four control subjects (40 males, four females), age range, 3–39 years (mean age, 19.8 years); 34 healthy and normal control subjects and nine medical control subjects with normal scans	Normal pons and midbrain

(*continued*)

Investigators	Autistic patients (number, gender, criteria, ages, etc.)	Control subjects	Findings
Posterior fossa (*continued*)			
Kleinman et al. (1992)	Thirteen patients (10 males, three females); range, 2–16 years (mean, 7.4 years); Vineland adaptive scores of 20–71; three patients with seizures	Twenty-eight medical control subjects (15 males, 13 females), age range, 1 month–12 years, 17 with seizures	Normal midsagittal areas of vermian lobules I–V and VI–VII, pons, and fourth ventricle
Murakami et al. (1989)	Ten patients (eight males, two females); DSM-III; range, 14–39 years; nine patients from study of Courchesne et al. (1988)	Eight control subjects (seven males, one female), age range, 19–33 years; of the eight, three normal control subjects and five medical control subjects	Smaller cerebellar hemispheres, correlated with vermian lobules VI–VII only in autistic subjects
Piven et al. (1992)	Fifteen males; DSM-III-R and Autism Diagnostic Interview; range, 8–53 years (mean, 27 years)	Thirty control subjects in two groups: 15 age- and nonverbal IQ-matched control subjects, mean age, 30 years, four with mental retardation; 15 age- and SES-matched, healthy normal control subjects from hospital staff	Smaller vermian lobules VI–VII only when compared with the normal control group. Normal pons and fourth ventricle. Larger midsagittal brain area
Both forebrain and posterior fossa			
Ekman et al. (1991)	Fifteen patients (10 males, five females); DSM-III-R; range, 2–13 years (mean, 8 years); seven patients with seizures	None (clinical evaluation)	No pathological changes in cerebrum, cerebellum, or brain stem
Gaffney et al. (1987)	Thirteen patients (10 males, three females); DSM-III; range, 5–22 years (mean, 11 years); IQs of 60–135; one patient with seizures; two patients with neurofibromatosis	Thirty-five medical control subjects (21 males, 14 females) with normal scans, age range, 4–19 years (mean age, 12 years)	Enlarged fourth ventricle. Normal corpus callosum, cerebellum, cerebrum, and cranium

(*continued*)

Investigators	Autistic patients (number, gender, criteria, ages, etc.)	Control subjects	Findings
Both forebrain and posterior fossa (*continued*)			
Gaffney and Tsai (1987)	Fourteen patients (11 males, three females); DSM-III; IQs of 60–135	None (clinical reading by neuroradiologist)	Six of 14 patients with varied abnormalities, including heterotopic gray matter, basal ganglia abnormalities, dilated lateral and fourth ventricles, and right temporal cystic mass
Nowell et al. (1990)	Fifty-three patients; modified DSM-III; range, 2–22 years (mean, 9 years); all but 6% with IQs of less than 81; 8% with seizures	Thirty-two institutionalized control subjects with normal MRIs, age range, 1–17 years (mean age, 8.5 years), 11 with seizures; 19 were studied for precocious puberty and used only for vermian measures	Normal vermian height and shape Of patients, 7.6% with significant vermian atrophy No abnormalities of amygdala or limbic system Other differences between patients and control subjects were not impressive

7

The Contribution of Neuroimaging to Behavioral Neurogenetics Research

Fragile X Syndrome, Turner Syndrome, and Neurofibromatosis-1

Allan L. Reiss and Martha Bridge Denckla

The neurobiological pathways leading to serious cognitive disability and behavioral dysfunction in children often are obscured by etiological heterogeneity within the group of individuals being studied. For example, several decades of research on behaviorally defined syndromes, such as autism and attention-deficit/hyperactivity disorder, suggest that rapid progress in understanding underlying genetic and neurobiological factors may be impeded by the etiological heterogeneity of individuals meeting the well-accepted diagnostic criteria that define these important pediatric disorders. Genetic and neurobiological heterogeneity in behaviorally defined disorders likely is a cause of dilution of or inconsistency in findings derived from groups of individuals with these conditions (Baumgardner et al., 1994; Reiss & Freund, 1990). Although etiological heterogeneity in neurobehavioral or developmental syndromes may impede rapid progress in understanding the pathogenesis of these disorders, it also reflects our admittedly early stage of scientific knowledge in this area.

Continued research efforts aimed at further subdividing behaviorally defined syndromes into etiologically meaningful subgroups are essential to our eventual understanding of the pathogenesis of childhood brain disorders. A complementary research strategy promoted at the Kennedy Krieger Institute, Baltimore, Maryland, and other research centers focuses on the study of individuals who have a known or suspected homogeneous genetic etiology of neurobehavioral and developmental dysfunction. This approach is similar to more traditional, neuroanatomically based lesion studies in neurology, with the exception that, in this case, the "lesion" begins at the level of DNA. Accordingly, the phrase *behavioral neurogenetics* has been coined to represent this new research approach (Baumgardner et al., 1994) (Figure 7.1).

Two important assumptions underlie behavioral neurogenetics research. The first assumption is that the complex pathway, beginning with one or more genetic factors affecting brain development or function and, ultimately, leading to behavioral or cognitive dysfunction, will be more accessible when studied in genetically homogeneous groups. The second assumption is that the information derived from such investigations will be directly relevant to our understanding of gene–brain–behavior associations in normal individuals. Despite the fact that behavioral neurogenetics research is a direct outgrowth of the relatively recent explosion in genetic knowledge, the research findings from our center and those of others already support the first of these assump-

This research was supported by National Institutes of Health Grants HD31715 (National Institute of Child Health and Human Development Human Brain Project), MH01142, and HD25806.

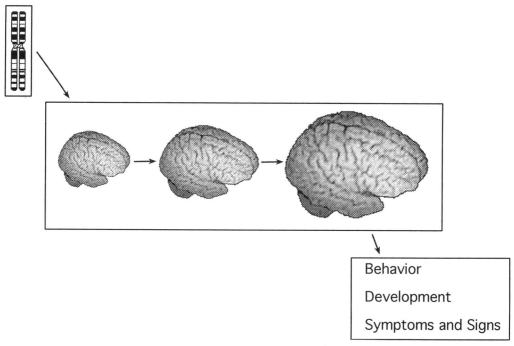

Figure 7.1.   Schematic of the theory underlying behavioral neurogenetics research. Genetic factors influence brain development and functioning, which ultimately is manifested as problems with learning and behavior.

tions. The second assumption awaits confirmation as our collective knowledge base in behavioral neuroscience matures.

Understanding the neurobiological pathways through which particular genetic factors produce abnormalities in brain development and neurobehavioral function is a critical step in the eventual design of more specific intervention strategies. Our ongoing research into three specific genetic etiologies of cognitive and behavioral dysfunction in children is the focus of this chapter.

FRAGILE X SYNDROME

Genetics

Recognized widely as a distinct clinical syndrome only in the late 1970s, fragile X syndrome is now known to be the most common heritable cause and at least the second-most common specific genetic etiology of cognitive and behavioral disability in humans. In 1991, it was determined that the clinical manifestations of the fragile X syndrome are caused by mutations in a gene, *FMR1*, that is located on the long arm (q27.3 band) of the X chromosome (Verkerk et al., 1991). Although the precise function of the protein product of *FMR1* is unknown, evidence suggests a role in RNA binding (Ashley et al., 1993; Siomi et al., 1994).

The most common mutation occurring within the *FMR1* locus involves expansion of a repetitive sequence of three DNA nucleotides (cytosine-guanine-guanine [CGG]) within a regulatory (promoter) region of the gene (Verkerk et al., 1991). The number of *FMR1* CGG repeats present in individuals in the general population ranges approximately from 6 to 54 (Fu et al., 1991). When 200 or more CGG repeats are present, components of the *FMR1* gene undergo hypermethylation, a phenomenon that is associated with silencing (inactivation) of the gene and the clinical manifestations of the fragile X syndrome (Hansen et al., 1992; Pai et al., 1994; Pieretti et al., 1991). This molecular state commonly is referred to as the FMR1 full mutation. An intermediate range of repeats (approximately 50–200 CGGs) is referred to as the premutation and is characterized by the presence of normal *FMR1* activation and normal phenotype (Reiss, Freund, Abrams, et al., 1993; Rousseau et al., 1994). Some individuals have a combination of methylated and unmethylated alleles of differing size (i.e., falling within both the full mutation and premutation categories, referred to as a mosaic status for the *FMR1* gene. A small number of individuals have been described as having large (i.e., more than 200 repeats) repeat lengths that may be partially unmethylated, referred to as methylation mosaics. A schematic representation of the molecular basis of the fragile X mutation is illustrated in Figure 7.2.

Males with fragile X are hemizygous—the mutation occurs on the only X chromosome present in each somatic cell. As is the case with many X chromosome-linked genetic diseases, males with the full mutation usually are more affected than are females with the full mutation, who are heterozygous (the mutation occurs only on one of the two X chromosomes present in a cell). However, unlike many X-linked conditions, the fragile X full mutation appears to be semidominant, because many females who are heterozygous are affected in the cognitive and behavioral domains. Because of the process of random X chromosome inactivation (Lyon, 1991), normal somatic tissue in females who are heterozygous for the fragile X mutation consists of two populations of cells, one population in which the fragile X chromosome retains full capacity for genetic expression and one population in which the unaffected X chromosome is active. Accordingly, the proportion of cells in which the fragile X versus the normal X is active also may be associated with phenotypic expression in females who are heterozygous for fragile X mutation. This phenomenon is thought to account, at least partially, for the range of effects of the full mutation in females—from severe to none at all.

The fragile X mutation is an important member of a growing family of genetic disorders in which the manifestations of the condition are associated with expansion of trinucleotide repeat sequences (Caskey et al., 1992). Other diseases in this category also have neurological or neurodevelopmental manifestations including FRAXE (a genetic condition resulting from a mutation in a gene close to *FMR1*), spinocerebellar ataxia-1, Huntington disease, myotonic dystrophy, and spinal muscular atrophy (Kennedy disease). The unique pattern of inheritance associated with the fragile X mutation also illustrates the notion of genetic anticipation, a concept referring to a change

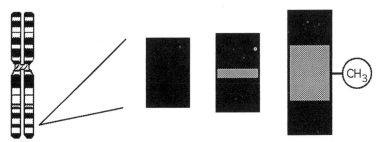

Figure 7.2.   A schematic of a normal X chromosome. To the right of this schematic are three blown-up representations of the fragile X region. From left to right these representations are of the normal allele, the premutation allele (small CGG repeat), and the full mutation allele (large CGG repeat with methylation at the CpG island).

for the worse in the effects of a genetic factor as it passes through successive genera-
tions (Sutherland & Richards, 1992). In the case of fragile X syndrome, a father who
has the premutation on his only X chromosome nearly always passes the premutation
to each of his daughters without significant change in the size of the repeat (Oberle et
al., 1991). When a mother who has the premutation on one of her two X chromosomes
passes that chromosome to her children, both sons and daughters can have either the
premutation or the full mutation. Children who inherit an X chromosome with the full
mutation from their mothers also will have the full mutation, usually increased in size.
Therefore, the condition in which the premutation develops the potential for conver-
sion to a full mutation occurs after it is passed from a mother to her children (Rousseau
et al., 1991).

Neurobehavioral Phenotype

Although fragile X syndrome has a broad range of phenotypic features, its effects on
the brain are the most important from the standpoint of the affected individual's daily
functioning. Nearly all males and approximately 50% of females with the full mutation
have mild to severe mental retardation. Descriptions of the cognitive, language, and
behavioral components of the syndrome also suggest enough consistency in the quality of dysfunction within these functional domains to characterize a fragile X neurobehavioral phenotype (Baumgardner et al., 1992; Baumgardner et al., 1995; Bregman et
al., 1988; Hagerman, 1991; Reiss & Freund, 1990, 1992).

In males, the behavioral component of the fragile X phenotype consists of social
problems with peers, language and communication impairments, unusual responses
to sensory stimuli, stereotypic behavior, and hyperactivity (Baumgardner et al., 1995;
Bregman et al., 1988; Cohen et al., 1988; Hagerman, 1991; Reiss & Freund, 1992; Sudhalter et al., 1991). Some investigators have conceptualized the behavior problems that
occur in males who have the fragile X full mutation as having features in common with
the behavioral syndrome of autism (Cohen et al., 1991; Reiss & Freund, 1992). Cognitive dysfunction in males who have fragile X syndrome includes deficits in short-term
memory, visuospatial ability, visual-motor coordination, processing of sequential information, and executive function (Crowe & Hay, 1990; Freund & Reiss, 1991, in press;
Kemper et al., 1988; Theobald et al., 1987). In addition, cross-sectional and longitudinal studies in males with fragile X syndrome indicate the possibility of progressive decline in IQ scores, which is most apparent during the transition between prepuberty
and puberty (Dykens et al., 1989; Hagerman et al., 1989; Hodapp et al., 1990; Lachiewicz et al., 1987).

Although less information is available about females who have fragile X syndrome, evidence suggests that females who are heterozygous for the full mutation
demonstrate behavior problems that are similar in quality but lesser in severity than
are those seen in males with this condition (Baumgardner et al., 1992; Freund et al.,
1993; Hagerman, 1991). Social disability, anxiety, depression, and stereotypic behavior
appear to be particularly important components of the female phenotype. The cognitive profile of relative strengths and weaknesses in females who have fragile X syndrome resembles that in males who have fragile X syndrome; this holds true for females with IQ scores in the normal range (Freund & Reiss, 1991, in press; Prouty et al.,
1988; Theobald et al., 1987).

Neuropathology

Neuroimaging investigations that focus on the neuroanatomy associated with particular conditions frequently draw on information derived from neuropathology studies to

help guide and confirm the focus of hypothesis-driven research. Unfortunately, the contribution of traditional neuropathological investigation to our understanding of neurobiological dysfunction in fragile X syndrome has been relatively limited because of the inaccessibility of the living brain in this nonfatal disease and the comparatively recent recognition of the syndrome and the gene that causes it. Anatomical and histological examination of the fragile X brain has been restricted to a small number of neuropathological studies with limited tissue sampling. These studies show nonspecific, subtle abnormalities in neuronal cell morphology in the neocortex (Hinton et al., 1991; Rudelli et al., 1985).

Neuroimaging

Findings from early imaging studies of fragile X syndrome were derived from qualitative analysis of computed tomography (CT) or magnetic resonance imaging (MRI) studies in males. These reports indicated the presence of increased size of the lateral ventricles in some individuals and other nonspecific findings (Wisniewski et al., 1991).

Our group began a series of quantitative imaging studies in both males and females with the FMR1 full mutation after early case reports suggested that abnormalities of the posterior fossa (in particular, the cerebellar vermis) may be associated with autism (Courchesne et al., 1988). Like others, we had noted that males with fragile X frequently manifested behaviors that fell within the autistic spectrum (Brown et al., 1982; Levitas et al., 1983; Meryash et al., 1982). Accordingly, the posterior fossa was our first neuroanatomical focus of interest. An initial study showed that the area of the cerebellar vermis was significantly smaller in four men who had mental retardation and fragile X syndrome compared with that in four unaffected men (Reiss et al., 1988). The smaller size of this structure appeared to be confined to the same vermal lobules (VI and VII) that were reported to be unusually small in a subgroup of individuals who had autism (Reiss, 1988). Two additional quantitative MRI studies were conducted to assess the neuroanatomy of the posterior fossa and other selected central nervous system (CNS) regions in 14 males and 12 females with fragile X, who ranged in age from 2 to 43 years (mean = 15 years) (Reiss, Aylward, et al., 1991; Reiss, Freund, et al., 1991). Compared with gender-, age-, and IQ-matched control subjects, both males and females with fragile X were shown to have a significantly decreased posterior cerebellar vermis area and increased fourth ventricle volume (Figure 7.3). Analyses of several other regions of interest, including total cerebellar hemisphere volume, showed no differences between the groups.

After conducting studies directed at the posterior fossa, we began to investigate cerebral morphology in individuals with fragile X. Our initial analyses focused on brain regions that potentially were implicated in the pathogenesis of cognitive and behavioral dysfunction in fragile X syndrome by virtue of the consistent pattern of neurobehavioral dysfunction revealed in affected males and females. These studies showed that individuals with the fragile X full mutation had both global and regional variations of cerebral anatomy that distinguished them from age-matched and age- and IQ-matched control subjects (Abrams & Reiss, 1995; Mazzocco et al., 1995; Reiss, Abrams, et al., 1995; Reiss et al., 1994).

The temporal lobe neuroanatomy of 15 subjects with fragile X (six male, nine female), who ranged in age from 6 to 27 years (mean = 13 years), was quantified from MRI results and compared with that of 26 age- and IQ-matched control subjects. Analyses showed that the right and left hippocampal volumes were significantly larger in the group with fragile X than in the control group. Of considerable interest was the finding that subjects with fragile X, but not control subjects, showed an age-related in-

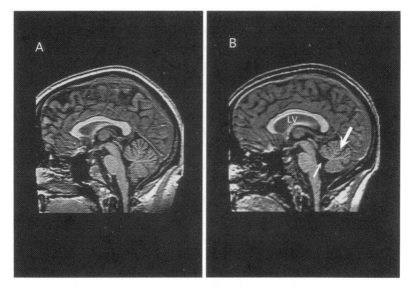

Figure 7.3.   Midsagittal images of 16-year-old twin girls with the fragile X full mutation who were discordant for mental retardation. Twin A has an IQ of 105 (normal), and twin B has an IQ of 47 (moderate mental retardation). Twin B has a relative reduction in size of her cerebellar vermis (large arrow) and increased volumes of her fourth ventricle (small arrow) and lateral ventricles (LV). (From Reiss, A.L., Abrams, M.T., et al. [1995]. Neurodevelopmental effects of the FMR-1 full mutation in humans. *Nature Medicine, 1,* 159; reprinted by permission.)

crease in hippocampal volume and decrease in superior temporal gyral volume. In a separate study, the cerebral neuroanatomy of 51 children and young adults with fragile X was evaluated (Reiss, Abrams, et al., 1995). Compared with age-, IQ-, and gender-matched control groups, both males and females with fragile X had significantly increased caudate nucleus volumes, and males also had significantly increased lateral ventricular volumes. Both caudate and lateral ventricular volumes were negatively correlated with IQ scores (i.e., larger [aberrant] volume was associated with lower IQ scores). Caudate volume also was negatively correlated with the methylation (activation) status of the *FMR1* gene, such that larger volume was associated with decreased activation of the unaffected X chromosome. Findings also suggested that aberrant (increased) ventricular volume in individuals with fragile X syndrome may be associated with maturation. In this study, the neuroanatomical features of 16-year-old identical twin girls who had the *FMR1* mutation and were discordant for mental retardation also were analyzed. Structural differences between the twins largely were consistent with results derived from our group studies and showed that the twin with mental retardation had a smaller cerebellar vermis area, significantly larger lateral ventricular volume, and moderately larger subcortical nuclei.

Summary

Little is known about the pathogenetic mechanism, developmental timing, and CNS localization of brain dysfunction resulting from the FMR1 full mutation. Our initial neuroimaging findings, however, indicate that the FMR1 full mutation has both a general effect on brain development, as shown by increased cerebral and ventricular volumes, and a selective effect on the growth and maintenance of specific brain regions, including the caudate nucleus, cerebellar vermis, hippocampus, superior temporal gyrus, and, possibly, thalamus. Neuroimaging results also indicate that alterations in the sizes of specific neuroanatomical regions in individuals with fragile X syndrome include both increases and decreases. The decreased size of a brain region often is viewed as indicating damage to and dysfunction of that region. Recent data suggest that the larger-than-normal size of a particular brain region also may be associated with neuropsychiatric disorders, such as schizophrenia or affective disorder (Breier et al., 1992; Swayze et al., 1992). Abnormally large size of a brain region could result from interference with normal pruning of particular neurons or synapses, a process that is thought to result in more specific and functional neuronal connectivity.

Dysfunction of neuroanatomical pathways involving particular brain regions could explain components of the fragile X neurobehavioral phenotype: For example, the finding of increased caudate nucleus volume in both males and females with the fragile X full mutation is of interest, because this subcortical nucleus functions as a component of neural systems reciprocally connected with the cerebral cortex. Although the caudate nucleus is recognized for involvement in voluntary control of eye movement, this nucleus also is thought to function as a zone of convergence for information processing related to emotional and cognitive control via reciprocal connections with nonmotor regions of the frontal cortex, including the dorsolateral prefrontal and lateral orbitofrontal regions (Cote & Crutcher, 1991; Cummings, 1993; Taylor et al., 1990). Reports describing the effect of lesions within these frontal-subcortical circuits suggest that profound disturbance in executive function, motor programming, regulation of affect, impulse control, and flexibility in response to environmental cues can occur when these regions are damaged (reviewed by Cummings, 1993). Abnormalities of brain circuits involving frontal-caudate connections, therefore, may be causally related to some of the neurobehavioral limitations observed in individuals with fragile X syndrome, including attention dysfunction, hyperactivity, and problems with impulse control (Hagerman, 1991; Reiss & Freund, 1992).

Similarly, abnormalities of other neuroanatomical regions observed to have aberrant size in our morphological studies of individuals with fragile X syndrome may contribute to the observed fragile X neurobehavioral phenotype. The cerebellar vermis normally is involved in processing sensory information and modulating attention and movement and may play a role in language (reviewed by Reiss, Aylward, et al., 1991). The hippocampus is involved in attention, learning, and memory, whereas the superior temporal gyrus is part of the neurofunctional system underlying language (Cummings, 1993; Mesulam, 1985; Reiss, Aylward, et al., 1991; Taylor et al., 1990). Of interest is the fact that the findings from our initial neuroimaging investigations are consistent with studies that show a nonrandom distribution of expression of the *FMR1* gene in the developing mammalian brain, with increased expression in the cerebellum, hippocampus, and specific cortical regions (Abitbol et al., 1993; Hinds et al., 1993).

Analyses that have examined the association of particular regions with age suggest the possibility of abnormal age-related volume changes associated with the fragile X full mutation. These findings may be relevant to the childhood decline in IQ scores that has been described for both males and females with the fragile X full mutation (Curfs et al., 1989; Fisch et al., 1994; Hagerman et al., 1989; Lachiewicz et al., 1987). Caution must be exercised, however, in the interpretation of statistical associations between age and neuroanatomy in individuals with fragile X syndrome because the analyses have been conducted on a relatively small number of subjects, findings available thus far have been derived exclusively from cross-sectional as opposed to longitudinal analyses, and the data do not point to a specific developmental epoch when dele-terious effects may be most significant.

Continued studies of brain morphology associated with the fragile X syndrome are under way in our laboratory. These studies focus on replicating the above-described initial findings, providing a fine-grained analysis of cortical morphology, and developing prospective longitudinal assessment of neuroanatomy in children and young adults with this important genetic condition.

TURNER SYNDROME

Genetics

The 46 chromosomes that comprise the normal human complement of genetic material are organized into 22 pairs of non–sex-determining chromosomes (autosomes) and 1 pair of sex-determining chromosomes. Complete absence of one X chromosome is the only monosomic (i.e., single-chromosome) condition compatible with life in humans. Turner syndrome is the clinical entity that arises in phenotypic females from partial or complete absence of one of the two X chromosomes (either the maternal or the pater-nal); approximately 60% of cases of Turner syndrome are caused by X monosomy (Lippe, 1990). This disorder, which occurs at birth in approximately 1 in 2,000 females, is associated with a well-documented physical phenotype that includes gonadal dys-genesis, lack of pubertal maturation, infertility, short stature, shield chest, webbing of the neck, coarctation of the aorta, and horseshoe kidney (Palmer & Reichmann, 1976; Park et al., 1983).

A typical female has two X chromosomes in each cell—one from her mother and one from her father. As a process of normal female embryonic development, *most* of the genes on one of the two X chromosomes in each cell are inactivated (Lyon, 1991). This process appears to be random in that it is equally probable that the maternally or the paternally derived X chromosome in a cell will be inactivated. Somatic tissue in typical females, therefore, consists of a mosaic of two populations of cells—one in which the paternal X chromosome retains full capacity for genetic expression and one in which the maternal X chromosome is active. It also is apparent that a small number of genes on the inactivated X chromosome escape the inactivation process and continue to be expressed (Goodfellow et al., 1984; Schneider-Gadicke et al., 1989). The typical female, therefore, has two working copies of these genes as opposed to one. Accordingly, the *genetic* differences that distinguish females with Turner syndrome from unaffected fe-males can be summarized as follows: 1) the presence of the hemizygous state (i.e., only one working copy) of genes on the X chromosome that normally escape inactivation, and 2) the lack of a somatic cell population containing an active X chromosome from either the paternal or the maternal line. Both of these differences are discussed below in the context of neuroimaging findings in females with Turner syndrome.

Neurobehavioral Phenotype

Although most females with Turner syndrome have IQs in the normal range, they also have been reported to be vulnerable to specific learning disabilities (Rovet, 1993). In particular, a common thread throughout studies of subjects with Turner syndrome is decreased performance IQ relative to verbal IQ and generalized difficulty in per-forming visuospatial tasks (Alexander et al., 1966; LaHood & Bacon, 1985; McCauley et al., 1987; Pennington et al., 1985; Rovet, 1993). Consistent with a previous report by Waber (1979), recent work undertaken at our research center indicates that visuo-spatial problems in girls with Turner syndrome appear in conjunction with poor planning and organization, suggesting a potential executive function component to these impairments.

Behavior problems, particularly hyperactivity and attention problems, have been reported in girls with Turner syndrome (McCauley et al., 1986; Rovet, 1993). Problems with social development and social functioning in females with Turner syndrome include delayed emotional maturity, difficulty understanding social cues, needing more structure to socialize, poor peer relations, shyness, and poor body image (McCauley, 1990; McCauley et al., 1986; Sonis et al., 1983).

Neuropathology

Measurable difficulties in learning or behavior in females with Turner syndrome reflect differences in brain development and function caused, directly or indirectly, by the monosomic state of X chromosome genes. Several neuropathology reports from females with Turner syndrome predate the beginning of neuroimaging studies in this population. In one early study, a 16-year-old girl with the 45,X karyotype (45 chromosomes, including only 1 X chromosome) was described as having abnormalities in cerebral cortical organization, including cortical dysplasia and neuronal heterotopias (Brun & Skold, 1968). This patient, however, was unrepresentative of the majority of females with Turner syndrome inasmuch as she had mental retardation, had a seizure disorder, and died as a result of complications from a medulloblastoma. Gullotta and Rehder (1974) reported bilateral clusters of neuroglia located in the upper temporal gyri and the island of Reil in a single female with Turner syndrome. No details about the age, neurobehavioral function, or method of diagnosis of this female were provided. Molland and Purcell (1974) described a newborn with the 45,X karyotype who was found to have abnormalities of the posterior fossa that were consistent with Dandy-Walker syndrome. Similar findings in a female with Turner syndrome of unspecified age and clinical status were reported by Urich (1979). A more recent study of a newborn with the 45,X karyotype also detected abnormalities of the posterior fossa, including cerebellar hypoplasia as well as neuronal heterotopias in cerebellar white matter and the medulla (Della Giustina et al., 1985). Less severe abnormalities in cellular organization also were found in the frontal cortex and hippocampus. Finally, Nielsen et al. (1977) described the neuropathological examination of two women with the Turner syndrome phenotype: A 52-year-old woman with X monosomy, normal IQ, seizures, diabetes, and psychosis was found to have abnormalities of the globus pallidus and perivascular fibrillar gliosis. A 24-year-old woman with a 45,X/46,X,i (Xq) karyotype and normal IQ was found to have small multiple infarcts secondary to atherosclerosis of the middle cerebral artery. No cytological abnormalities were observed in either of these adult cases.

In summary, as is the case for fragile X syndrome, data revealing the neuropathology of Turner syndrome are limited to a small number of autopsy studies yielding heterogeneous findings, including abnormalities of cerebral cortical organization and developmental deviation of structures in the posterior fossa, particularly midline cerebellum. Much of the neuropathological data concerning females with Turner syndrome also are derived from the examination of newborns or of females with Turner syndrome who have medical or cognitive features that, in general, are uncharacteristic of the majority of individuals who have this condition. The relative lack of information from neuropathology studies underscores the importance of in vivo neuroimaging to attempts to understand the complex interrelations among the genetic, neurobiological, and behavioral components of Turner syndrome.

Neuroimaging

Brain imaging studies of females with Turner syndrome include studies of both brain function and structure. One positron emission tomography study of five women with Turner syndrome and varying chromosomal constitutions suggested that there was bilaterally decreased glucose metabolism in the parietal and occipital cortices (Clark et al., 1990). Initial structural brain imaging studies of females with Turner syndrome include two reports of agenesis of the corpus callosum detected by CT in 14- and 19-year-old females with mental retardation and the 45,X karyotype (Araki et al., 1987; Kimura et al., 1990). Several MRI studies of females with Turner syndrome also have been reported. Murphy et al. (1993) collected MRI data from 18 women with Turner syndrome, including 9 mosaic and 9 nonmosaic subjects, and from 19 control women. Compared with control women, women with Turner syndrome had significantly smaller volumes of the cerebral hemispheres, and smaller region-to-whole-brain proportions for the parietal-occipital brain region, hippocampus, lenticular nucleus, and thalamus. All differences were reported as bilateral. Women with Turner syndrome also were reported to have greater asymmetry (the left side was larger than the right) in the parietal-occipital region and increased volume of the third ventricle compared with control women. No differences were observed between the groups in amygdala, parahippocampal gyrus, and lateral ventricular volumes. Psychological data obtained from this study showed the expected group differences (performance IQ lower than verbal IQ) on the Wechsler Adult Intelligence Scale–Revised (WAIS–R) (Wechsler, 1981), suggesting that the group with Turner syndrome was representative of women with this condition. The women with Turner syndrome had lower scores on all cognitive measures except verbal comprehension, a WAIS–R factor for which no group difference emerged. Women with a mosaic Turner syndrome genotype manifested differences that fell between those of women in the control and nonmosaic groups on nearly all measures of brain structure and cognitive performance.

Researchers in our laboratory have completed two studies of female children with Turner syndrome. In an initial report, Reiss, Freund, Plotnick, et al. (1993) reported on the results of a comprehensive assessment of prepubertal identical female twins who were *discordant* for Turner syndrome. The unusual nature of this naturally occurring genetic phenomenon provided an opportunity to elucidate more fully the neurobehavioral and neuroanatomical phenotypes associated with Turner syndrome. Zygosity for the twins was established with the use of DNA fingerprinting, and no evidence of chromosomal mosaicism was seen in either twin. Physical features seen in the affected twin were relatively mild with respect to the full spectrum of physical malformations and disabilities associated with Turner syndrome. The neurobehavioral phenotypes of the twins also were compared. Although both girls scored in the superior range of intelligence, the affected twin's performance IQ was disproportionately affected; her score was 18 points lower than was that of her sister, whereas their verbal IQs differed by only 3 points. Other relative differences were noted in the executive, visuospatial, and visual-motor domains of function. A behavioral evaluation indicated greater problems with attention, hyperactivity, and anxiety in the affected twin. A quantitative analysis of brain anatomy revealed evidence of both general and regional effects of X monosomy on neurodevelopment. Cerebrospinal fluid (CSF) volume was increased by 25% with a corresponding decrease in gray matter volume in the affected twin compared with her sister. The right frontal, right parietal-occipital, and left parietal regions showed the greatest discrepancy between the sisters with respect to increased CSF and decreased gray matter volumes in the twin with X monosomy. Differences in the posterior fossa also were noted; there was a 50% relative increase in the volumes of the fourth ventricle and cisterna magna and a 10%–15% relative reduction in size of the cerebellar vermis, pons, and medulla in the affected twin.

Reiss, Mazzocco, et al. (1995) completed a separate MRI study of 30 girls with Turner syndrome and 30 individually age-matched control girls. The cognitive and behavioral features of the girls with Turner syndrome in this investigation were characteristic of those found in previous studies of females with this genetic condition, and the average age (±standard deviation) of the two groups was approximately 11 ± 3 years. Unlike Murphy et al.'s 1993 study of women with Turner syndrome, no group differences in overall cerebral or subcortical volumes or degrees of asymmetry in any brain region were observed. Consistent with the findings of Murphy et al. (1993), evaluation of the regional distribution of gray and white matter revealed consistent group differences in both the right and left parietal regions. Specifically, differences in tissue volume ratios were seen for both the right and left parietal areas, but differences in individual gray and white matter ratios were seen in the right parietal regions exclusively. In general, girls with Turner syndrome had a smaller proportion of brain tissue (both gray and white matter) in the right and left parietal regions and a suggestion of a larger proportion of tissue in the right inferior parietal-occipital region than did girls in the control group. Among girls with Turner syndrome, volumes of neuroanatomical regions for which group differences emerged were not correlated with performance on cognitive tests.

Summary

Coupled with data obtained from studies of behavioral and cognitive function, neuroimaging studies of females with Turner syndrome suggest abnormalities of particular regions of the brain that may underlie the neurobehavioral-cognitive phenotype. A consistent finding thus far is the presence of an abnormally small proportion of tissue (Murphy et al., 1993; Reiss, Freund, Plotnick, et al., 1993; Reiss, Mazzocco, et al., 1995) and, perhaps, decreased brain function (Clark et al., 1990) in the parietal-occipital region of the brain in females with Turner syndrome. Abnormal brain function in the parietal-occipital region is an intriguing finding given that cognitive evaluation of females with Turner syndrome consistently shows relative weaknesses in functions subserved by this area of the brain, particularly in the right hemisphere (i.e., visuospatial abilities). Despite the fact that convincing correlations between brain imaging findings and measures of cognitive or behavioral functioning have not been demonstrated in the same females with Turner syndrome, initial neuroimaging studies suggest that more refined analyses of posterior brain regions in females with Turner syndrome are needed. Findings from Reiss, Freund, Plotnick, et al.'s 1993 study of monozygotic twins who were discordant for Turner syndrome and the limited collection of neuropathology reports also suggest that additional investigation of posterior fossa neuroanatomy is warranted.

It is also important to note the discrepancies in study results between the report on 30 children with Turner syndrome (Reiss, Mazzocco, et al., 1995) and the study of affected women (Murphy et al., 1993) with respect to overall cerebral volume and proportional volume (i.e., region-to-brain ratio) of specific subcortical structures. It is possible that these discrepancies may be explained by differences in subject ascertainment (e.g., Murphy et al. [1993] included more mosaic subjects), genetic status (e.g., parental origin of the single X chromosome), or methods of image processing or analysis. Alternatively, undetected direct or indirect effects of X monosomy could be responsible for changes in brain morphology over time in females with Turner syndrome. Age-related volume changes in females with Turner syndrome could arise directly from decreased levels of protein for X chromosome genes that normally escape inactivation and are present in a single copy only in a female with Turner syndrome or indirectly from the absence of a normal endogenous hormonal environment, particularly during puberty. These possibilities can be investigated only through research that incorporates longitudinal imaging analysis of larger numbers of pre- and postpubertal females with Turner syndrome.

Equally important is the investigation of possible effects of imprinting as a cause of neurobiological variance within the population of females with Turner syndrome. As noted previously, females with Turner syndrome lack a set of either maternally or paternally derived X chromosome genes in each cell. It is clear that some genetic diseases occur because of the absence of either the maternal or the paternal member of a gene pair (Hall, 1990). Preliminary investigations into the effects of parental origin of the single X chromosome in females with Turner syndrome have indicated that, from the standpoint of selected physical characteristics, such as birth weight, height, or cardiovascular and renal abnormalities, females with Turner syndrome who have a single, paternally derived X chromosome do not differ from females who have a single, maternally derived X chromosome (Mathur et al., 1991). However, the broad range of severity in neurobehavioral and neuropsychological abnormalities occurring in females with Turner syndrome raises unanswered questions about possible effects of genetic imprinting on brain structure and function in this condition.

NEUROFIBROMATOSIS-1

Genetics and Neurobehavioral Phenotype

Neurofibromatosis-1 (NF-1), also known as von Recklinghausen disease, is the most common of the neurocutaneous syndromes. It is inherited in an autosomal dominant fashion with an incidence of approximately 1 in 4,000 among all ethnic groups. CNS involvement can take the form of a nerve sheath or meningeal tumor or of a tumor arising from glial cells from within the substance of the brain and spinal cord. In addition to these specific pathological lesions, CNS involvement also can take the form of cognitive impairment (National Institutes of Health Consensus Development Conference, 1988). Compared with an estimated frequency of 15% in the general population, the frequency of learning disabilities among children with NF-1 ranges from 29% to 37% (Riccardi, 1995) and can be responsible for significant lifetime morbidity.

There is a general consensus (Riccardi, 1995) that children with NF-1, compared with the general population and with their own siblings, have lower IQs (low to average) and lower scores on tests of spatial ability. Beyond these two widely accepted statements, the NF-1-associated profile for language, attentional, and learning disabilities has not been refined.

Neuroimaging and Neuropathology

When structural neuroimaging with MRI became a widely used clinical assessment in the late 1980s, reports appeared indicating that, in the studies of patients with NF-1,

T2-weighted hyperintensities (brain tissue that appears abnormally bright on MRIs) often were seen (Brown et al., 1987; Duffner et al., 1989; Dunn & Roos, 1989). These T2-weighted hyperintensities seen on MRIs are not visible on CT scans. Because they are not enhanced by gadolinium on T1-weighted images and do not exhibit a significant mass effect, these "lesions" appear to be unrelated to the occurrence of brain tumors (coincident in less than 5%); they are, however, seen so frequently (in 60%) that many clinicians would opt to include them, along with café au lait spots (CLS) and Lisch nodules (LN), among the criteria for the diagnosis of NF-1. As is explained below, these lesions cannot be considered pathognomonic evidence of NF-1. One particular subclass of brain tumors, optic glioma, itself a frequent (and frequently asymptomatic) manifestation of NF-1, is reported to be associated with the presence of T2-weighted hyperintensities, particularly in younger patients (less than 28 years of age) (Sevick et al., 1992). The T2-weighted hyperintensities have come to be called unidentified bright objects (UBOs) because of their perceived resemblance to MRI findings in multiple sclerosis and other common neurological disorders (Figure 7.4). Among neurodevelopmental disorders, only phenylketonuria has been reported to be associated with similar UBOs (Cleary et al., 1994). In location, UBOs are most frequently found in the basal ganglia, followed by the brainstem and cerebellum with equal frequency; UBOs appear less frequently in the subcortical cerebral white matter (Bognanno et al., 1988). Whether the optic tract hyperintensities should be grouped with UBOs or with asymptomatic optic gliomas remains under discussion (Riccardi, 1995). The UBOs in the globus pallidus, which usually are larger, have been thought by some investigators to represent a distinct type of lesion (Aoki et al., 1989); this view, based on the very early years of MRI data concerned with UBOs in NF-1, is less widely held because large brainstem and cerebellar UBOs also have been seen (Itoh et al., 1994). Similarly, T1-weighted hyperintense appearance, once thought to be limited to UBOs in the basal ganglia, now is well documented elsewhere (Riccardi, 1995), although this is a rare phenomenon.

The underlying nature of the anomalous tissue that gives rise to UBOs remains a mystery. Clinical researchers hold varying views on this matter, with dysmyelination,

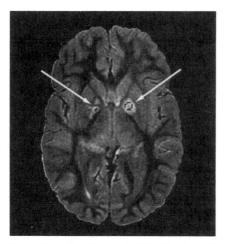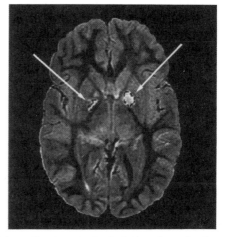

Figure 7.4. Semiautomated identification of hyperintense tissue appearing in the basal ganglia of a 7-year-old boy with NF-1. The image on the left shows rater-designated "seed values" (identified by the arrows) surrounding tissue that is clearly hyperintense. A computer-executed algorithm then finds and selects all of the connected tissue with like intensity (image on the right). This "region grow" is done in three dimensions, although only a two-dimensional case is shown here.

hamartoma (a mass that resembles a tumor but actually represents anomalous development of tissue that belongs within the organ within which it is found), and heterotopia
being etiological candidates (Riccardi, 1995). Heterotopia UBO may be heterogeneous—some represent gray matter abnormalities and some represent white matter
abnormalities. Some appear to be rotund and merit the term *objects*, whereas others appear to be more linear, streaky, or diffuse and, therefore, are better characterized as *unidentified bright signals* (UBS). For the remainder of this chapter, the term UBS is
adopted (see Riccardi, 1995).

Neuropathological evidence regarding the nature of UBS is limited to one abstract
(Zimmerman et al., 1992) in which these lesions were correlated with same-site postmortem histology in the brains of two children with NF-1; the pathology was reported
to be consistent with dysplastic glial proliferation. Five areas (two consisting of globus
pallidus tissue and three from midbrain peduncles) were examined and found to exhibit infiltration with glial cells, characterized by bizarre hyperchromatic nuclei, perivascular gliosis associated with foci of microcalcification, and (at the periphery of the
lesions) spongy alterations of white matter. It is to be emphasized that each such lesion
localized to a site on MRI where, during life, typical UBS were visualized. This study
was interpreted by its first author to indicate that the dysplastic gliosis relates to aberrant myelination (Zimmerman et al., 1992).

An additional complication in the endeavor to understand the pathology of UBS is
that their natural history is one of change in signal over time. By using various age cut-
offs ("younger/older" at 15, 20, and 28 years), investigators have agreed that younger
patients with NF-1 are more likely than are older patients with NF-1 to exhibit UBS on
MRIs (Aoki et al., 1989; Itoh et al., 1994). A longitudinal study has revealed stable or
diminishing UBS in patients who were followed from the first into the second decade
of life (Sevick et al., 1992); the decrease or disappearance of UBS in a few patients who
were evaluated twice between the ages of 8 and 17 years hints at the same trend with
age (Itoh et al., 1994). Transiency of the lesions seen as UBS implies support for the
dysmyelination interpretation, because malformation (e.g., as hamartoma, heterotopia) or abnormality (e.g., neoplasia) would not be expected to be transient. Because
most postmortem pathology reports are of adult brains, the difficulty of understanding
what underlies UBS (if, in fact, these are things of the past) is magnified.

If the UBS represent disordered myelination or myelin maturation caused by abnormal or delayed glial cell differentiation, this pathogenesis may be traced to neurofibromin, the protein encoded by the *NF-1* gene. Neurofibromin is not clearly defined in terms of its function, but it may act as an effector of the *rasGTP* oncogene,
sending a signal that is instrumental in cell proliferation and differentiation (Riccardi,
1995). In any event, UBS are seen far less often in parents who have NF-1 than in their
children who also have NF-1 (Hofman et al., 1994; Itoh et al., 1994).

The significance of UBS in terms of cognitive impact remains a matter of considerable controversy. Two early MRI studies (Duffner et al., 1989; Dunn & Roos, 1989)
found no cognitive impact attributable to the presence of UBS; neither study used specific formal cognitive assessment of the subjects with NF-1 and neither used family
control subjects. Two subsequent MRI studies (Hofman et al., 1994; North et al., 1994)
strongly suggested that those children with NF-1 whose MRIs revealed evidence of
UBS were cognitively impaired in relation to those children with NF-1 whose MRIs revealed no UBS. These two studies, although sharing the feature of formal and extensive evaluations of cognitive and academic functions of subjects, differ in design.
North et al. (1994) reported data on 40 children with NF-1 and confined their use of

MRI data to the dichotomy of the presence versus the absence of UBS. North et al. (1994) concluded that those children with NF-1 who did not have UBS (38% of 40 subjects) did not differ significantly in any respect from the general population, whereas those who did have UBS (62% of 40 subjects) had lower IQ, language, motor, and academic scores. Hofman et al. (1994) used a family-based design with sibling controls and reported that, compared with the siblings' scores, children with NF-1 had lower IQs and visuospatial ability that were predicted by the number of locations in which UBS were identified. These two studies are, therefore, convergent but address issues at different levels: 1) dichotomous versus continuous with respect to UBS parameter, and 2) comparison with the general population versus comparison with siblings with respect to cognitive parameters.

Others have reported attempts to replicate the finding of North et al. (1994) that the presence of UBS was associated with learning problems. Reporting on small samples, some poster presentations and abstracts have refuted this association; in an abstract involving 84 children with NF-1 (ages 8–16 years), however, Moore et al. (in press) reported that UBS involvement of a particular location (diencephalon, more specifically, either thalamus or hypothalamus) was associated with significantly lower IQ, memory, motor, and attentional scores. Moore et al. (in press) examined each location separately and reported no cognitive impact with heterotopias (their interpretive term for UBS) in the cerebral hemispheres, basal ganglia, brainstem, or cerebellum. Moore et al. (in press), unlike North et al. (1994), did not have any UBS involving the optic tracts in their sample population, whereas 64% (16 children) of the 25 subjects with UBS in North et al.'s (1994) sample population had optic tract involvement. Both studies report the basal ganglia to be a common site at which UBS are found.

In the only two studies to date that have reported using sibling control designs, UBS have been found to bear a highly significant relationship to the cognitive impairments found in children with NF-1. In both studies, cognitive impairments were defined in relation to sibling scores by means of pairwise analyses of IQ and other more specific neuropsychological task scores. Hofman et al. (1994) found that those scores showing the greatest pairwise discrepancy were found in a sample of 12 sibships to be significantly correlated with the number of locations in which UBS were seen. For full-scale IQ, this correlation was at the significance level $p < 0.0003$; for judgment of line orientation (JLO) (Benton et al., 1976), it was significant when $p < 0.02$. In a follow-up study to these findings, Denckla et al. (1996) used an enlarged sample (19 sibships) to pursue a multiple regression model in which not only number of UBS-occupied locations, but also the age of the child with NF-1, the mode of inheritance of NF-1 (familial versus sporadic), and the volume of brain tissue occupied by total volume of all UBS tissue were considered as potential predictors of the sibling-referenced lowering of IQ associated with NF-1. The findings of the Hofman et al. (1994) study were confirmed in that the number of UBS-occupied locations accounted for 42% of the variance in NF-1–associated reduction in IQ; none of the other variables considered, including UBS volume in relation to brain tissue volume, added significantly to the prediction of the effect of UBS on IQ. The most common locations of UBS, when present, were as follows: always in the basal ganglia, followed in frequency in the brainstem, and less frequently in the cerebellum. Most UBS were bilateral in distribution. Of the 16 subjects with basal ganglia UBS, 11 had additional brainstem UBS, and 7 had cerebellar UBS. In addition, a few subcortical, peduncular, and thalamic UBS were visualized. No subjects with optic tract involvement of UBS were admitted to the study. It is to be emphasized that in all cases in which there were any UBS at all, the basal ganglia always were the site of UBS (even if there was only one such hyperintensity); most UBS-positive scans exhibited a bilateral distribution of UBS.

The significance of these findings is illustrated by the fact that two boys with familial NF-1, in whom no UBS were found, had IQs virtually identical to those of their solidly average brothers. Equally illustrative is the case in which, against a background of superior parental and sibling IQs, a boy with sporadic NF-1 and in whom four brain regions were occupied by UBS was, although still in the average IQ range, significantly less intelligent than would be expected. The sibling and family design reveals one possible source of the apparently contradictory literature regarding UBS and IQ: Without data from which to derive a non—NF-1–associated expectation for IQ, the impact of UBS may disappear into a comparison with population means. Furthermore, there may be hidden or unanticipated sampling biases within a general population of families with NF-1 members such that impact of UBS may be obscured; compare the average IQ of the boy with sporadic NF-1 and UBS (whose family members have high IQs) with the IQ of another child with NF-1 (but no UBS) from a family in which the members have low to average IQs, and the possibilities become clear.

Furthermore, because UBS, when present, invariably appeared in basal ganglia, JLO, a visuospatial task, was the most impaired NF-1–associated cognitive finding, and because the basal ganglia are the second-most common brain region to give rise to spatial impairments (including JLO scores), Mott et al. (1995) attempted to predict JLO impairments (relative to siblings) in the 19 children with NF-1 by age, mode of inheritance, UBS volume in the basal ganglia, and UBS volume across all other locations. The JLO impairments were highly correlated with greater UBS volume occurring along a pathway that ran from the right basal ganglia to the left cerebellum; in contrast, UBS that preponderantly occupied the opposite pathway (left basal ganglia to right cerebellum) failed to correlate with JLO impairments (Mott et al., 1995).

Summary

In summary, it is clear that, in NF-1, discrete lesions occur at both the DNA and neuroanatomical levels. Evidence has been accumulated that UBS are relevant to the lowering of IQ in children with NF-1; furthermore, a "connectionist" or "network" model is supported by the role of the number, rather than the volume, of UBS. UBS volume may emerge as important in a more specific set of brain–behavior relationships. Larger samples from several sites are required to replicate this still-controversial conclusion. The ages and UBS localizations of the subjects, as well as control for general familial cognitive factors, must be specified if the controversy is to be resolved.

The authors believe that quantitative neuroimaging will play an increasingly important role in providing a much-needed window into the neurodevelopmental pathways leading to learning and behavior problems in children. Intensive study of the three conditions described in this chapter and other specific courses of learning and behavior problems is ongoing at the Kennedy Krieger Institute, Baltimore, Maryland; the emphasis of this research is on the elucidation of links between gene, brain, and behavior.

REFERENCES

Abitbol, M., Menini, C., Delezoide, A.L., Rhyner, T., Vekemans, M., & Mallet, J. (1993). Nucleus basalis magnocellularis and hippocampus are the major sites of FMR-1 expression in the human fetal brain. *Nature Genetics, 4,* 147–153.

Abrams, M., & Reiss, A. (in press). Quantitative brain imaging studies of fragile X syndrome. *Developmental Brain Dysfunction*.

Alexander, D., Ehrardt, A.A., & Money, J. (1966). Defective figure drawing, geometric and human, in Turner's syndrome. *Journal of Nervous and Mental Disease, 152*, 161–167.

Aoki, S., Barkovich, A.J., Nishimura, K., Kjos, B.O., Machida, T., Cogen, P., Edwards, M., & Norman, D. (1989). Neurofibromatosis types 1 & 2: Cranial MR findings. *Radiology, 172*, 527–534.

Araki, K., Matsumoto, K., Shiraishi, T., Ogura, H., Kurashige, T., & Kitamura, I. (1987). Turner's syndrome with agenesis of the corpus callosum, Hashimoto's thyroiditis and horseshoe kidney. *Acta Paediatrica (Japanese Overseas Edition), 29*, 622–626.

Ashley, C.J., Wilkinson, K.D., Reines, D., & Warren, S.T. (1993). FMR1 protein: Conserved RNP family domains and selective RNA binding. *Science, 262*, 563–6.

Baumgardner, T.L., Green, K., & Reiss, A.L. (1992). The psychological effects associated with fragile X syndrome. *Current Opinion in Pediatrics, 4*, 609–615.

Baumgardner, T.L., Green, K.E., & Reiss, A.L. (1994). A behavioral neurogenetics approach to developmental disabilities: Gene–brain–behavior associations. *Current Opinion in Neurology, 7*, 172–178.

Baumgardner, T.L., Reiss, A.L., Freund, L., & Abrams, M. (1995). Specification of the neurobehavioral phenotype in males with fragile X syndrome. *Pediatrics, 95*(5), 744–752.

Benton, A., Varney, N., & Hamsher, K.S. (1976). *Judgment of line orientation*. Iowa City: Department of Neurology, University of Iowa.

Bognanno, J.R., Edwards, M.K., Lee, T.A., Dunn, D.W., Roos, K.L., & Klatte, E.C. (1988). Cranial MR imaging in neurofibromatosis. *American Journal of Neuroradiology, 9*, 461–468.

Bregman, J.D., Leckman, J.F., & Ort, S.I. (1988). Fragile X syndrome: Genetic predisposition to psychopathology. *Journal of Autism and Developmental Disorders, 18*, 343–354.

Breier, A., Buchanan, R.W., Elkasher, A., Munson, R.C., Kirkpatrick, B., & Gellad, F. (1992). Brain morphology and schizophrenia. *Archives of General Psychiatry, 49*, 921–926.

Brown, E.W., Riccardi, V.M., Mawad, M., Handel, S., Goldman, A., & Bryan, R.N. (1987). MR imaging of optic pathways in patients with neurofibromatosis. *American Journal of Neuroradiology, 9*, 1031–1036.

Brown, W.T., Jenkins, E.C., Friedman, E., Brooks, J., Wisniewski, K., Raguthu, S., & French, J. (1982). Autism is associated with the fragile-X syndrome. *Journal of Autism and Developmental Disorders, 12*, 303–308.

Brun, A., & Skold, G. (1968). CNS malformations in Turner's syndrome. *Acta Neuropathologica Scandinavica, 10*, 159–161.

Caskey, C.T., Pizzuti, A., Fu, Y.H., Fenwick R.J., & Nelson, D.L. (1992). Triplet repeat mutations in human disease. *Science, 256*, 784–789.

Clark, C., Klonoff, H., & Hayden, M. (1990). Regional cerebral glucose metabolism in Turner syndrome. *Canadian Journal of Neurology Science, 17*, 140–144.

Cleary, M., Walter, J., & Wraith, J. (1994). MRI in phenylketonuria. *Lancet, 344*, 87–90.

Cohen, I.L., Fisch, G.S., Sudhalter, V., Wolf, S.E., Hanson, D. Hagerman, R., Jenkins, E.C., & Brown, W.T. (1988). Social gaze, social avoidance, and repetitive behavior in fragile X males: A controlled study. *American Journal of Mental Retardation, 92*, 436–446.

Cohen, I.L., Sudhalter, V., Pfadt, A., Jenkins, E.C., Brown, W.T., & Vietze, P.M. (1991). Why are autism and the fragile-X syndrome associated?: Conceptual and methodological issues. *American Journal of Human Genetics, 48*, 195–202.

Cote, L., & Crutcher, M.D. (1991). The basal ganglia. In E.R. Kandel & J.H. Schwartz (Eds.), *Principles of neural science* (pp. 647–659). New York: New York University Press.

Courchesne, E., Young-Courchesne, R., Press, G.A., Hesselink, J.R., & Jernigan, T.L. (1988). Hypoplasia of cerebellar vermal lobules VI and VII in autism. *New England Journal of Medicine, 318*, 1349–1354.

Crowe, S.F., & Hay, D.A. (1990). Neuropsychological dimensions of the fragile X syndrome: Support for a non-dominant hemisphere dysfunction hypothesis. *Neuropsychologia, 28*, 9–16.

Cummings, J.L. (1993). Frontal-subcortical circuits and human behavior. *Archives of Neurology, 50*, 873–880.

Curfs, L.M., Borghgraef, M., Wiegers, A., Schreppers, T.G., & Fryns, J.P. (1989). Strengths and weaknesses in the cognitive profile of fra(X) patients. *Clinical Genetics, 36*, 405–410.

Della Giustina, E., Forabosco, A., Botticelli, A.R., & Pace, P. (1985). Neuropathology of the Turner syndrome. *Pediatria Medica e Chirurgica, 7*, 49–55.

Denckla, M.B., Hofman, K., Mazzocco, M.M.M., Melhem, E., Reiss, A.L., Bryan, R.N., Harris, E.L., Lee, J., Cox, C.S., & Schuerholz, L.J. (1996). Relationship between T2-weighted hyperintensities (unidentified bright objects) and lower IQs in children with neurofibromatosis-1. *American Journal of Medical Genetics (Neuropsychiatric Genetics), 67,* 98–102.

Duffner, P.K., Cohen, M.E., Seidel, G., & Shucard, D.W. (1989). The significance of MRI abnormalities in children with NF-1. *Neurology, 39,* 373–378.

Dunn, D.W., & Roos, K.L. (1989). Magnetic resonance imaging evaluation of learning difficulties and incoordination in neurofibromatosis. *Neurofibromatosis, 2,* 1–5.

Dykens, E.M., Hodapp, R.M., Ort, S., Finucane, B., Shapiro, L.R., & Leckman, J.F. (1989). The trajectory of cognitive development in males with fragile X syndrome. *Journal of the American Academy of Child and Adolescent Psychiatry, 28,* 422–426.

Fisch, G.S., Simensen, R., Arinami, T., Borghgraef, M., & Fryns, J.P. (1994). Longitudinal changes in IQ among fragile X females: A preliminary multicenter analysis. *American Journal of Medical Genetics, 51,* 353–357.

Freund, L.S., & Reiss, A.L. (1991). Cognitive profiles associated with the fra(X) syndrome in males and females. *American Journal of Medical Genetics, 38,* 542–547.

Freund, L.S., & Reiss, A.L. (in press). A neurocognitive phenotype of young males and females with fragile X. *Developmental Neuropsychology.*

Freund, L.S., Reiss, A.L., & Abrams, M.T. (1993). Psychiatric disorders associated with fragile X in the young female. *Pediatrics, 91,* 321–329.

Fu, Y.H., Kuhl, D.P., Pizzuti, A., Pieretti, M., Sutcliffe, J.S., Richards, S., Verkerk, A.J., Holden, J.J., Fenwick, R.G., Warren, S.T., Oostra, B.A., Nelson, D.L., & Caskey, C.T. (1991). Variation of the CGG repeat at the fragile X site results in genetic instability: Resolution of the Sherman paradox. *Cell, 67,* 1047–1058.

Goodfellow, P.N., Pym, B., Mohandas T., & Shapiro, L.J. (1984). The cell surface antigen locus, MIC2X, escapes X-inactivation. *American Journal of Human Genetics, 36,* 777–782.

Gullotta, F., & Rehder, H. (1974). Chromosomal anomalies and central nervous system. *Beitrage zur Pathologie, 152,* 74–80.

Hagerman, R.J. (1991). Physical and behavioral phenotype. In R.J. Hagerman & A.C. Cronister (Eds.), *Fragile X syndrome* (pp. 3–68). Baltimore: Johns Hopkins University Press.

Hagerman, R.J., Schreiner, R.A., Kemper, M.B., Wittenberger, M.D., Zahn, B., & Habicht, K. (1989). Longitudinal IQ changes in fragile X males. *American Journal of Medical Genetics, 33,* 513–518.

Hall, J.G. (1990). Genomic imprinting: Review and relevance to human diseases. *American Journal of Human Genetics, 46,* 857–873.

Hansen, R.S., Gartler, S.M., Scott, C.R., Chen, S.H., & Laird, C.D. (1992). Methylation analysis of CGG sites in the CpG island of the human FMR1 gene. *Human Molecular Genetics, 1,* 571–578.

Hinds, H.L., Ashley, C.T., Sutcliffe, J.S., Nelson, D.L., Warren, S.T., Housman, D.E., & Schalling, M. (1993). Tissue specific expression of FMR-1 provides evidence for a functional role in fragile X syndrome. *Nature Genetics, 3,* 36–43.

Hinton, V.J., Brown, W.T., Wisniewski, K., & Rudelli, R.D. (1991). Analysis of neocortex in three males with the fragile X syndrome. *American Journal of Medical Genetics, 41,* 289–294.

Hodapp, R.M., Dykens, E.M., Hagerman, R.J., Schreiner, R., Lachiewicz, A.M., & Leckman, J.F. (1990). Developmental implications of changing trajectories of IQ in males with fragile X syndrome. *Journal of the American Academy of Child Adolescent Psychiatry, 29,* 214–219.

Hofman, K.J., Harris, E.L., Bryan, R.N., & Denckla, M.B. (1994). Neurofibromatosis type 1: The cognitive phenotype. *Journal of Pediatrics, 124,* S1–S8.

Itoh, T., Magnaldi, S., White, R.M., Denckla, M.B., Hofman, J.J., Naidu, S., & Bryan, R.N. (1994). Neurofibromatosis type 1: The evolution of deep gray and white matter MR abnormalities. *American Journal of Neuroradiology, 15,* 1–7.

Kemper, M.B., Hagerman, R.J., & Altshul, S.D. (1988). Cognitive profiles of boys with the fragile X syndrome. *American Journal of Medical Genetics, 30,* 191–200.

Kimura, M., Nakajima, M., & Yoshino, K. (1990). Ullrich-Turner syndrome with agenesis of the corpus callosum. *American Journal of Medical Genetics, 37,* 227–228.

Lachiewicz, A.M., Gullion, C.M., Spiridigliozzi, G.A., & Aylsworth, A.S. (1987). Declining IQs of young males with the fragile X syndrome. *American Journal of Mental Retardation, 92,* 272–278.

LaHood, B., & Bacon, G. (1985). Cognitive abilities of adolescent Turner's syndrome patients. *Journal of Adolescent Health Care, 6,* 358–364.

Levitas, A., Hagerman, R.J., Braden, M., Rimland, B., McBogg, P., & Matus, I. (1983). Autism and the fragile X syndrome. *Journal of Developmental and Behavioral Pediatrics, 4*, 151–158.

Lippe, B. (1990). Primary ovarian failure. In S.A. Kaplan (Ed.), *Clinical pediatrics*. Philadelphia: W.B. Saunders.

Lyon, M.F. (1991). The quest for the X-inactivation centre. *Trends in Genetics, 7*, 69–70.

Mathur, A., Stekol, L., Schatz, D., MacLaren, N.K., Scott, M.L., & Lippe, B. (1991). The parental origin of the single X chromosome in Turner syndrome: Lack of correlation with parental age or clinical phenotype. *American Journal of Human Genetics, 48*, 682–686.

Mazzocco, M., Freund, L., Baumgardner, T., & Reiss, A. (1995). The neurobehavioral and neuro-anatomical effects of the FMR-1 full mutation: Monozygotic twins discordant for the fragile X syndrome. *Neuropsychology, 9*(4), 470–480.

McCauley, E. (1990). Psychosocial and emotional aspects of Turner syndrome. In D.B. Berch & B.G. Bender (Eds.), *Sex chromosome abnormalities and human behavior* (pp. 78–99). Boulder, CO: Westview.

McCauley, E., Ito, J., & Key, T. (1986). Psychosocial functioning in girls with Turner's syndrome and short stature: Social skills, behavior problems, and self-concept. *Journal of the American Academy of Child Psychiatry, 25*, 105–112.

McCauley, E., Kay, T., Ito, J., & Treder, R. (1987). The Turner syndrome: Cognitive deficits, affective discrimination, and behavior problems. *Child Development, 58*, 464–473.

Meryash, D.L., Szymanski, L.S., & Gerald, P.S. (1982). Infantile autism associated with the fragile X syndrome. *Journal of Autism and Developmental Disorders, 12*, 295–301.

Mesulam, M. (1985). Patterns in behavioral neuroanatomy: Association areas, the limbic system, and hemispheric specialization. In M. Mesulam (Ed.), *Principles of behavioral neurology* (pp. 1–70). Philadelphia: F.A. Davis Co.

Molland, E.A., & Purcell, M. (1974). Biliary atresia and the Dandy-Walker anomaly in a neonate with 45,X Turner's syndrome. *Journal of Pathology, 115*, 227–230.

Moore, B.D., Slopis, J.M., Schomer, D., Jackson, E., & Levy, B. (in press). Neuropsychological significance of areas of high signal intensities on brain MRI of children with neurofibromatosis. *Neurology.*

Mott, S.H., Skryja, P.A., Baumgardner, T.L., Colli, M.J., Reiss, A.L., Hofman, K., Mazzocco, M.M.M., & Denckla, M.B. (1995). Neurofibromatosis type 1 (NF-1): Correlation between volumes of T2 weighted high intensity signals (UBOs) within neural pathways and impaired performance on judgment of line orientation (JLO). *Annals of Neurology, 38*, 509.

Murphy, D., DeCarli, C., Daly, E., Haxby, J., Allen, G., White, B., McIntosh, A., Powell, C., Horwitz, B., Rapoport, S., & Schapiro, M. (1993). X-chromosome effects on female brain: A magnetic resonance imaging study of Turner's syndrome. *Lancet, 342*, 1197–1200.

National Institutes of Health Consensus Development Conference. (1988). Neurofibromatosis: Conference statement. *Archives of Neurology, 45*, 575–578.

Nielsen, J., Nyborg, H., & Dahl, G. (1977). *Turner's syndrome: A psychiatric-psychological study of 45 women with Turner's syndrome compared with their sisters and women with normal karyotypes, growth retardation and primary amenorrhea*. Aarhus, Denmark: Acta Jutlandica XLV, Medicine Series.

North, K., Joy, P., Yuille, B., Cocks, N., Mobbs, E., Hutchins, P., McHugh, K., & DeSilva, M. (1994). Specific learning disability in children with neurofibromatosis type 1: Significance of MRI abnormalities. *Neurology, 44*, 878–883.

Oberle, I., Rousseau, F., Heitz, D., Kretz, C., Devys, D., Hanauer, A., Boue, J., Bertheas, M.F., & Mandel, J.L. (1991). Instability of a 550-base pair DNA segment and abnormal methylation in fragile X syndrome. *Science, 252*, 1097–1102.

Pai, J.T., Tsai, S.F., Horng, C.J., Chiu, P.C., Cheng, M.Y., Hsiao, K.J., & Wuu, K.D. (1994). Absence of FMR-1 gene expression can be detected with RNA extracted from dried blood specimens. *Human Genetics, 93*, 488–493.

Palmer, C.G., & Reichmann, A. (1976). Chromosomal and clinical findings in 110 females with Turner syndrome. *Human Genetics, 35*, 35–49.

Park, E., Bailey, J.D., & Cowell, C.A. (1983). Growth and maturation of patients with Turner's syndrome. *Pediatrics Research, 17*, 1–7.

Pennington, B.F., Heaton, R.K., Karzmar, P., Pendleton, M.G., Lehman, R., & Schucard, D.W. (1985). The neuropsychological phenotype in Turner syndrome. *Cortex, 21*, 391–404.

Pieretti, M., Zhang, F.P., Fu, Y.H., Warren, S.T., Oostra, B.A., Caskey, C.T., & Nelson, D.L. (1991). Absence of expression of the FMR-1 gene in fragile X syndrome. *Cell, 66*, 817–822.

Prouty, L.A., Rogers, R.C., Stevenson, R.E., Dean, J.H., Palmer, K.K., Simensen, R.J., Coston,

G.N., & Schwartz, C.E. (1988). Fragile X syndrome: Growth, development, and intellectual function. *American Journal of Medical Genetics, 30*, 123–142.

Reiss, A., & Freund, L. (1990). Neuropsychiatric aspects of fragile X syndrome. *Brain Dysfunction, 3*, 9–22.

Reiss, A., Mazzocco, M., Greenlaw, R., Freund, L., & Ross, J. (1995). Neurodevelopmental effects of X monosomy: A volumetric imaging study. *Annals of Neurology, 38*, 731–738.

Reiss, A.L. (1988). Cerebellar hypoplasia and autism. *New England Journal of Medicine, 319*, 1152–1153.

Reiss, A.L., Abrams, M.T., Greenlaw, R., Freund, L., & Denckla, M. (1995). Neurodevelopmental effects of the FMR-1 full mutation in humans. *Nature Medicine, 1*, 159–167.

Reiss, A.L., Aylward, E., Freund, L.S., Joshi, P.K., & Bryan, R.N. (1991). Neuroanatomy of fragile X syndrome: The posterior fossa. *Annals of Neurology, 29*, 26–32.

Reiss, A.L., & Freund, L. (1992). Behavioral phenotype of fragile X syndrome: DSM-III-R autistic behavior in male children. *American Journal of Medical Genetics, 43*, 35–46.

Reiss, A.L., Freund, L., Abrams, M.T., Boehm, C., & Kazazian, H. (1993). Neurobehavioral effects of the fragile X premutation in adult women: A controlled study. *American Journal of Human Genetics, 52*, 884–894.

Reiss, A.L., Freund, L., Plotnick, L., Baumgardner, T., Green, K., Sozer, A.C., Reader, M., Boehm, C., & Denckla, M.B. (1993). The effects of X monosomy on brain development: Monozygotic twins discordant for Turner's syndrome. *Annals of Neurology, 34*, 95–107.

Reiss, A.L., Freund, L. Tseng, J.E., & Joshi, P.K. (1991). Neuroanatomy in fragile X females: The posterior fossa. *American Journal of Human Genetics, 49*, 279–288.

Reiss, A.L., Lee, J., & Freund L. (1994). Neuroanatomy of fragile X syndrome: The temporal lobe. *Neurology, 44*, 1317–1324.

Reiss, A.L., Patel, S., Kumar, A.J., & Freund, L. (1988). Preliminary communication: Neuroanatomical variations of the posterior fossa in men with the fragile X (Martin-Bell) syndrome. *American Journal of Medical Genetics, 31*, 407–414.

Riccardi, V. (1995, March). Consensus conference on learning disabilities and cognitive impairments in children with neurofibromatosis, Houston, TX.

Rousseau, F., Heitz, D., Biancalana, V., Blumenfeld, S., Kretz, C., Boue, J., Tommerup, N., Van Der Hagen, C., DeLozier-Blanchet, C., Croquette, M.F., Gilgenkrantz, S., Jalbert, P., Voelckel, M.A., Oberle, I., & Mandel, J.L. (1991). Direct diagnosis by DNA analysis of the fragile X syndrome of mental retardation. *New England Journal of Medicine, 325*, 1673–1681.

Rousseau, F., Heitz, D., Tarleton, J., MacPherson, J., Malmgren, H., Dahl, N., Barnicoat, A., Mathew, C., Mornet, E., Tejada, I., Maddalena, A., Spiegel, R., Schinzel, A., Marcos, J.A.G., Schwartz, C., & Mandel, J.L. (1994). A multicenter study on genotype-phenotype correlations in the fragile X syndrome, using direct diagnosis with probe StB12.3: The first 2,253 cases. *American Journal of Human Genetics, 55*, 225–237.

Rovet, J. (1993). The psychoeducational characteristics of children with Turner syndrome. *Journal of Learning Disabilities, 26*, 333–341.

Rudelli, R.D., Brown, W.T., Wisniewski, K., Jenkins, E.C., Laure, K.M., Connell, F., & Wisniewski, H.M. (1985). Adult fragile X syndrome: Clinico-neuropathologic findings. *Acta Neuropathologica (Berlin), 67*, 289–295.

Schneider-Gadicke, A., Beer Romero, P., Brown, L.G., Nussbaum, R., & Page, D.C. (1989). ZFX has a gene structure similar to ZFY the putative human sex determinant and escapes X inactivation. *Cell, 57*, 1247–1258.

Sevick, R.J., Barkovich, A.J., Edwards, M.S.B., Koch, T., Berg, B., & Lempert, T. (1992). Evolution of white matter lesions in neurofibromatosis type 1: MR findings. *American Journal of Radiology, 159*, 171–175.

Siomi, H., Choi, M., Siomi, M.C., Nussbaum, R.L., & Dreyfuss, G. (1994). Essential role for KH domains in RNA binding: Impaired RNA binding by a mutation in the KH domain of FMR1 that causes fragile X syndrome. *Cell, 77*, 33–39.

Sonis, W.A., Levine Ross, J., Blue, J., Cutler, G.B., Loriaux, P.L., & Klein, R.P. (1983, October). *Hyperactivity and Turner's syndrome.* Paper presented at the Meeting of the American Academy of Child Psychiatry, San Francisco.

Sudhalter, V., Scarborough, H.S., & Cohen, I.L. (1991). Syntactic delay and pragmatic deviance in the language of fragile X males. *American Journal of Medical Genetics, 38*, 493–497.

Sutherland, G.R., & Richards, R.I. (1992). Anticipation legitimized: Unstable DNA to the rescue [Editorial]. *American Journal of Human Genetics, 51*, 7–9.

Swayze, V.W., Andreasen, N.C., Alliger, R.J., Yuh, W.T.C., & Ehrhardt, J.C. (1992). Subcortical and temporal structures in affective disorder and schizophrenia: A magnetic resonance imaging study. *Biological Psychiatry, 31*, 221–240.

Taylor, A.E., Saint, C.J., & Lang, A.E. (1990). Subcognitive processing in the frontocaudate "complex loop": The role of the striatum. *Alzheimer Disease and Associated Disorders, 4*, 150–160.

Theobald, T.M., Hay, D.A., & Judge, C. (1987). Individual variation and specific cognitive deficits in the fra(X) syndrome. *American Journal of Medical Genetics, 28*, 1–11.

Urich, H. (1979). Cerebellar malformations: Some pathogenic considerations. *Clinical and Experimental Neurology, 16*, 119–131.

Verkerk, A.J., deVries, B.B., Niermeijer, M.F., Fu, Y.H., Nelson, D.L., Warren, S.T., Majoor, K.D., Halley, D.J., & Oostra, B.A. (1992). Intragenic probe used for diagnostics in fragile X families. *American Journal of Medical Genetics, 43*, 192–196.

Verkerk, A.J., Pieretti, M., Sutcliffe, J.S., Fu, Y.H., Kuhl, D.P., Pizzuti, A., Reiner, O., Richards, S., Victoria, M.F., Fuping Zhang, M.F.V., Eussen, B.E., van Ommen, G.J.B., Blonden, L.A.J., Riggins, G.J., Chastain, J.L., Kunst, C.B., Galjaard, H., Caskey, C.T., Nelson, D.L., Oostra, B.A., & Warren, S.T. (1991). Identification of a gene (FMR-1) containing a CGG repeat coincident with a breakpoint cluster region exhibiting length variation in fragile X syndrome. *Cell, 65*, 905–914.

Waber, D.P. (1979). Neuropsychological aspects of Turner's syndrome. *Developmental Medicine and Child Neurology, 21*, 58–70.

Wechsler, D. (1981). *Wechsler Adult Intelligence Scale–Revised*. New York: The Psychological Corporation.

Wisniewski, K.E., Segan, S.M., Miezejeski, C.M., Sersen, E.A., & Rudelli, R.D. (1991). The fra(X) syndrome: Neurological, electrophysiological, and neuropathological abnormalities. *American Journal of Medical Genetics, 38*, 476–480.

Zimmerman, R.A., Yachnis, A.T., Rorke, L.B., Rebsamen, S.L., Bilaniuk, L.T., & Zackal, E. (1992). Pathology of findings of high signal intensity findings in neurofibromatosis type 1: Abstract from 78th scientific assembly and annual meeting of the Radiological Society of North America. *Radiology, 186*(P), 123.

8

Neuroimaging Studies
of Children with Epilepsy
William D. Gaillard

Neuroimaging has evolved since the early 1980s to encompass a set of instrumental and powerful tools in the evaluation and management of children with epilepsy. Computed tomography (CT) and, to an even greater extent, magnetic resonance imaging (MRI) are able to discern brain structure, often with great detail; these methods, however, confer no information on neuronal function or physiological processes. Functional imaging is designed to assess some of many possible physiological functions. Functional imaging most commonly is performed with positron emission tomography (PET) or single photon emission computed tomography (SPECT), but new advances in MRI technology allow functional application with the use of conventional scanners. This chapter begins with a brief review of the epilepsies, then reviews the use of CT and MRI in the evaluation of children with epilepsy, and, finally, discusses the use of functional imaging, PET, and SPECT in adults and in children. The chapter closes with a consideration of advances in using MRI for functional mapping of cognitive processes.

THE EPILEPSIES

Epilepsies are classified into three groups: the partial epilepsies, the primary generalized epilepsies, and the epilepsy syndromes (e.g., infantile spasms, Lennox-Gastaut syndrome, Landau-Kleffner syndrome) (Commission on Classification and Terminology of the International League Against Epilepsy, 1981). Imaging studies are used first to determine a cause and then to identify a seizure focus. Structural imaging studies (i.e., MRI) are routinely performed in all children with epilepsy except those who have primary generalized epilepsy without focal features. Functional imaging more commonly has been performed in children who have partial epilepsy or an epilepsy syndrome.

A partial seizure is one with a known or suspected cortical focus. A partial seizure may be limited in neuronal involvement and time, thereby remaining focal without alteration of consciousness; this is a simple partial seizure. A partial seizure that originates in, or spreads to involve, the limbic system, thereby causing consciousness to be altered, is a complex partial seizure. A partial seizure that spreads to involve the whole brain is secondarily generalized. Additional descriptive terms applied to partial seizures usually define their clinical onset, which, in turn, identifies their manifestation and origin; for example, a focal-motor seizure has its focus in the motor strip; an olfactory seizure, in the olfactory cortex; and a gelastic (laughing) seizure, in the hypothalamus. Partial seizures may be associated with focal pathology, such as tumor, vascular malformation, stroke, cortical dysplasia, contusion, or mesial temporal sclerosis. Such abnormalities often can be seen on structural imaging studies or are associated with focal physiological dysfunction identified by functional imaging. Intractable partial seizures that are refractory to medical anticonvulsant treatment may be amenable to surgical alleviation; this accounts for the burgeoning of functional imaging and its application to patients with intractable partial seizures. The temporal lobe is a common site of origin for seizure(s) in patients with chronic partial epilepsy. Temporal structures are more prone to generate seizures than are other brain regions. In addition, it is easier to resect a unilateral temporal lobe focus, the likelihood of surgical success is greatest (approximately 80%–85% are seizure-free after surgery), and the chance of neurological impairment is lower. In patients with seizure foci outside the temporal lobe (extratemporal), the likelihood of surgical success is closer to 50%. Before surgery can be considered an option, the seizure origin must reliably be identified to one operable focus: one lobe on one side of the brain (Engel, 1993; Wyllie, 1993).

Many of the epilepsy syndromes, although apparently clinically generalized, are thought to have a focal component. Two examples are infantile spasms—characterized by serial myoclonic seizures, a hypsarrhythmic pattern on an electroencephalogram (EEG), and, often, mental retardation—and the Lennox-Gastaut syndrome—characterized by myoclonic, tonic, and atypical absence seizures; an EEG demonstrating slowed background rhythms and slow spike and wave patterns; and, often, mental retardation. Children with such syndromes often are devastated by their disease; they frequently develop cognitive decline variably attributed to continual seizures, antiepileptic drug toxicity, or the underlying etiology. Functional imaging technology has been used in an effort to better understand the phenomenology of these syndromes as well as to search for a focus. When a focus can be found, some investigators argue that children with some epilepsy syndromes may benefit from resective surgery. Because most epilepsy syndromes occur during childhood, presumably reflecting an age-dependent manifestation of neuronal maturation, cerebral development has been another topic of pediatric functional imaging research.

The primary generalized epilepsies, such as absence seizures and juvenile myoclonic epilepsy, by definition have no known cortical focus but may originate in deep subcortical structures; as a result, such epilepsies are not amenable to surgical treatment. Those imaging studies that have been performed on patients with generalized epilepsies have been undertaken to achieve greater understanding of the physiology of these epilepsies rather than to treat individual patients.

CT AND MRI STUDIES IN CHILDREN WITH EPILEPSY

A structural imaging study using either CT or MRI should be performed on any child with a partial epilepsy or a catastrophic epilepsy syndrome to examine brain structure, which may explain the etiology and focus of seizures. CT is less expensive than is MRI, and access to CT scanners is more widespread than is that for MRI scanners. In addition, sedation often is required to perform an MRI on a child. CT also is able to better discern a recent central nervous system (CNS) bleed or an old calcification. The anatomical resolution of CT, however, is considerably lower than is that of MRI, performed at 1.5-tesla (1.5-T, magnetic field strength), and thus will not detect the majority of structural abnormalities associated with epilepsy (Kuzniecky et al., 1987; Sperling et al., 1986; Theodore, Carson, et al., 1992). Because CT detects only gross structural abnormalities and those causes that require urgent intervention (e.g., CNS bleed, large stroke), it is best reserved to evaluate a child with acute onset of seizures, in the setting of a history of either a focal seizure, focal examination, or prolonged alteration in mental status, or when MRI is unavailable.

High-resolution (1 mm–2 mm) 1.5-T MRI is the structural imaging study of choice when evaluating a child with epilepsy (i.e., recurrent, unprovoked seizures). Tumors (e.g., ganglioglioma, astrocytoma, oligodendroglioma), vascular malformations, and strokes, all occasional causes of epilepsy, are readily discerned by MRI (Kuzniecky et al., 1987). Another common etiology for seizures in children are neuronal migration disorders, which range from the catastrophic disorders of cortical lamination (e.g., lissencephaly [smooth brain], pachygyria, polymicogyria), to regional migrational disorders (e.g., schizencephally), and to small cortical areas of microdysgenesis (e.g., aberrantly formed cortex) and neuronal heterotopia (e.g., misplaced neurons) (Kuzniecky et al., 1993). Cortical dysplasia characteristic of tuberous sclerosis and neurofibromatosis can be seen, as can evidence for congenital infection (e.g., cytomegalovirus, toxoplasmosis) or antenatal ischemia (e.g., periventricular leukomalacia) (Kuzniecky, Garcia, et al., 1991). Evidence for some infectious etiologies, such as cysticercosis in patients from areas in which it is endemic, also can be seen. The advent of thin-cut coronal images of the hippocampus (2 mm–5 mm) makes possible the identification of mesial temporal sclerosis, a common cause of complex partial seizures in adolescents and young adults, and small areas of microdysgenesis and gliosis (see Figure 8.1) (Grattan-Smith et al., 1993; Jack et al., 1990; Jackson et al., 1990; Kuzniecky, Garcia, et al., 1991; Kuzniecky et al., 1987; Kuzniecky, Suggs, et al., 1991). Gadolinium contrast does not increase the yield of MRI appreciably unless tumor or infection is strongly considered. Any of the above-mentioned findings can explain the reason for seizures. It is only the more focal abnormalities, however, that help to identify seizure focus: Such abnormalities include microdysgenesis, mesial temporal sclerosis, stroke, vascular malformation, and tumor. A retrospective study of children who were considered candidates for epilepsy surgery at the University of Alabama at Birmingham found that, of children with abnormal MRI, 25% had tumors, 25% had mesial temporal sclerosis, and 25% had cortical dysgenesis (Kuzniecky et al., 1993).

In the population of children with epilepsy, however, structural imaging often is normal. As one would expect, children with normal development and normal physical examinations are more likely to have normal studies. The greater the cognitive impairment, abnormal development, and abnormality of the neurological examination, the more likely MRI will be abnormal.

Clinical functional neuroimaging in epilepsy has been centered about surgical considerations and, hence, directed in the following three broad areas: 1) to identify or confirm the ictal focus, usually in preparation for epilepsy surgery; 2) to help determine the prognosis of surgical benefit; and 3) to locate critical cerebral function (e.g., language, but also the primary motor/sensory cortex) relative to the ictal focus so that eloquent function is not lost as a result of surgery. During epilepsy surgery evaluation, any imaging modality, be it structural MRI or functional modalities, such as PET or SPECT, that confirms the ictal source identified by clinical phenomenology and EEG lessens the need for invasive monitoring and increases the likelihood of correct identification and, therefore, surgical success (Cascino et al., 1991; Engel et al., 1990; Jack et al., 1992; Rowe et al., 1991; Theodore, Sato, et al., 1992). When tests are discordant the noninvasive identification of the seizure origin becomes uncertain; in this case, caution is warranted, and invasive monitoring almost always is necessary before resection is performed (Cascino et al., 1991; Engel et al., 1990; Jack et al., 1992; Theodore, Sato,

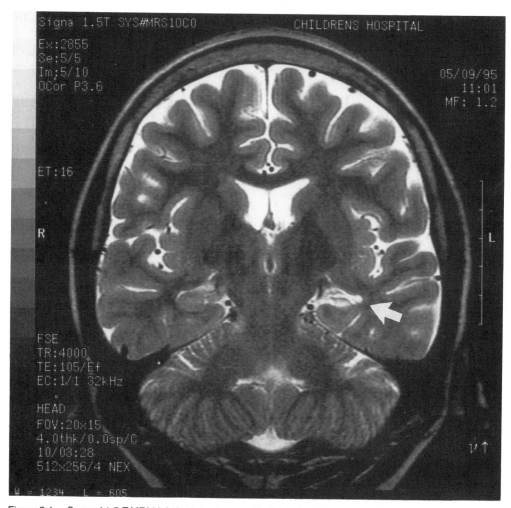

Figure 8.1.   Coronal 1.5-T MRI (right brain is shown on the left) of an 11-year-old child with left mesial temporal lobe seizure focus. The left hippocampus is atrophied and has increased signal, as seen in this T2-weighted image (arrow). These findings are pathognomonic for mesial temporal sclerosis.

et al., 1992). Invasive monitoring involves the placement of intracranial depth or subdural grid electrodes; these electrodes can remain in place for up to 3 weeks. Confirmation is sought because scalp ictal telemetry can be misleading and sometimes cannot be clearly interpreted. Functional imaging studies, therefore, are performed either to reduce the need for invasive monitoring or to direct better placement of electrodes for additional monitoring (Engel et al., 1990; Theodore, Sato, et al., 1992). Other issues of greater research than clinical interest also have been explored. Examples of such issues are normal patterns of cerebral metabolism during development, the natural history of the effect of epilepsy on cerebral metabolism, the effect of epilepsy and drug therapy on metabolism and receptor binding, the effect of epilepsy on the organization of cognitive processes, and the relation between metabolism and blood flow in epileptogenic tissue (Chugani, Phelps, & Mazziotta, 1987; Frost et al., 1988; Gaillard et al., 1995; Henry, Frey, et al., 1993; Theodore, 1988; Theodore et al., 1989; Theodore, Carson, et al., 1992; Zametkin et al., 1993).

FUNCTIONAL IMAGING STUDIES IN ADULTS AND CHILDREN WITH EPILEPSY: PET, SPECT, AND fMRI

Of the many functional imaging modalities available for the evaluation of epilepsy patients, the one with which investigators have had the most experience is interictal (between seizures) [^{18}F]fluorodeoxyglucose (FDG) PET, a measure of glucose utilization (Abou-Khalil et al., 1987; Engel et al., 1982; Hajek et al., 1993; Henry, Massiota, & Engel, 1993; Radtke et al., 1993, 1994; Ryvlin et al., 1992; Sackallares et al., 1990; Theodore et al., 1988; Theodore et al., 1990; Theodore, Sato, et al., 1992). Its use is best established in adults, but these findings appear to apply to children as well (Gaillard, White, et al., 1995; Hosokawa et al., 1989; Maeda et al., 1992). In adult patients with partial epilepsy originating from the temporal lobe, FDG PET reveals focal abnormalities—a region of decreased glucose utilization or hypometabolism—in approximately 70%–90% of patients. The variability in the percentage reflects the generation of the scanner (old scanners have 8-mm resolution, new scanners have 5-mm resolution) and patient selection bias. The hypometabolic area often is larger than is the electrical ictal focus, as determined by subdural grid studies, and may extend into the adjacent cortex in the frontal, parietal, or occipital lobe (Theodore et al., 1988). In approximately 10%–20% of patients, the subcortical structures—caudate or thalamus— also may be hypometabolic (Henry, Massiota, & Engel, 1993). Usually, but not always, the most profound hypometabolism is found in the temporal lobe (80%–90%) (Theodore et al., 1988). Some investigators have observed greater lateral than mesial temporal lobe hypometabolism even when there was a mesial temporal seizure focus (Hajek et al., 1993; Sackallares et al., 1990). On occasion, regional hypometabolism is found only in lobar cortex adjacent to the ictal lobe. FDG PET, therefore, is an excellent lateralizing test but not necessarily as excellent of a localizing test (Theodore et al., 1988; Theodore, Sato, et al., 1992). In one large study undertaken at the University of California, Los Angeles, PET was never falsely lateralizing, and, when FDG PET regional hypometabolism was found to be concordant with ictal-scalp EEG, invasive depth studies did not provide additional information (Engel et al., 1990). When regional hypometabolism, defined as greater than 15% asymmetry in brain regions ipsilateral to the focus compared with the analogous contralateral region, is present, then there is a significantly higher prospect of surgical success (Radtke et al., 1993; Theodore, Sato, et al., 1992). Measures of asymmetry are important because visual differences are detected by the unaided eye at approximately 10% asymmetry, but outcome is not measurably different unless asymmetry is greater than 15%.

If an MRI abnormality (e.g., tumor, infarct, encephalomalacia, cerebral dysgenesis, vascular malformation) is present, then PET is less likely to provide additional information (Gaillard, Bhatia, et al., 1995). As a result of improvements in MRI, principally hippocampal volume measurement and detection of signal abnormalities in the hippocampus, mesial temporal sclerosis can more readily be detected (Grattan-Smith et al., 1993; Jack et al., 1990; Jackson et al., 1990; Lencz et al., 1992). Mesial temporal sclerosis commonly is associated with complex partial seizures of temporal lobe origin (70% of young adults). When found, it almost invariably identifies the seizure focus correctly and is associated with an 85%–95% likelihood of an excellent result from surgery (Cascino et al., 1991; Jack et al., 1990). An excellent surgical result is defined as the patient being seizure free, or having aurae and/or rare nocturnal seizures only, which means the patient is able to drive. FDG PET is superior to MRI in detecting focal cerebral abnormalities, including the hypometabolism associated with mesial temporal sclerosis (Gaillard, Bhatia, et al., 1995; Sperling et al., 1986; Theodore et al., 1990). In a recent series of studies involving 18 patients at the National Institutes of Health, Bethesda, Maryland, if mesial temporal sclerosis was seen with MRI, then FDG PET did not provide additional localizing information (Gaillard, Bhatia, et al., 1995). PET provided additional information to structural MRI in 20% of the 18 patients.

What the zone of hypometabolism represents is unclear (Engel et al., 1982). In some patients, it is a reflection of neuron loss in the hippocampus and resultant loss of neuronal projections and synaptic connections. In other patients, it represents cortical dysplasia in which malformed connections utilize less glucose. In still other patients, it seems to be a purely functional phenomenon, representing either a regional neuronal effect to suppress aberrant neuronal activity or a widespread cortical effect of impaired circuitry caused by epileptogenic activity.

In extratemporal lobe epilepsy, FDG PET has proved to be less useful. In the absence of a clear structural lesion, FDG PET is focal in 33%–50% of cases, although, when focal hypometabolism is present, the localizing value of PET is of greater value (more specific) than is that in the evaluation of temporal lobe epilepsy. When scalp EEG is either nonlateralizing or bilateral and MRI is normal, then FDG PET shows focal abnormalities in fewer than 33% of patients, and these findings are of uncertain clinical significance (Radtke et al., 1994).

In children with partial seizures, the findings are the same as for adults; this should not be surprising because more than 80% of adult patients evaluated for epilepsy surgery have experienced seizure onset during childhood. In temporal lobe epilepsy, focal abnormalities are present in approximately 67%–75% of patients (see Figure 8.2 on p. *xxxii*) (Grattan-Smith et al., 1993; Kuzniecky et al., 1993). The longer the duration of the epilepsy, the greater the likelihood that focal regional hypometabolism will be found. Of children who have had epilepsy for fewer than 5 years, 30% have focal metabolic abnormalities; of those who have had epilepsy for 10 years, 65% have focal abnormalities; and of those who have had epilepsy for 15 years, 75% have focal abnormalities. The greater likelihood of finding metabolic abnormalities in patients who have had epilepsy longer suggests that, in some patients, intractable partial seizures of temporal lobe origin are associated with increasing cerebral dysfunction. Uncontrolled seizures, furthermore, may cause ongoing cerebral injury, thereby supporting the argument for early surgical intervention. It is not clear, however, whether the presence of hypometabolism early in the course of epilepsy is of prognostic value. FDG PET is of similar usefulness in children as in adults for detecting extratemporal partial epilepsy (Gaillard, White, et al., 1995; Maeda et al., 1992). FDG PET may be more sensitive than MRI, especially in patients younger than 2 years of age, in detecting small areas of cerebral dysgenesis (Chugani et al., 1988; Chugani et al., 1990; Lee et al., 1994). MRI is less sensitive in younger children because white matter myelination is incomplete, which results in the blurring of the demarcation of gray matter. Cerebral dysgenesis is a common etiology of seizures in children, especially those with early onset seizures.

Children and adults with primary generalized epilepsies do not show focal abnormalities when FDG PET studies are undertaken. Children with Lennox-Gastaut syndrome and those with infantile spasms have demonstrated somewhat different results. In children with Lennox-Gastaut syndrome, FDG PET revealed abnormalities in 40%–45% of cases, but, of these, 25% showed global hypometabolism, and the other 15%–20% showed focal hypometabolism (Chugani, Mazziotta, et al., 1987; Theodore et al., 1987). The significance of focal PET abnormalities is unclear in these children because they have not undergone epilepsy surgery. Most of the children with focal PET abnormalities had either an abnormal MRI or a history of partial seizures. Those children with global metabolic abnormalities had an earlier age of seizure onset (younger than 1 year of age) and more severe mental retardation. The metabolic PET abnormalities, therefore, may reflect the severity of the etiology rather than that of the seizures themselves. Patients with infantile spasms who were found to have regions of focal hypometabolism usually also had focal EEG abnormalities or asymmetries of neurological examinations and, often, but not always, had focal MRI (Chugani et al, 1990). The metabolic abnormalities usually are seen in the posterior quadrant, and, when structural MRI is grossly normal, the area of hypometabolism usually reflects cortical dysplasia.[1] Given such findings, infantile spasms may be better viewed as a focal seizure disorder manifested at an early age by clinical spasms. Surgery in this group seems to be beneficial, but controlled studies, rigorous categorization, and long-term follow-up studies are lacking.

PET also has been used in the evaluation of children for hemispherectomy. Most children considered for this procedure have Rasmussen's encephalitis (progressive unilateral hemispheric inflammation), Sturge-Weber syndrome, hemimegalancephally (unilateral cerebral dysgenesis), extensive unilateral cerebral infarcts, or widespread cerebral dysgenesis (Chugani et al., 1988). Children with these conditions have a hemiparesis, are incapacitated by focal seizures often with secondary generalization, and may exhibit an epileptic encephalopathy in which the incessant seizures from the damaged hemisphere interfere with the functioning of the intact hemisphere. The affected hemisphere invariably exhibits widespread cortical hypometabolism, as one would expect from the clinical examination and MRI. Some investigators also maintain that, in patients who are being considered for hemispherectomy, the presence of regional metabolic abnormalities contralateral to the affected hemisphere is a poor prognostic sign both for functional development and seizure control (Chugani et al., 1988).

Ictal (during seizures) studies with FDG PET have not been useful. The half-life of the FDG ligand (90 min) and the period of ligand uptake (30 min) are considerably longer than is the period of the ictus (usually 30 s to 5 min). The regional abnormalities seen have varied considerably. A region of hypermetabolism sometimes is seen to correspond to the seizure focus and sometimes is a remote effect of a focal seizure. In addition, the ensuing postictal depression sometimes is so profound that focal hypometabolism is seen at the seizure origin. Ictal studies, therefore, are not useful clinical tools in evaluating epilepsy patients.

The use of ^{11}C-flumazenil as a marker of central benzodiazepine receptors has shown a decrease in binding in the mesial temporal lobe and normal neocortical binding in adults with mesial temporal sclerosis (Henry, Frey, et al., 1993). These abnormalities are more restricted than are FDG abnormalities in the same patients and may reflect the selective loss of CA1 and CA3 neurons (the pathological hallmarks of mesial temporal sclerosis) and their γ-aminobutyric acid receptors. Binding studies with opiate ligands have demonstrated a relative increase in μ opiate receptors (i.e., increased binding) in lateral temporal cortex ipsilateral to the ictal focus (Frost, Mayberg, Fisher, et al., 1988). No changes have been detected in the other opiate receptor subtypes, δ and $\varkappa$ (Table 8.1) (Theodore, Carson, et al., 1992). These ligands are not readily available for clinical use.

The other common ligand used for PET studies is [15]O water (^{15}O PET), a marker of blood flow. A study comparing [15]O PET and FDG PET in patients with temporal lobe epilepsy found interictal regional (usually temporal) hypoperfusion ipsilateral to the ictal focus in 35% of patients and falsely lateralizing information in 10% of patients. In

---

[1]This observation has yet to be confirmed by other investigators.

Table 8.1.   PET findings in temporal lobe epilepsy

Ligand	Physiological marker	Findings
[18]FDG	Cerebral metabolism	Decreased uptake in mesial and lateral temporal lobe (70%–90%); extratemporal hypometabolism seen less commonly
[11]C-flumazenil	Central benzodiazepine receptors	Decreased benzodiazepine receptor binding in mesial temporal lobe
[11]C-carfentanil	Central opiate receptors	Increased μ receptor binding in mesial temporal lobe; no change in δ or $\varkappa$ receptor binding
[18]F-cyclofoxy		
[15]O water	Cerebral blood flow	Occasional decreased cerebral perfusion in temporal lobe (30%–40%)

Note: Studies were performed predominantly in patients with mesial temporal focus. All findings are in tissue ipsilateral to the epileptic focus.

contrast, FDG PET was focal in 80% of these patients without false localization (Gaillard, Fazilat, et al., 1995). These findings suggest that the relationship between perfusion and metabolism is altered in epileptogenic tissue and that this alteration accounts for the poor efficacy and unreliability of interictal perfusion studies, including those in which SPECT is used.

SPECT, which is similar in principle to PET, is both less expensive and more widely available than is PET, but has the disadvantages of lower resolution and of providing data that are not quantifiable (Harvey & Berkovic, 1994; Rowe et al., 1991). The principal SPECT ligands used in epilepsy are markers of blood flow (^{99m}Tc-labeled hexamethyl-propyleneamine [HMPAO] is the most common, followed by the iodinated compounds isopropyl idoamphetamine and trimethyl-hydroxymethyl-iodobenzyl-propanediamine). HMPAO is a lipophilic compound, and 80% of HMPAO is taken up during its first pass through the cerebral vascular space. Once taken up, because of differences in pH, HMPAO loses its lipophilic abilities, becomes trapped, and is unable to redistribute itself thereafter. The relatively long half-life of [99m]Tc (6 h) allows for greater time in performing the scan to acquire the brain images (Harvey & Berkovic, 1994).

Interictal HMPAO SPECT studies are in agreement with [15]O PET studies: Properly lateralizing focal hypoperfusion is seen in approximately 35%–50% of patients, and falsely lateralizing abnormalities are seen in another 10% of patients with proven temporal lobe epilepsy (Harvey & Berkovic, 1994; Rowe et al., 1991). Ictal SPECT studies, however, have proved to be valuable for seizure localization in children and adults (Harvey, Bowe, et al., 1993; Harvey, Hopkins, et al., 1993). In temporal lobe epilepsy, the initial blood flow change at ictal onset is local hyperperfusion, most marked in the temporal tip, followed by a zone of hypoperfusion in middle and posterior temporal lobe (Rowe et al., 1991). Shortly thereafter a more profound lobar hypoperfusion is seen in the immediate postictal state. Within 30 min of seizure cessation, the typical interictal pattern of perfusion can be seen. In patients with temporal lobe epilepsy, ictal HMPAO SPECT—similar to FDG PET—has been proven to localize properly in greater than 70%–80% of cases and also is reputedly similar in extratemporal seizure disorders when structural lesions are not present (Marks et al., 1992; Rowe et al., 1991). There are limitations: To be valid, injection must occur within 30 s of the ictal cessation. The best results are obtained with injection at ictal onset because spread of seizure theoretically may lead to falsely localizing hyperperfusion. When generalization of the ictus occurs, success in detecting a focal abnormality is less likely. When more than one seizure type is present, then ictal SPECT obviously gives information only for that one seizure type during which HMPAO was injected. The ligand availability is very short: There is an approximately 30-min window in which a patient can have a seizure after the ligand is made. The half-life of the ^{99m}Tc, however, is long (greater than 6 h); as a result, there is more time to arrange SPECT scanning after injection. In PET scanning, in contrast, the short half-life of ligands requires image acquisition soon after injection. New SPECT ligands will further extend this window of opportunity for injection to several hours.

Just as it is desirable to excise the seizure focus, it is undesirable to injure a region of brain that performs a critical function, such as motor movement, sight, or language. The current method for identifying the hemispheric dominance of language, the intra-carotid injection of amytal, which effectively anesthetizes one hemisphere for a brief period (intracarotid amytal test [IAT] or Wada procedure), is somewhat crude (Wada & Rasmussen, 1960). Localization of the receptive and expressive language cortex can be performed only by cortical stimulation, either in the operating room or with the use of subdural electrode grids (Ojemann et al., 1989; Wyllie et al., 1988). These methods are difficult to perform and have measurable risk and discomfort. It is noteworthy that markers of blood flow also can be used in cortical mapping. The underlying premise is that increased neuronal activity engendered while a person is performing a task is associated with anatomically restricted specific increases in blood flow (Ginsburg et al., 1988; Peterson et al., 1988; Peterson et al., 1989). In other words, if a task, such as naming words, is performed while blood flow is being assessed, then the areas of brain in which blood flow is increased during the task are presumably the cortical areas subserving that task. By applying this premise, the visual, motor, and sensory cortex can be mapped in an individual noninvasively (Ginsburg et al., 1988). For purposes of epilepsy evaluation and research, such methods can be used to identify higher order cognitive functions, such as language (Pardo & Fox, 1993). ^{15}O PET studies have been performed for some time and have used established paradigms to study different aspects of language (e.g., Demonet et al., 1992; Howard et al., 1992; Peterson et al., 1988; Peterson et al., 1989; Price et al., 1992; Wise et al., 1991). Blood flow patterns during reading of single words, object recognition (pictures), auditory response naming, and word generation are now known and can be used to identify the receptive language cortex (Wernicke's area) and the expressive language cortex (Broca's area). Because of constraints of radiation exposure and the low signal-to-noise ratio, however, these studies usually are performed in cohorts with group analysis. This method of data analysis averages out individual differences in activation. Simply put, all individuals have a Broca's area, usually in the left inferior frontal gyrus, but it is not in the exact same place in all individuals. Advances in ^{15}O PET design and data analysis make possible potential single-subject studies, but these are not universally available. The use of ^{15}O PET to identify the language cortex in individual patients has been confirmed by the converse phenomenon—disruption by cortical stimulation through subdural grids placed for ictal focus identification and cortical mapping.

In pediatrics, the limitations of radiation exposure make these options unavailable for patient evaluation or research. Advances in MRI technology, however, allow for the application of these principles with the use of conventional scanners with fast imaging techniques. The greater spatial resolution of MRI (1 mm–2 mm) and temporal resolution (1–2 s), as well as the ability to repeat paradigms without risk of radiation exposure, make functional MRI (fMRI) a promising tool for pediatric use, not only in evaluating epilepsy patients, but also in exploring normal cognitive development and its pathological variants in developmental learning disorders, such as dyslexia, attention deficit disorder, and learning disabilities. By taking advantage of the paramagnetic properties of deoxyhemoglobin as an endogenous contrast agent, alterations in blood flow in activated tissue can be detected (Cohen & Bookheimer, 1994). Activation is accompanied by an increase in blood flow with an increase in oxygenated hemoglobin, as oxygen extraction is less; the change in ratio of oxyhemoglobin to deoxyhemoglobin results in a detectable change in MRI signal. As a result, while a given section of the brain is imaged every 2–5 s during a task, the temporal organization of physiological response also can be mapped.

fMRI has been used in adults and children to identify the primary motor and sensory cortex, including the primary occipital cortex (Belliveau et al., 1991; Kwong et al., 1992; Turner et al., 1993). fMRI methods also can be applied to mapping cognitive function (Binder et al., 1994; Hinke et al., 1993; McCarthy et al., 1993; Rueckert et al., 1994). Studies in children that used a silent verbal fluency paradigm, designed to activate Broca's area, have successfully identified Broca's areas in 10 of 11 children with partial seizures. When, upon command, children generate a list of words that fall into a specific category (e.g., animals, foods) or begin with a specific letter (e.g., c, r, w) (Gaillard et al., 1994), there is region-specific increase in MRI signal of approximately 1.5%–3%, in the inferior frontal gyrus and premotor areas in the language-dominant hemisphere (Figure 8.3 on p. *xxxii*). Some activation also is seen in nondominant hemispheres, but this is of a considerably lesser extent. Confirmation of these findings is available in six children who underwent IATs (Gaillard et al., 1994). Similar fMRI paradigms have been used to successfully lateralize Broca's area in adults and also have been confirmed by IATs. In 1996, therefore, it appears as though amytal tests to lateralize language and cortical stimulation to identify eloquent cortex may become obsolete.

As with any new technology, however, there are practical and interpretive limitations to fMRI (Cohen & Bookheimer, 1994). Imaging often identifies draining veins, which may be millimeters removed from the truly activated cortex. In addition it is unclear to what extent the activated cortex is essential to performing the function in question. Behavior modification programs to improve compliance in some children and computer software advances to improve the correction of some head motion in the scanner and to compensate for the scan fMRI limitations must be developed. Successful fMRI studies require subject cooperation in performing tasks and remaining still, because data analysis is sensitive to the slightest head motion. These limitations of cooperation and motion are related to patient age and intelligence.

MRI spectroscopy provides another noninvasive means of examining markers of metabolic activity and cellular health in epileptogenic and healthy neuronal tissue. In an epileptogenic temporal cortex, usually mesial temporal sclerosis, the spectroscopy signal of N-acetyl-aspartate (NAA), a marker of neurons, is decreased. The signals for choline and creatinine are increased, presumably reflecting greater membrane surface area (i.e., gliosis); as a result, the NAA-to-choline ratio is decreased (Hugg et al., 1993; Prichard & Rosen, 1994). The inorganic phosphate (P_i) signal is increased, whereas, the phosphomonoester (PME) and phosphocreatinine (PCr) signals are decreased. The decrease in the PME-to-P_i and PCr-to-P_i ratios suggests reduced high-energy phosphate metabolism and, therefore, decreased oxidative phosphorylation in epileptogenic tissues (Hugg et al., 1992; Kuzniecky et al., 1992). These findings support metabolic data from FDG PET studies. Changes in interictal lactate have not been found, and some investigators describe an alkaline pH. These observations reflect gliosis and loss of functional neurons. In 1996, application of these techniques to other epilepsies is in progress.

SUMMARY

In the evaluation of a child with epilepsy, the imaging test of choice is a high-resolution MRI. If structural abnormalities are not found, then a functional imaging study may be helpful. In instances of suspected temporal lobe epilepsy or cortical dysplasia in a young child, an FDG PET should be performed. When PET is unavailable (or the result is normal) or an extratemporal focus is suspected, then an ictal SPECT study should be considered. When the data from imaging and electrical studies point to the same source or side for the epileptogenic focus, the likelihood of surgical success is highest; when the results are discordant, caution is warranted. When imaging studies are not focal, invasive studies usually are necessary, but the probability of surgical success is reduced. When EEG and functional imaging are localizing, the need for invasive monitoring for ictal focus determination may be eliminated; when studies are lateralizing, electrode placement may be directed so as to reduce the extent of electrode placement and, thereby, lessen surgical morbidity and mortality. When this book went to press in mid-1996, functional imaging did not eliminate the need for cortical mapping of function; new applications of fMRI in the near future, however, will make possible the non-invasive assessment of cortical function.

REFERENCES

Abou-Khalil, B.W., Siegel, G.J., Sackellares, J.C., Gilman, S., Hichwa, R., & Marshal, R. (1987). Positron emission tomography studies of cerebral glucose metabolism in chronic partial epilepsy. *Annals of Neurology, 22*, 480–486.

Belliveau, J., Kennedy, D., McKinstry, R., Buchbinder, B., Weisskoff, R., Cohen, M., Vevea, J., Brady, T., & Rosen, B. (1991). Functional mapping of the human visual cortex by magnetic resonance imaging. *Science, 254*, 716–719.

Binder, J.R., Rao, S.M., Hammeke, T.A., Yetkin, F.Z., Jesmanowicz, A., Bandettini, P.A., Wong, E.C., Estkowski, L.D., Goldstein, M.D., Haughton, V.M., & Hyde, J.S. (1994). Functional magnetic resonance imaging of human auditory cortex. *Annals of Neurology, 35*, 662–672.

Cascino, G.D., Jack, C.R., Parisi, J.E., Sharbough, F., Hirschorn, K., Meyer, F., Marsh, W., & O'Brien, P. (1991). Magnetic resonance imaging-based volume studies in temporal lobe epilepsy: Pathological correlations. *Annals of Neurology, 30*, 31–36.

Chugani, H.T., Mazziotta, J., Engel, J., & Phelps, M. (1987). The Lennox Gastaut syndrome: Metabolic subtypes determined by 2-deoxy-2[[18]f]luoro-D-glucose positron emission tomography. *Annals of Neurology, 21*, 4–13.

Chugani, H.T., Phelps, M., & Mazziotta, J. (1987). Positron emission tomography study of human brain functional development. *Annals of Neurology, 22*, 487–497.

Chugani, H.T., Shewmon, D.A., Peacock, W.J., Shields, W.D., Mazziotta, J.G., & Phelps, M.E. (1988). Surgical treatment of intractable neonatal-onset seizures: The role of positron emission tomography. *Neurology, 38*; 1178–1188.

Chugani, H.T., Shields, W., Shewmon, D., Olson, D., Phelps, M., & Peacock, W. (1990). Infantile spasms. I. PET identifies focal cortical dysgenesis in cryptogenic cases for surgical treatment. *Annals of Neurology, 27*, 406–413.

Cohen, M.S., & Bookheimer, S.Y. (1994). Localization of brain function using magnetic resonance imaging. *Trends in Neuroscience, 17*, 268–277.

Commission on Classification and Terminology of the International League Against Epilepsy. (1981). Proposal for revised clinical and electroencephalographic classification of epileptic seizures. *Epilepsia, 22*, 489–501.

Demonet, J.F., Chollet, F., Ramsay, S., Cardebat, D., Nespoulous, J.L., Wise, R., Rascol, A., & Frackowiak, R. (1992). The anatomy of phonological and semantic processing in normal subjects. *Brain, 115*, 1769–1782.

Engel, J., Jr. (Ed.). (1993). *Surgical treatment of the epilepsies* (2nd ed.). New York: Raven Press.

Engel, J., Jr., Henry, T.R., Risinger, M.W., Mazziotta, J., Sutherling, W., Levesque, M., & Phelps, M. (1990). Presurgical evaluation for partial epilepsy: Relative contributions of chronic depth-electrode recordings versus FDG-PET and scalp-sphenoidal ictal EEG. *Neurology, 40*, 1670–1677.

Engel, J., Phelps, M., Mazziotta, J., & Crandal, P. (1982). Findings underlying focal temporal lobe hypometabolism in partial epilepsy. *Annals of Neurology, 12*, 518–528.

Frost, J.J., Mayberg, H.S., Fisher, R.S., Douglass, K.H., Dannals, R.F., Links, J.M., Wilson, A.A., Ravert, H.T., Rosenbaum, A.E., Snyder, S.H., & Wagner, H.N. (1988). Mu opiate receptors measured by PET are increased in temporal lobe epilepsy. *Annals of Neurology, 23*, 231–237.

Gaillard, W.D., Bhatia, S., Bookheimer, S.Y., Fazilat, S., Sato, S., & Theodore, W.H. (1995). FDG-PET and volumetric MRI in the evaluation of patients with partial epilepsy. *Neurology, 45*, 123–126.

Gaillard, W.D., Fazilat, S., White, S., Malow, B., Sato, S., Reeves, P., Herscovitch, P., & Theodore, W.H. (1995). Interictal metabolism and blood flow are uncoupled in temporal lobe cortex of patients with complex partial epilepsy. *Neurology, 45*, 1841–1847.

Gaillard, W.D., Hertz-Pannier, L., Mott, S., Weinstein, S., Conry, J., Kolodgie, M., Theodore, W.H., & Le Bihan, D. (1994). Identification of cortical language areas using 1.5 T functional MRI in children with epilepsy. *Annals of Neurology, 36*, 504.

Gaillard, W.D., White, S., Malow, B., Flamini, R., Weinstein, S., Sato, S., Kufta, C., Schiff, S., Devinsky, O., Fazilat, S., Reeves, P., & Theodore, W.H. (1995). FDG-PET in children and adolescents with partial seizures: Role in epilepsy surgery evaluation. *Epilepsy Research, 20*, 77–84.

Ginsburg, M., Chang, J., Kelley, R., Yoshii, F., Barker, W., Ingenito, G., & Boothe, T. (1988). Increases in both cerebral glucose utilization and blood flow during execution of a somatosensory task. *Annals of Neurology, 23*, 152–160.

Grattan-Smith, J.D., Harvey, A.S., Desmond, P.M., & Chow, C.W. (1993). Hippocampal sclerosis in children with intractable temporal lobe epilepsy: Detection with MR imaging. *American Journal of Radiology, 161*, 1045–1048.

Hajek, M., Antonini, A., Leenders, K.L., & Wieser, H.G. (1993). Mesiobasal versus lateral temporal lobe epilepsy: metabolic differences in the temporal lobe shown by interictal 18-F-FDG positron emission tomography. *Neurology, 43*, 79–86.

Harvey, A.S., & Berkovic, S.F. (1994). SPECT imaging of regional CBF in children with partial epilepsy. *Acta Neuropediatrica, 1*, 8–27.

Harvey, A.S., Bowe, J.M., Hopkins, I.J., Shield, L.K., Cook, D.J., & Berkovic, S.F. (1993). Single photon emission computed tomography in children with temporal lobe epilepsy. *Epilepsia, 34*, 869–877.

Harvey, A.S., Hopkins, I.J., Bowe, J.M., Cook, D.J., Shield, L.K., & Berkovic, S.F. (1993). Frontal lobe epilepsy: Clinical seizure characteristics and localization with ictal 99mTc-HMPAO SPECT. *Neurology, 43*, 1966–1980.

Henry, T.R., Frey, K.A., Sackellares, J.C., Gilman, S., Kueppe, R.A., Brunberg, J.A., Ross, D.A., Berent, S., Yang, A.B., & Kuhl, D.E. (1993). In vivo cerebral metabolism and central benzodiazepine receptor binding in temporal lobe epilepsy. *Neurology, 43*, 1998–2005.

Henry, T.R., Massiota, J.C., & Engel, J., Jr. (1993). Interictal metabolic anatomy of mesial temporal lobe epilepsy. *Archives of Neurology, 50*, 582–589.

Hinke, R.M., Hu, X., Stillman, A.E., Kim, S.G., Merkle, H., Salmi, R., & Ugurbil, K. (1993). Functional magnetic resonance imaging of Broca's area during internal speech. *Cognitive Neuroscience and Neuropsychology, 4*, 675–678.

Hosokawa, S., Kato, M., Otsuka, M., Kuwabara, Y., Ichiya, Y., & Goto, I. (1989). Positron emission tomography in epilepsy: Correlative study. *Japanese Journal of Psychiatry and Neurology, 43*, 349–353.

Howard, D., Patterson, K., Wise, R., Brown, W.D., Friston, K., Weiller, C., & Frackowiak, R. (1992). The cortical localization of the lexicons. *Brain, 115*, 1769–1782.

Hugg, J.W., Laxer, K.D., Matson, G.B., Maudsle, A.A., Husted, C.A., & Weiner, M.W. (1992). Lateralization of human focal epilepsy by 31-P magnetic resonance spectroscopic imaging. *Neurology, 42*, 2011–2018.

Hugg, J.W., Laxer, K.D., Matson, G.B., Maudsle, A.A., & Weiner, M.W. (1993). Neuron loss localizes human temporal lobe epilepsy by in vivo proton magnetic spectroscopy imaging. *Annals of Neurology, 34*, 788–794.

Jack, C.R., Sharbrough, F.W., Cascino, G.D., Hirschorn, K., O'Brien, P., & Marsh, W. (1992). Magnetic resonance image-based hippocampal volumetry: Correlation with outcome after temporal lobectomy. *Annals of Neurology, 31*, 138–146.

Jack, C.R., Sharbrough, F.W., Twomey, C.K., Cascino, G., Hirschorn, K., O'Brien, P., Marsh, W., Zinsmeister, A., & Scheithauer, B. (1990). Temporal lobe seizures: Lateralization with MR volume measurements of the hippocampal formation. *Radiology, 175*, 423–429.

Jackson, G.D., Berkovic, S.F., Tress, B.M., Kalnins, R., Fabinyi, G., & Bladin, P. (1990). Hippocampal sclerosis can be reliably detected by magnetic resonance imaging. *Neurology, 40*, 1869–1875.

Kuzniecky, R., Elaavish, G.A., Hetherington, H.P., Evanochko, W.T., & Pohost, G.M. (1992). In vivo 31-P nuclear magnetic resonance spectroscopy of human temporal lobe epilepsy. *Neurology, 42*, 1586–1590.

Kuzniecky, R., Garcia, J., Faught, E., & Morawetz, R. (1991). Cortical dysplasia in temporal lobe epilepsy: MRI correlations. *Annals of Neurology, 29*, 293–298.

Kuzniecky, R., Murro, A., King, D., Morawetz, R., Smith, J., Powers, R., Yaghmai, F., Faught, E., Gallagher, B., & Snead, O.C. (1993). Magnetic resonance imaging in childhood intractable partial epilepsies: Pathologic correlations. *Neurology, 43*, 681–687.

Kuzniecky, R., Sayette, V. de la, Ethier, R., Melanson, D., Andermann, F., Berkovic, S., Robitaille, Y., Olivier, A., Peters, T., & Feindel, W. (1987). Magnetic resonance imaging on temporal lobe epilepsy: Pathological correlations. *Annals of Neurology, 22*, 341–347.

Kuzniecky, R., Suggs, S., Gaudier, J., & Faught, E. (1991). Lateralization of epileptic foci by MRI in temporal lobe epilepsy. *Journal of Neuroimaging, 1*, 163–167.

Kwong, K., Belliveau, J., Chesler, D., Goldberg, I., Weisskoff, R., Poncelet, B., Kennedy, D., Hoppel, B., Cohen, M., Turner, R., Cheng, H., Brady, T., & Rosen, B. (1992). Dynamic magnetic resonance imaging of human brain activity during primary sensory stimulation. *Proceedings of the National Academy of Sciences of the United States of America, 89*, 5675–5679.

Lee, N., Radtke, R.A., Gray, L., Burger, P.C., Montine, T.J., DeLong, G.R., Lewis, D.V., Oakes, W.J., Friedman, A.H., & Hoffman, J.M. (1994). Neuronal migration disorders: Positron emission tomography correlations. *Annals of Neurology, 35*, 290–297.

Lencz, T., McCarthy, G., Bronen, R., Scott, T., Inserni, J., Sass, K., Novelly, R., Kim, J., & Spenser, D. (1992). Quantitative magnetic resonance imaging in temporal lobe epilepsy: Relationship to neuropathology and neuropsychological function. *Annals of Neurology, 31*, 629–637.

Maeda, N., Watanabe, K., Negroro, T., Aso, K., Haga, Y., Kito, M., Shylaja, N., Ohki, T., Sakuma, S., Ito, K., Tadokoro, M., & Kato, T. (1992). Usefulness of PET scan in child with mesial frontal lobe epilepsy. *Brain Development, 14*, 161–164.

Marks, D.A., Katz, A., Hoffer, P., & Spenser, S.S. (1992). Localization of extratemporal epileptic foci during ictal single photon emission computed tomography. *Annals of Neurology, 31*, 250–255.

McCarthy, G., Blamire, A.M., Rothman, D.L., Gruetter, R., & Shulman, R.G. (1993). Echoplanar magnetic resonance imaging studies of frontal cortex activation during word generation in humans. *Proceedings of the National Academy of Sciences of the United States of America, 90*, 4952–4956.

Ojemann, G., Ojemann, J., Lettich, E., & Berger, M. (1989). Cortical language localization in left dominant hemisphere: An electrical stimulation mapping investigation in 117 patients. *Journal of Neurosurgery, 71*, 316.

Pardo, J.V., & Fox, P.T. (1993). Preoperative assessment of the cerebral dominance for language with CBF PET. *Human Brain Mapping, 1*, 57–68.

Peterson, S., Fox, P., Posner, M., Mintun, M., & Raichle, M. (1988). Positron emission tomographic studies of the cortical anatomy of single word processing. *Nature, 331*, 585–589.

Peterson, S., Fox, P., Posner, M., Mintun, M., & Raichle, M. (1989). Positron emission tomographic studies of processing of single words. *Journal of Cognitive Neuroscience, 1*, 153–170.

Price, C., Wise, R., Ramsay, S., Friston, K., Howard, D., Patterson, K., & Frackowiak, R. (1992). Regional response differences within the human auditory cortex when listening to words. *Neuroscience Letters, 146*, 179–182.

Prichard, J.W., & Rosen, B.R. (1994). Functional study of the brain by NMR. *Journal of Cerebral Blood Flow and Metabolism, 14*, 365–372.

Radtke, R.A., Hanson, M.W., Hoffman, J.M., Crain, B.J., Walczak, T.S., Lewis, D.V., Beam, C., Coleman, R.E., & Friedman, A.H. (1993). Temporal lobe hypometabolism on PET: Predictor of seizure control after temporal lobectomy. *Neurology, 43*, 1088–1092.

Radtke, R.A., Hanson, M.W., Hoffman, J.M., Heinz, E.R., Walczak, T.S., Lewis, D.V., Coleman, R.E., & Friedman, A.F. (1994). Positron emission tomography: Comparisons of clinical utility in temporal lobe and extratemporal epilepsy. *Journal of Epilepsy, 7*, 27–33.

Rowe, C.C., Berkovic, S.F., Austin, M.C., McKay, W.J., & Bladru, P.F. (1991). Patterns of postictal cerebral blood flow in temporal lobe epilepsy: Qualitative and quantitative analysis. *Neurology, 41*, 1096–1103.

Rueckert, L., Appollonio, I., Graffman, J., Jezzard, P., Johnson, R., Le Bihan, D., & Turner, R. (1994). Magnetic resonance imaging functional activation of left frontal cortex during covert word production. *Journal of Neuroimaging, 4*, 67–70.

Ryvlin, P., Philippon, B., Cinotti, L., Froment, J.C., LeBar, D., & Mauquirere, F. (1992). Functional neuroimaging strategies in temporal lobe epilepsy: A comparative study of 18-FDG-PET and 99m-Tc-HMPAO-SPECT. *Neurology, 31*, 650–656.

Sackallares, I.L., Siegel, G.J., Abou-Khalil, B.W., Hood, T.W., Gilman, S. McKeever, P.E., Hichwa, R.D., & Hutchins, G.D. (1990). Differences between lateral and mesial temporal metabolism interictally in epilepsy of mesial temporal origin. *Neurology, 40*, 1420–1426.

Sperling, M., Wilson, G., Engel, J., Babb, T., Phelps, M., & Bradley, W. (1986). Magnetic resonance imaging in intractable partial epilepsy: Correlative studies. *Annals of Neurology, 20*, 57–62.

Theodore, W.H. (1988). Antiepileptic drugs and cerebral glucose metabolism. *Epilepsia, 29* (Suppl. 2), S48–S55.

Theodore, W., Bromfield, E., & Onorati, L., (1989). The effect of carbamazepine on cerebral glucose metabolism. *Annals of Neurology, 25*, 516–520.

Theodore, W.H., Carson, R.E., Andersen, P., Zametkin, A., Blasberg, R., Leiderman, D.B., Rice, K., Newman, A., Channing, M., Dunn, B., Simpson, N., & Herscovitch, P. (1992). PET imaging of opiate receptor binding in human epilepsy using ^{18}F cyclotoxy. *Epilepsy Research, 13*, 124–139.

Theodore, W.H., Fishbein, D., & Dubinsky, R. (1988). Patterns of cerebral glucose metabolism in patients with partial seizures. *Neurology, 38*, 1201–1206.

Theodore, W.H., Katz, D., Kufta, C., Sato, S., Patronas, N., Smothers, H., & Bromfeld, E. (1990). Pathology of temporal lobe foci: Correlation with CT, MRI, and PET. *Neurology, 40*, 797–803.

Theodore, W.H., Rose, D., Patronas, N., Sato, S., Holmes, M., Bairamian, D., Porter, R., DeChiro, G., Larson, S., & Fishbein, D. (1987). Cerebral glucose metabolism in the Lennox-Gastaut syndrome. *Neurology, 21*, 14–21.

Theodore, W.H., Sato, S., Kufta, C., Balish, M.B., Bromfield, E.B., & Leiderman, D. (1992). Temporal lobectomy for uncontrolled seizures: The role of positron emission tomography. *Annals of Neurology, 32*, 789–794.

Turner, R., Jezzard, P., Wen, H., Kwong, K.K., Le Bihan, D., Zeffiro, T., & Balaban, R.S. (1993). Functional mapping of the human visual cortex at 4 and 1.5 tesla using deoxyhemoglobin contrast EPI. *Magnetic Resonance in Medicine, 29*, 277–279.

Wada, J., & Rasmussen, T. (1960). Intracarotid injection of sodium amytal for the lateralization of cerebral speech dominance: Experimental and clinical observations. *Journal of Neurosurgery, 17*, 266–282.

Wise, R., Chollet, F., Hadar, U., Friston, K., Hoffner, E., & Frackowiak, R. (1991). Distribution of cortical neural networks involved in word comprehension and word retrieval. *Brain, 114*, 1803–1817.

Wyllie, E. (Ed.). (1993). *The treatment of epilepsy: Principles and practice.* Philadelphia: Lea & Febiger.

Wyllie, E., Luders, H., Morris, H., Lesser, R., Dinner, D., Rothner, A., Erenberg, G., Cruse, R., & Friedman, D. (1988). Subdural electrodes in the evaluation of epilepsy surgery in children and adults. *Neuropediatrics, 19*, 80–86.

Zametkin, A., Liebenauer, L., Fitzgerald, G., King, A., Minkunas, D., Herscovitch, P., Yamada, E., & Cohen, R. (1993). Brain metabolism in teenagers with attention-deficit hyperactivity disorder. *Archives of General Psychiatry, 50*, 333–340.

9

Brain Structure and Function in Pediatric Acquired Immunodeficiency Syndrome

Pim Brouwers,
Charles DeCarli, and Lucy A. Civitello

Infection with the human immunodeficiency virus type-1 (HIV-1), the virus that causes acquired immunodeficiency syndrome (AIDS), has become a major source of morbidity and mortality in infants and children as well as adults. As of December 31, 1994, the Centers for Disease Control and Prevention, Atlanta, Georgia, had received reports of 6,209 cases of AIDS in children younger than 13 years of age and 1,964 cases in adolescents between 13 and 19 years of age in the United States (Centers for Disease Control and Prevention, 1994); several thousand more children and adolescents are believed to be infected. Although pediatric AIDS cases account for only approximately 2% of the reported AIDS cases, the number of infected infants and children with maternally transmitted HIV-1 is expected to continue to rise (Rogers et al., 1987). Infants and children with AIDS are at high risk for developing severely disabling neurological and neuropsychological abnormalities (Belman et al., 1985; Epstein et al., 1985; Ultmann et al., 1985) predominantly as a direct effect of HIV-1 infection on the brain (Brouwers et al., 1990; Epstein et al., 1987; Sharer et al., 1986).

This chapter summarizes the applications of neuroimaging techniques to HIV-1–related brain disease in infants and children and their relation to clinical neurological, neuropsychological, and pathological findings and outcome.

PEDIATRIC HIV IN THE UNITED STATES

Transmission

Most infants and children (more than 88%) who acquire the infection do so from a mother who is HIV-1 positive (vertical transmission); the remaining infants and children with HIV-1 (fewer than 12%) acquire it directly from transfusion of blood or blood products. Children with vertically acquired HIV infection are becoming more prevalent, even in smaller cities and rural areas, as more women of childbearing age become infected (Oxtoby, 1990; Rogers et al., 1987). More than 70% of the cases of vertical transmission are associated with intravenous drug abuse by either the mother or her sexual partner (Curran et al., 1988; Rogers et al., 1987). Transfusion of blood or blood products to the mother or unprotected sex with a non–intravenous drug–abusing, HIV-1–positive male (e.g., hemophiliac, bisexual) accounts for the remaining determined cases of vertically transmitted pediatric HIV-1 infection. Because the U.S. blood supply has been essentially safe since early spring of 1985, children infected as a result of transfusion account for a decreasing proportion of pediatric cases.

A mother can transmit HIV-1 to her child via three routes: 1) in utero, by transplacental passage throughout gestation; 2) during the intrapartum period, through exposure to maternal blood or other fluids; or, 3) more rarely, through breast-feeding. As of 1996, it has not been determined in which stage of pregnancy vertical transmission of HIV-1 is most likely to occur. Cumulative evidence suggests that the vertical transmission rate via all three routes in the United States is approximately 25%–30% (Andiman et al., 1990; Connor et al., 1994; Goedert et al., 1989; Rogers et al., 1987). These estimates, however, may need to be adjusted because, in a recent study, maternal transmission rates were reduced from 25% to 8% with the use of aggressive antiretroviral therapy with azidothymidine (AZT) to pregnant women and their newborn offspring (Conner et al., 1994).

Clinical Course

The latency between infection and the first signs of HIV disease in vertically infected children varies widely, ranging from children who become symptomatic as soon as a few months after birth to those who do not show symptoms until 7–10 years later (Rogers et al., 1987). The interval between infection and the onset of symptoms, on average, tends to be longer in children who acquired the virus by transfusion, and it also is longer in adults than in children (Medley et al., 1987; Rogers et al., 1987).

Several studies have indicated a bimodal distribution in the latency to onset of HIV-1 symptoms and in the course of the illness among vertically infected children, which suggests the presence of two distinct subgroups (Auger et al., 1988; Blanche et al., 1990; DePaula et al., 1991; Scott et al., 1989). One subgroup, comprising approximately one third of vertically infected patients, has an onset of symptoms at approximately 4–6 months of age, frequent severe progression of disease exhibiting opportunistic infections and encephalopathy (degenerative disease of brain) before the first birthday, and short survival time. The other subgroup, in contrast, develops symptoms at approximately 4–8 years of age or later and has neither opportunistic infections nor encephalopathy in the first years of life. Age at first symptomatic event, therefore, may be an important prognostic factor for rate of progression of disease and survival time and may identify children who are at risk for developmental delay and encephalopathy.

INVOLVEMENT OF THE CNS

The central nervous system (CNS) in patients with HIV-1 can be affected either by HIV-1 itself or by other infections or neoplastic disease. This occurs because HIV-1 significantly reduces the host's ability to fight infection or cancer. This chapter first addresses the more common non—HIV-1–related causes of CNS dysfunction.

Non—HIV-1–Related CNS Infections

Opportunistic infections of the CNS are uncommon in children with HIV-1 infection and AIDS (Civitello et al., 1993; Gayle & D'Angelo, 1991; Krupp et al., 1985; Miller & Remington, 1991), whereas, in adults with AIDS, opportunistic infections are the most common neuropathological finding (Levy et al., 1985; Porter & Sande, 1992). In a multicenter autopsy study of 114 cases of pediatric AIDS, only 11 children were found to have opportunistic CNS infections (Kozlowski et al., 1990). One of the reasons that opportunistic infections are so rare in children is that such infections principally are reactivations of infections acquired earlier in life that have become latent. Infants and children may not have been exposed to these organisms at this young age. Bacterial CNS infections also are uncommon (4%–11% incidence rate) in children with AIDS (Belman et al., 1988; Frank et al., 1989; Pelton & Klein, 1991).

CNS Tumors

Highly malignant CNS lymphoma was the most common cause of CNS mass lesions found in an autopsy study of 31 patients who had had pediatric AIDS (Dickson et al., 1990). Clinically, children with pediatric AIDS may present with mental status changes, behavior changes, seizures, and the onset of focal neurological signs. Neurological deterioration usually is more rapid than is HIV-1–related encephalopathy. Primary tumors commonly are multifocal and occur in deep gray structures (i.e., basal ganglia and thalamus). Computed tomography (CT) brain scans reveal isodense or hyperdense lesions that enhance with contrast and usually are accompanied by surrounding edema. Metastatic lymphomas, however, may be located more peripherally in the CNS and may have extensive meningeal involvement. The long-term prognosis for patients with metastatic lymphomas is poor (Epstein, DiCarlo, et al., 1988).

Stroke

Stroke was the most common cause of the focal neurological deficits that were seen in 10 of 31 autopsies of pediatric AIDS patients (Dickson et al., 1990). Intracerebral hemorrhage, in particular, was common in children with bleeding disorders. Massive dilatation of arteries of the circle of Willis has led to stroke in some cases (Husson et al., 1992; Park et al., 1990). Cells of the vessel wall have been found to contain HIV-1 antigen. It is possible that direct infection of endothelial cells may be responsible for some cases of cerebrovascular disease. Infarctions also may be associated with meningeal infections, which cause inflammation of the vessels and subsequent stroke (Dickson et al., 1990; Frank et al., 1989).

HIV-1–Related CNS Manifestations

Pathology

HIV-1 is known to enter the CNS shortly after systemic infection (Davis et al., 1992) and to infect brain microglia and macrophages but not neurons (Dickson et al., 1994). Release of various neurotoxic factors are postulated as the primary cause of neurological damage (Epstein & Gendelman, 1993).

The pathological spectrum of CNS HIV-1 infection is different in children than in adults (Kure et al., 1991). When examined clinically, children often are found to have acquired microcephaly, and they also are found to have low brain weight at autopsy (Burns, 1992). When a child has had encephalopathy, symmetrical ventricular enlargement and sulcal widening are seen (Belman et al., 1988). Microscopically, the regions of the deep gray matter and central white matter are most affected (Epstein, Sharer, & Goudsmit, 1988). Mineralization of the wall of blood vessels in the basal ganglia and frontal white matter is the most common pathological abnormality (Kure et al., 1991). Myelin pallor is the second-most common abnormality (Burns, 1992). Inflammatory infiltrates and multinucleated giant cells also are common in children with progressive encephalopathy (Dickson et al., 1989; Epstein, Sharer, & Goudsmit, 1988; Kure et al., 1991); these occur mostly in central white matter and deep gray matter, but can be seen in the neocortex, accompanied by neocortical cell loss (Masliah et al., 1994). In children, the pathological manifestations of HIV-1 parallel, in general, the clinical and neuropsychological severity of the disease (Wiley et al., 1990). Finally, spinal cord involvement also is common in children. In a study conducted by Dickson et al. (1989), 15 of 20 spinal cords sampled revealed corticospinal tract degeneration; in 6 of 15 spinal cords, this reflected delayed myelination, but, in the remaining 9, there was axonal injury.

Clinical Course

The true incidence of HIV-1–related CNS disease in infants and children remains unknown. It is estimated that between 30% and 65% of children with advanced symptomatic HIV-1 disease may develop progressive encephalopathy (Belman et al., 1988; Belman et al., 1985; Butler et al., 1991; Civitello et al., 1993; Epstein, Sharer, & Goudsmit, 1988; Epstein et al., 1985; Epstein et al., 1986; Oleske et al., 1983). In European studies that included children with asymptomatic, mildly symptomatic, and advanced HIV-1 disease, incidence rates of 9%–20% have been reported; however, the follow-up of these patients has been relatively short (Blanche et al., 1989; Blanche et al., 1990; Cogo et al., 1990). The incidence of severe neurobehavioral impairments appears to be declining, likely because of earlier and more widespread antiretroviral treatment (Portegies et al., 1989).

At least three mutually exclusive patterns of cognitive dysfunction exist in infants and children with HIV-1 (Working Group of the American Academy of Neurology AIDS Task Force, 1991)—encephalopathy, neuropsychological impairments, and apparently normal functioning. The severity of HIV-1–related CNS disease and clinical findings appears, in part, to depend on a patient's age and stage of systemic disease.

Encephalopathy   Encephalopathy in children with AIDS can be either progressive or static. Progressive encephalopathy may be either subacute, with a rapid, relentless course, or indolent, with a plateau course (Belman et al., 1988; Epstein et al., 1985; see Figure 9.1).

The most severe form of encephalopathy is the subacute progressive course and is most common in infants and young children (Belman et al., 1988; Belman et al., 1985; Epstein et al., 1985; Epstein et al., 1986). Children with subacute progressive encephalopathy progressively lose previously acquired cognitive, motor, language, and adaptive skills. They show decreased gestures and vocalizations and may develop a characteristic mask-like facial appearance with an alert, wide-eyed expression and a paucity of spontaneous facial movements (i.e., a facial diplegia) (Belman et al., 1988). Some of these patients may show increased hyperactivity and emotional lability, whereas others may exhibit symptoms common in autism (see Chapter 6), such as flattened affect, lack of social responsiveness, severe language delay or mutism, apathy and withdrawal, and minimal interest in one's environment (Belman et al., 1988; Belman et al., 1985; Epstein et al., 1986; Moss et al., 1994; Ultmann et al., 1985). The level of psychological functioning of children with progressive encephalopathy, in general, is pervasively and globally impaired (Brouwers, Moss, Wolters, et al., 1992). If he or she has begun walking, a child with encephalopathy may begin toe walking or may stop walking. Many children develop spastic quadriplegia or spastic diplegia, accounting for their motor decline. Older childen may present with long tract signs, such as increased tone and hyperreflexia in the lower extremities and gait disturbances. Movement disorders, however, are less frequent. Eye movement abnormalities are common and include an impaired up gaze and slow saccades and pursuits (Civitello et al., 1993).

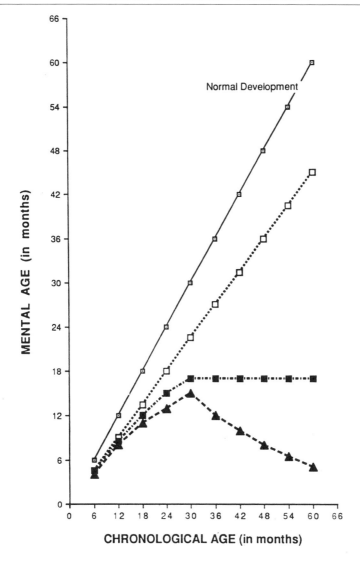

Figure 9.1. Schematic representation of the different encephalopathic courses. (--□-- = static course; --■-- = plateau course; --▲-- = subacute course.). (From Brouwers, P., Belman, A.L., & Epstein, L. [1991]. Central nervous system involvement: Manifestations and evaluation. In P.A. Pizzo & C.M. Wilfert [Eds.], *Pediatric AIDS: The challenge of HIV infection in infants, children, and adolescents*, p. 323. Baltimore: Williams & Wilkins; reprinted by permission.)

Seizures also are infrequent in children with AIDS. In a study of 121 children with symptomatic HIV-1 disease, only 20 (16%) had seizures, most of which were not associated with HIV-1 factors (i.e., febrile seizures, acute CNS disorders [e.g., meningitis, stroke], prematurity) (Civitello et al., 1993). Only 3 of 121 children developed seizures, along with altered mental status, before death secondary to progressive HIV-1 CNS disease and/or encephalitis. In addition, only 4 of 121 children (all younger than 4 years of age) had generalized myoclonic jerks without epileptiform discharges, as demonstrated by electroencephalography, as a presenting feature of their progressive encephalopathy.

A more frequent, but less severe, form of encephalopathy has an indolent plateau course. Development reaches a plateau, resulting in a decline in age-normed scores, but previously acquired skills are not lost. New milestones are acquired in an abnormally slow manner or not at all (Belman, 1990; Belman et al., 1988; Diamond et al., 1987; Ultmann et al., 1987). Motor involvement, particularly long tract signs, is common, and there may be acquired microcephaly. This course may be followed by either deterioration or improvement.

Approximately 25% of children with symptomatic HIV-1 have evidence of static or nonprogressive encephalopathy (Belman et al., 1988; Brouwers, Belman, & Epstein, 1994). They continue to acquire skills and abilities at rates that are consistent with their initial impaired levels of functioning, albeit below the rate expected without their illness (Belman et al., 1985; Epstein et al., 1986). The children's motor impairments (typically long tract signs) are stable, as are their rates of brain growth. Attention-deficit/ hyperactivity disorder also may be present. Initial levels of functioning range from moderate mental retardation to low-average intelligence, and these levels remain stable over time (Belman et al., 1988; Epstein et al., 1986; Ultmann et al., 1985). The cause of static encephalopathy and its relationship to CNS HIV-1 infection remains uncertain. In utero exposure to alcohol and/or other drugs (e.g., cocaine); prematurity; nutritional, metabolic, and endocrinological abnormalities; chronic infections; chronic hypoxia; psychosocial issues; and genetic factors all are confounding risk factors that could account for the impairments in functioning (Belman et al., 1988; Bose et al., 1994; Epstein et al., 1986; Ultmann et al., 1985; Ultmann et al., 1987). In some patients, static encephalopathies may stem from past active HIV-1 replication in the brain (i.e., in intrauterine or early postnatal life), which presumably leads to structural brain damage and then becomes quiescent and inactive.

Neuropsychological Impairments   Cognitive impairments associated with HIV-1 in children without encephalopathy are heterogeneous. Children with symptomatic HIV-1 disease may function globally within the normal range, but some will show more accentuated profiles between compromised and preserved cognitive abilities. Selective weaknesses in perceptual motor functioning (Epstein et al., 1986), gait and motor coordination (Diamond et al., 1987), attentional functioning (Brouwers et al., 1989; Hittelman et al., 1991), and expressive language (Belman et al., 1985; Wolters et al., 1989) have been described. Most studies, however, have focused on a specific disability. Few investigators have conducted comprehensive evaluations and within-study comparisons of the different abilities.

Nonetheless, two domains of cognitive function stand out as particularly vulnerable in HIV-1 infection in children: attentional processes and expressive behavior. Attention deficits and hyperactivity have been recognized widely in patients with pediatric HIV-1 disease. Behavior ratings and assessments have indicated increased distractibility, excitability, and impulsiveness (Hittelman et al., 1991; Moss et al., 1994). In an analysis of the factors of the Wechsler Intelligence Scale for Children–Revised (Wechsler, 1974), a relative weakness on freedom from distractibility factor subtests has been documented (Brouwers et al., 1989). Many children who exhibit these features in the hospital or testing setting exhibit learning and behavior problems in school, and some have repeated one or two grades, despite having above average to high IQs. It is unclear, however, to what degree attentional problems are attributable directly to HIV-1. In a study of children who were HIV-1–positive and those who were HIV-1–negative, all of whom had hemophilia, deficits were found on tasks requiring sustained attention; these measures, however, did not discriminate between the two groups (Whitt et al., 1993). Similarly, in a comparison between school-age children with symptomatic HIV-1 infection and long-term survivors of acute lymphoblastic leukemia, approximately equal proportions of the two groups were classified as having attention impairments (Brouwers, Moss, & Poplack, 1992). Other etiologies, including those related to medical, genetic, and psychosocial variables, therefore, also may be factors in these impairments.

Across several modalities of behavior, including language functioning, social skills, and affect, expressive behavior seems to be disproportionately affected in children with pediatric HIV-1 (Belman et al., 1988; Epstein et al., 1986; Hittelman, 1990; Hittelman et al., 1991; Moss et al., 1994; Moss et al., in press). Speech and language frequently become impaired. Impairments in expressive language are common, whereas receptive language often is only mildly delayed or is normal (Epstein et al., 1986; McCardle et al., 1991; Ultmann et al., 1985; Ultmann et al., 1987; Wolters et al., 1994).

Wolters et al. (1994) have further investigated the specific vulnerability of expressive language to the effects of HIV-1 infection in children, as indicated by parental report, with standardized psychometric measures of verbal functioning that assess the children themselves (Wolters et al., 1995). Receptive language abilities were found to be significantly higher than were expressive abilities in both children with encephalopathy and those without encephalopathy who had symptomatic HIV-1. Moreover, unaffected siblings of the patients showed no significant discrepancy, thereby ruling out the influence of environmental factors. Social adaptive skills and affect also are influenced. Children with HIV-1 may become more socially withdrawn, show loss of initiative and decreased interest in participating in school and peer activities, and have difficulty expressing their feelings and emotions both verbally and nonverbally (Belman et al., 1988; Bose et al., 1994; Moss et al., 1994; Moss et al., in press; Ultmann et al., 1987; Wolters et al., 1994).

Apparently Normal Functioning Some children with HIV-1 appear to be unimpaired when they undergo neuropsychological evaluations and have no neurological abnormalities, even when previous opportunistic infections or chronic bacterial infections are present. Two subgroups may be identified. In the first, subjective changes in psychomotor speed, fatigue, and mood have been reported by parents and caregivers (Cohen et al., 1991; Pizzo et al., 1988). Some of these patients with average IQs (ranging from 85 to 115) have shown significant improvements with the use of AZT therapy (Brouwers et al., 1990). These children, therefore, may have incorrectly been considered to be noncompromised, because their previous levels of functioning may have been in the high-average or high range.

The second subgroup, comprising patients who are not thought to be CNS compromised, are patients who score more than 1 standard deviation above their age norm (i.e., full scale IQs greater than 115) and have no history of decline. In a study evaluating the benefits of didanosine, an antiretroviral drug, these patients failed to show changes in neurocognitive performance (Butler et al., 1991) over 6–12 months of follow-up (Wolters et al., 1991). This may suggest that, at baseline, the CNS of these patients was not measurably affected by HIV-1 infection, and, as a result, they did not show CNS benefits of antiretroviral therapy or deterioration in function over time.

NEUROIMAGING FINDINGS

Structural Brain Imaging

Computed Tomography

Interest in cerebral X-ray CT developed early in studies of pediatric HIV-1 infection (Belman et al., 1986; Epstein et al., 1985; Epstein et al., 1986). These studies, as well as those that followed (Belman et al., 1988; Chamberlain et al., 1991; DeCarli et al., 1993; Epstein, Sharer, & Goudsmit, 1988; Kauffman et al., 1992; Price et al., 1988; Roy et al., 1992), have shown remarkably consistent findings. In general, cerebral atrophy is the most common abnormality. The brain atrophy appears to be global (see Figure 9.2), in-

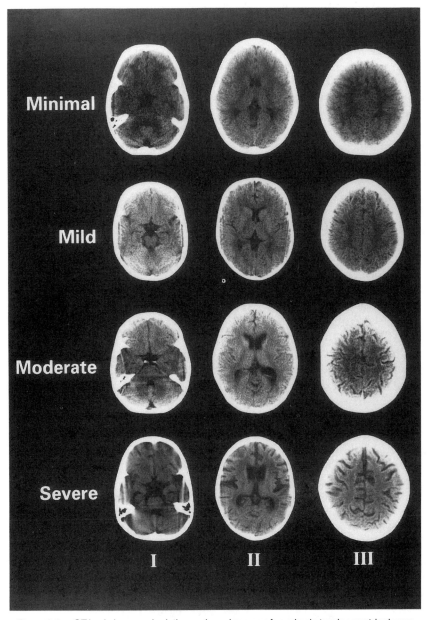

Figure 9.2.   CT brain images depicting various degrees of cerebral atrophy, ventricular en-largement, and leukoaraiosis. I) CT images at the level of the circle of Willis. II) CT images at the level of the foramen of Monro. III) CT images at the level of the centrum semiovale. (From DeCarli, C., Civitello, L.A., Brouwers, P., & Pizzo, P.A. [1993]. The prevalence of computed tomographic abnormalities of the cerebrum in 100 consecutive children symp-tomatic with the human immunodeficiency virus. *Annals of Neurology, 34*, p. 200; reprinted by permission.)

cluding both enlargement of cerebral ventricles and sulcal prominence, although De-Carli et al. (1993) found disproportionate frontal atrophy when overall atrophy measures were mild. Attenuation of cerebral white matter is the second-most common finding and correlates with the degree of cerebral atrophy (Belman et al., 1988; DeCarli et al., 1993).

Cerebral calcifications (see Figure 9.3) occur less frequently and, in general, are seen symmetrically in the basal ganglia and, in more severe cases, in the white matter of the frontal lobes (Belman et al., 1986; Belman et al., 1988; Epstein et al., 1986; Price et al., 1988). Early in the course of basal ganglia calcifications, the injection of contrast agents resulted in enhancement of those structures (Belman et al., 1986; Epstein et al., 1986), which suggests that cerebral calcifications follow the local breakdown of blood–brain barrier integrity consistent with the pathological findings of perivascular inflammation and mineralizations seen at autopsy (Burns, 1992).

The frequency of brain abnormalities revealed by CT of children with symptomatic HIV-1 disease was systematically examined by DeCarli et al. (1993) in 100 consecutive children for whom CT scans had been obtained as part of comprehensive intake evaluation for enrollment into antiretroviral treatment protocols. Of the initial group of 100, 17 children were excluded from the analysis because of confounding coincidental medical illnesses or congenital anomalies. Brain atrophy was identified in 65 of the remaining 83 children and was minimal in 22 of those 65 children. White matter attenuation was found in 22 children and was rated as minimal in 11 of the 22. Cerebral calcification was present in 16 children, all of whom had been vertically infected with HIV-

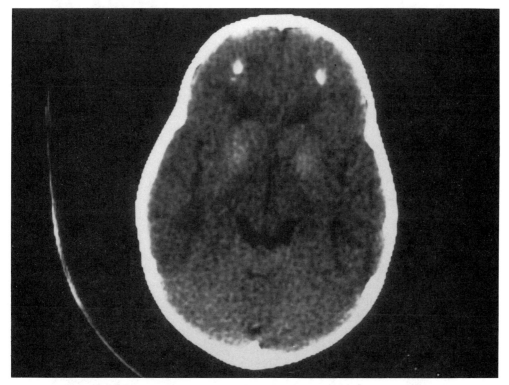

Figure 9.3.   CT image of the brain showing the presence of bilateral symmetric cerebral calcifications in the basal ganglia, as well as the periventricular white matter of the frontal lobe in a young patient with encephalopathy and vertically acquired, symptomatic HIV-1 disease.

1. Cerebellar atrophy, a previously unreported abnormality in children, was found in 10 patients. The severity of cerebral white matter attenuation correlated significantly with the severity of cerebral atrophy, but the presence or severity of cerebral calcification did not.

Magnetic Resonance Imaging

Cerebral magnetic resonance imaging (MRI) studies of children with HIV-1 have generally been comparative with CT studies. Cerebral MRIs were compared with CTs in three studies of small groups of children (Chamberlain, 1993; Chamberlain et al., 1991; Kauffman et al., 1992). Degrees of cerebral atrophy were identified equally in CT and MRI studies, but CT was better than MRI at identifying cerebral calcification, and MRI was slightly better than CT at identifying the presence of white matter abnormalities. The increased sensitivity of MRI to white matter lesions, such as patchy white matter abnormalities (see Figure 9.4), which has been confirmed in a larger study of adults with AIDS (Chrysikopoulos et al., 1990), is of uncertain clinical significance (Mitchell

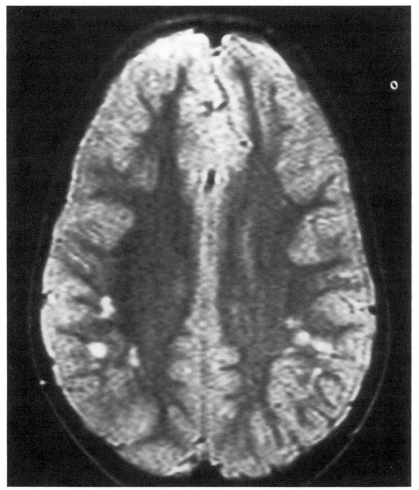

Figure 9.4.   MRI brain scan of a 10-year-old boy with transfusion-acquired, symptomatic HIV-1 disease, showing the presence of patchy white matter abnormalities on this T2-weighted spin echo at a level 7 mm above the lateral ventricle.

et al., 1993). Chamberlain (1993) also found no difference in identification of brain changes between CT and MRI in a longitudinal study.

The above-cited comparative studies of CT and MRI were performed primarily in children with neurological symptoms. Such comparisons may not fully utilize the potential sensitivity of MRI. In an MRI study of 310 children with hemophilia (Mitchell et al., 1993), brain atrophy was noted in only 8 of 124 children who were HIV-1 seronegative. In the HIV-1–seropositive group, composed of children who were asymptomatic and those who were symptomatic, the rate of abnormality was significantly higher: 28 of 186 children had atrophy. In children who were symptomatic, MRI does not appear to offer much more than CT with regard to the documentation of CNS involvement. MRI, however, may offer the probability of presymptomatic detection of CNS infection in children who are asymptomatic or only mildly symptomatic, whereas clinical markers of the disease may sometimes be insensitive to detecting infection in these children. Quantitation of brain volumes and cerebral tissue types, such as gray and white matter, may serve to strengthen our understanding of structure–function relations in children with HIV-1, in whom the direct effects of the virus are the primary mechanism for CNS manifestations.

Functional Brain Imaging

Magnetic Resonance Spectroscopy

Magnetic resonance spectroscopy (MRS) offers the ability to measure various hydrogen and phosphorus metabolites. Unfortunately, as of 1996, the authors are not aware of any studies in pediatric HIV-1 patients. A few studies of adults with AIDS have been published, and these are reviewed briefly in the hope that comparative studies in children will be forthcoming.

It generally is believed that HIV-1 disproportionally affects cerebral white matter, although cerebral atrophy is a prominent manifestation of cerebral HIV-1 infection (Brouwers, van der Vlugt, et al., 1995; Civitello et al., 1993). Neuroimaging findings support the association between cerebral atrophy and white matter disease (Belman et al., 1988; DeCarli et al., 1993). Localized proton MR spectra obtained from normal-looking white matter of patients with AIDS dementia have shown a decrease in the N-acetyl-aspartate (NAA)-to-creatine ratio and an increase in relative choline concentration (Jarvik et al., 1993; Menon et al., 1992). It was concluded that the reduction in NAA is evidence of neuronal loss or dysfunction within normal-looking cerebral white matter.

Phosphorus spectra were examined in brains of patients with AIDS dementia (Bottomley et al., 1992; Bottomley et al., 1990). Phosphocreatine and nucleoside triphosphate concentrations were found to be significantly reduced, which is consistent with the notion of a toxic process that affects brain cell function. This finding appears to be indicative of a process other than cell loss, because phosphorus MRS studies of patients with Alzheimer's disease essentially are normal (Murphy et al., 1993).

These preliminary MRS studies suggest that HIV-1 infection leads to neuronal dysfunction, even in normal-looking white matter. The suspected toxic action of HIV-1–related cytokines is supported by the novel finding of reduced concentrations of high-energy phosphates. Both findings await confirmation and extension by future MRS research.

PET and SPECT

Regional abnormalities of glucose metabolism at rest associated with AIDS dementia in adults were first described by Rottenberg et al. (1987). A total of 12 patients with

AIDS were compared with 18 healthy volunteers, and two patterns of metabolic activity were found: In patients with mild dementia, glucose metabolism in the basal ganglia increased; in patients with moderate and severe dementia, basal ganglia metabolism decreased and was associated with a global decrease in neocortical metabolism. These metabolic patterns correlated significantly with two measures of frontal lobe neuropsychological function. Rottenberg et al. (1987) confirmed these initial observations in a second study that included adults with AIDS but without dementia. Temporal lobe hypometabolism appeared to be more prominent in the patients with dementia in this study, and the degree of temporal lobe hypometabolism correlated with a number of neuropsychological tests of memory and attention (Rottenberg et al., 1987). A third study of homosexual men who were seropositive for HIV-1 but were asymptomatic showed a slight, but significant, reduction in prefrontal glucose utilization metabolism when compared with homosexual control subjects who were seronegative (Pascal et al., 1991).

Single photon emission computed tomography (SPECT) studies primarily have focused on sensitivity to early brain dysfunction in AIDS dementia (Ajmani et al., 1991; Pohl et al., 1992; Pohl et al., 1988; Rosci et al., 1992; Tatsch et al., 1990). Each of these studies showed significant increases in sensitivity over MRI and CT structural imaging. Abnormalities primarily consisted of asymmetric perfusion. In one study, there was a positive association between the decreased blood flow and the clinical severity of dementia (Ajmani et al., 1991). Focal uptake deficits were associated with focal neurological findings in all patients but one (Pohl et al., 1988).

Positron emission tomography (PET) and SPECT studies show early and frequent focal abnormalities of cerebral blood flow and metabolism in adults with HIV. The increased basal ganglia metabolism early in the infection suggests a possible pathophysiological role to the CNS expression of the virus. Motor signs and a subcortical type of dementia are common in adults with AIDS (Martin, 1994). Unfortunately, PET and SPECT studies have not been reported in children with AIDS, although the authors have performed a few PET scans and found focal, as well as generalized, hypometabolism (see Figure 9.5 on p. *xxxiii*). Future systematic investigations of children with PET or SPECT may offer new insights into the pathophysiology of AIDS and its effect on the developing nervous system.

UTILITY OF NEUROIMAGING FINDINGS

Relation to Timing of Infection

It is not known at which stage of pregnancy vertical transmission of HIV-1 most frequently occurs—in utero throughout gestation by transplacental passage or during the birth process through exposure to maternal blood or other fluids. The timing of the infection and the entry of HIV into the immature CNS may have significant repercussions for the integrity of the CNS and could be a critical factor in neuropathogenesis and neuropathology.

Most CT brain scan abnormalities in DeCarli et al.'s (1993) study of previously untreated children with symptomatic HIV-1 disease (i.e., ventricular enlargement, cortical atrophy, white matter abnormalities) were found with equal frequency in vertically infected and transfusion-infected patients. Relatively independent of brain atrophy, intracerebral calcifications were noted in 16 of 87 children (18%) with symptomatic HIV-1. Calcifications were seen only in vertically infected patients in this study and were not observed in patients who acquired HIV-1 through transfusions ($n=26$). In fact, 16 of 58 (28%) of the patients with vertically acquired disease demonstrated calcifications (DeCarli et al., 1993), and most of these were the younger (younger than 5 years of age) patients, which suggests that a maternal factor may be responsible for HIV-1–associated cerebral calcification.

The incidence and development of intracerebral calcifications and the possible relation to the timing of the infection were evaluated further. In a second study, Civitello et al. (1994) rated the most recent noncontrast CT scans of all patients with vertically acquired HIV-1 from the original study ($n=58$). In addition, the last available scan of all patients seen in the Pediatric Branch of the National Cancer Institute, National Institutes of Health, Bethesda, Maryland, who had acquired HIV-1 through a transfusion before 1 year of age ($n=34$) were rated. When calcifications were noted on a patient's most recent scan, all previous scans for that patient were also rated to determine the age at which calcifications were first detected.

Calcifications were more likely in vertically infected children (36%) than in transfusion-infected patients (14%; $p<0.02$), and the age at which calcifications were detected was lower in the vertically infected group (mean age, 1.9 years; range, 0.5–6 years) than in the transfusion-infected group (mean age, 7.6 years; range, 4.7–10.5 years). Of the five transfusion-infected patients with calcifications, four received transfusions as premature infants (at a median gestational age of 27 weeks versus a median gestational age of 34 weeks for those without calcifications), and one received a transfusion at 6 months of age. This last patient was the oldest patient to develop calcifications (at 10.5 years). None of the patients who were older than 6 months of age when they received transfusions and none of the patients with hemophilia had calcifications, as determined by CT scans (Civitello et al., 1994). This suggests a selective vulnerability of the basal ganglia in the developing brain to the effects of HIV-1. It also suggests that the brain may be invaded early by the virus in at least a subset of children with vertically acquired HIV-1. Calcifications in these patients may indicate intrauterine infection rather than intra- or postpartum infection because calcifications developed even earlier in the vertically infected patients than in premature infants who received transfusions as early as 27 weeks of gestation.

Relation to Neurobehavioral Function

A number of studies have examined the relation between brain imaging abnormalities and the presence of encephalopathy and its different clinical courses. The prevalence of various CT findings in the above-described clinical subtypes were compared. Brain scan abnormalities tended to be most frequent, as well as most severe, in children with subacute progressive encephalopathy. Cerebral atrophy, white matter attenuation, and basal ganglia calcification with associated frontal white matter calcifications all were observed (Belman et al., 1986; Epstein et al., 1986). Abnormalities for patients in the plateau phase of the illness were less frequent and less severe. For example, calcifications when present tend to be restricted to the basal ganglia (Belman et al., 1988). For patients classified with static encephalopathy the most common abnormality was mild cerebral atrophy, and in some white matter abnormalities (Belman et al., 1986; Chamberlain et al., 1991; Chatkupt et al., 1989; Epstein et al., 1987; Epstein et al., 1986; Kauffman et al., 1992; Price et al., 1988). It is important to note, however, that these studies may be biased because many patients in this study were referred specifically for possible ongoing neurological events. These data show a strong association between the presence of clinically identified HIV encephalopathy and abnormal brain imaging. Moreover, when there is clinical evidence of a progressive encephalopathy and an abnormal CT, the prognosis for survival beyond 2 years is poor (Epstein et al., 1986).

DeCarli et al. (1993) evaluated the clinical significance of various CT brain scan abnormalities in a study of consecutive children with symptomatic HIV-1. An extensive serial neuropsychological evaluation also was obtained for each patient, and change in neuropsychological function (i.e., deterioration, significant therapy-related improvement) was used to assist in the diagnosis of encephalopathy. All CT abnormalities were more severe in those children judged to have encephalopathy, and all children with cerebral calcifications had encephalopathy. The prevalence of CT abnormalities, however, did not significantly differ between children with encephalopathy and without encephalopathy; only the magnitude differed. A discriminant analysis then was used to assess the diagnostic efficacy of rated CT abnormalities to detect the presence of encephalopathy at the time of CT acquisition in this group. Age and overall rating of cerebral abnormality were identified as the significant discriminators, resulting in a 76% sensitivity and a 76% specificity (DeCarli et al., 1993). These results support the notion that HIV-1 infection of the brain occurs early in the course of disease and often may be asymptomatic or presymptomatic. The potential clinical implications of identifying children who are presymptomatic and have CNS HIV-1 infection remain to be studied.

Few studies have systematically evaluated whether structural brain changes observed in children with symptomatic HIV-1 are associated with specific behavior problems. By using a semiquantitative CT brain scan rating technique, Brouwers, DeCarli, et al. (1995) correlated abnormality ratings with both cognitive and socioemotional dysfunction.

Cognition

Brain abnormalities revealed by CT are highly predictive of cognitive functioning in children with symptomatic HIV-1 before antiretroviral treatment particularly in vertically infected children. CT brain scan abnormality measures accounted for most (more than 65%) of the intersubject variance in behavioral function in these children, which suggests that structural cerebral injury underlies these impairments. Brain imaging abnormalities, such as cortical atrophy, tend to be symmetrical and global and are consistent with the global nature of the neurocognitive impairments. In fact, no differential associations were found between specific verbal and/or perceptual-spatial impairments derived from the IQ tests of older children (older than 3 years of age) and CT abnormalities. Intracerebral calcifications, independent of the degree of brain atrophy, were associated with significant developmental abnormalities and additional delays in neurocognitive development (Brouwers, DeCarli, et al., 1995).

Brouwers, van der Vlugt, et al. (1995) also investigated the specific effect of white matter abnormalities, controlling for degree of cortical atrophy on cognitive functioning. Children with white matter abnormalities showed greater degrees of cognitive dysfunction than did children with only global cortical atrophy. Again, verbal-linguistic and perceptual-motor functioning were affected equally (Brouwers, van der Vlugt, et al., 1995).

Language

In children with symptomatic HIV-1, speech and language abilities frequently are impaired. Receptive language often is more intact than are expressive skills (Wolters et al., 1994). Language dysfunction, both receptive and expressive, was significantly correlated with the overall CT brain scan abnormality rating for both patients with encephalopathy and those without encephalopathy. Moreover, the magnitude of the discrepancy between receptive and expressive language scores was related to the degree of abnormality revealed by CTs in children with encephalopathy (Wolters et al., 1995). Preliminary data also point to the possible significance of basal ganglia abnormalities (i.e., calcifications on CT brain scans) for expressive language difficulties in patients with encephalopathy. In addition, poorer immune status was associated with more impaired language functioning (Wolters et al., 1995).

Behavior

Brain imaging abnormalities also were related to aberrant socioemotional behaviors. A more highly rated overall abnormality on CT was associated with higher ratings of symptoms of depression and autism (Brouwers, DeCarli, et al., 1995; Moss et al., 1994). Similarly, in another sample, children with white matter abnormalities, when compared with children without white matter abnormalities, exhibited more symptoms reminiscent of autism and showed lower adaptive functioning. Activities of daily living, particularly those requiring adaptive skills, and socialization were most affected (Brouwers, van der Vlugt, et al., 1995). The lack of a correlation with immune depletion indicated that these autistic behaviors were not significantly associated with end-stage disease.

Elevated hyperactivity and attention difficulty scores, however, were associated with more normal overall ratings on CTs (Brouwers, DeCarli, et al., 1995; Moss et al., 1994). This may reflect the activity-limiting motor abnormalities in severe encephalopathy. In contrast, in another sample, children with white matter abnormalities exhibited more pronounced attention deficits and hyperactivity symptoms than did those without white matter abnormalities (Brouwers, van der Vlugt, et al., 1995). It also is of interest that, on the one hand, the attention deficit and hyperactivity ratings did not correlate with the autistic scales of the Q sort (Moss et al., 1994) or any other socioemotional and cognitive scores. The autism rating, on the other hand, correlated with almost all other measures, both in the behavioral-cognitive domain and in the degree of white matter abnormality. This may indicate that these attention abnormalities are not specifically related to HIV-1 encephalopathy (Brouwers, Moss, Wolters, et al., 1992; Moss et al., 1994), a finding that is further supported by a positive correlation between hyperactivity rating and immune status (Brouwers, van der Vlugt, et al., 1995).

In summary, in children with symptomatic HIV-1, abnormalities on CTs are common, and, even when mild, these are clinically significant, which suggests that the CNS compromise associated with HIV-1 is a continuous process. These lesions, however, are correlated more closely with cognitive function in younger children with vertically acquired infection than in older children with transfusion-acquired infection, who may have had varying periods of normal brain development before HIV-1 infection.

Relation to Severity and Outcome

The relation between brain imaging abnormalities and disease progression also was evaluated with respect to AIDS severity, which is reflected in a number of markers of disease stage and progression, and with respect to outcome variables, such as length of survival.

Severity

Neurological and neuropsychological impairments are more frequent in the later stages of HIV-1 infection (Brouwers, Belman, & Epstein, 1994; Persaud et al., 1992; Tovo et al., 1992), although they have been reported as the first, and sometimes only, signs of HIV-1 infection in children (Scott et al., 1989).

The most widely used markers to define disease stage or progression in symptomatic HIV-1 disease have been evaluations of CD4 cell counts, as a measure of immune depletion, and of serum p24 antigen levels, as a measure of viral load (Butler et al., 1992; Tsoukas & Bernard, 1994). Early in HIV-1, in the asymptomatic stages, markers of immune activation, such as β_2-microglobulin and neopterin, may be useful and predictive of disease progression.

In an MRI study of 310 children with hemophilia (Mitchell et al., 1993), the HIV-seropositive group (mean age, 13.2 years) was divided into children with CD4 cell counts (a marker of the degree of immunosuppression in HIV) greater than 200 ($n = 135$) and those with CD4 cell counts less than 200 ($n = 51$). Cerebral atrophy was significantly more common in children with more advanced disease and low CD4 cell counts (17 of 51, or 33%) than in patients with more intact immune systems (11 of 135, or 8%), even after controlling for group-related age differences. Moreover, diffuse atrophy on MRI was associated with presumed HIV-related muscle weakness.

Studying the relation between CD4 and brain measures has been difficult in children with vertically acquired HIV-1 infection, because, in the first years of life, age-related, rapid physiological changes take place in absolute CD4 counts and in percentages of CD4. Studies that relate CD4, as a continuous measure, with CNS manifestations in infants and children became possible only in the 1990s, when formulae were developed to correct for age-related changes (European Collaborative Study, 1992). These formulae were used to calculate age-corrected z-scores for CD4 leukocyte measures and to demonstrate that more advanced immune depletion (i.e., low CD4) was associated with a more severe degree of abnormality on CT brain scans, as well as a greater level of cognitive dysfunction. Elevations of serum p24 antigen, another measure that reflects disease stage, also were related to CT brain scan abnormalities (Brouwers, Tudor-Williams, et al., 1995). Previous investigators had reported a relationship between cerebrospinal fluid p24 antigen and the presence of encephalopathy (Belman et al., 1988; Epstein et al., 1987).

The relationships established between the immunological and virological markers of HIV-1 disease progression and CNS function and structure were not discrete and compartmentalized. Correlations between CD4 and neurocognitive measures, as well as CT brain scan abnormalities, were based on relatively continuous distributions of CD4 percentages, the general cognitive index, and CT brain scan measures.

Systemic disease markers, such as CD4 values and p24 values, therefore, are related to neurological functioning, reflected by CT brain scan abnormalities and neurobehavioral impairments. It is clear, however, that these associations do not establish a causal relationship; in fact, the authors have hypothesized that all of these measures probably indirectly reflect the same underlying variable: the progression of HIV-1 disease. Furthermore, the progression of HIV-1 disease probably also leads to increases in the concentrations of the neuropathogenic factors responsible for HIV-1–associated CNS disease (Brouwers, Tudor-Williams, et al., 1995; Epstein & Gendelman, 1993).

The associations between CT brain scan ratings and CD4 percentages were robust but of similar magnitudes for the different types of lesions (i.e., atrophy, calcifications, white matter abnormalities), which suggests a global process. These findings (Brouwers, Tudor-Williams, et al., 1995) support the notion of early viral entrance into the CNS leading to subtle cerebral damage. This study also noted that immune markers of HIV-1 progression, in this case, CD4 cell counts, also may be associated with CNS disease. The relation between markers of HIV-1 disease progression and lesions identified by CT suggests that these CNS abnormalities are associated with HIV-1 infection. These findings further support the notion that the interaction between systemic disease progression and CNS abnormalities is continuous rather than discrete (Brouwers, DeCarli, et al., 1995).

Correlations between physiological markers and neuropsychological functioning tend to be stronger in children with HIV-1 than in adults with HIV-1. This may be because adult patients with HIV-1 are more heterogeneous with respect to previous medical history. Adults also are more likely to have other current (i.e., subclinical) CNS infections and are subject to a greater cumulative effect of the social, emotional, and academic environments on cognitive function over time (Brouwers, DeCarli, et al., 1995). The effect of environment also may play a role in that correlations of CD4 and p24 with CT measures were stronger than were those with neurocognitive scores. It is clear that the relation between immune and viral markers and the CNS is more direct than is the relation between immune and viral markers with cognitive functioning.

Advanced immune dysfunction and elevated viral burdens, markers of disease progression, place children at increased risk for the development of HIV-1–related CNS manifestations. Careful monitoring of neurological and psychological function in these patients, therefore, is warranted.

HIV-1 infection of the brain may lead to progressive encephalopathy in many cases. Clinical decline suggests progressive brain damage, and a number of studies have evaluated repeated CT measures over time in children with HIV-1 infection. Epstein et al. (1985) first noted progressive cerebral atrophy in two children with subacute progressive encephalopathy for whom multiple CTs were obtained. Follow-up studies, which had a median duration of 19 months, showed that of 20 children identified as having encephalopathy, 13 had died (Epstein et al., 1986). None of those identified as being normal or in the plateau phase of encephalopathy had died (Epstein et al., 1986). Similar findings were reported by Belman et al. (1988), who also documented progression of cerebral atrophy in 5 of 12 children in the plateau phase of encephalopathy. In another study, cerebral calcification was noted to worsen with time, as was the previously noted cerebral atrophy (Price et al., 1988).

Outcome

Markers of HIV-1 disease stage can be broadly classified as viral, immune, clinical, and laboratory. Changes in these disease markers have been related to clinical outcome measures, such as survival, and, therefore, can be considered surrogate markers of therapeutic response. These measures tend to be correlated, thereby indicating that, in some way, they all reflect the underlying progressive disease. Neuroimaging can be considered an adjunct laboratory measure for therapy-related brain changes.

Brain changes in response to continuous intravenous AZT treatment, as well as significant improvements in general levels of cognitive functioning, have been reported for patients with encephalopathy (DeCarli et al., 1991). Ventricular brain ratios (ventricular size-to-head size ratios) were significantly larger than age-corrected norms at induction of AZT therapy. In seven of eight children, ventricular brain ratios decreased toward normal, resulting in a significant overall treatment effect (see Figure 9.6). Correlations between the magnitude of brain changes and the magnitude of the IQ improvement were not significant. A second longitudinal brain imaging study supported the original observation (Chamberlain, 1993). A total of 14 children, 12 with abnormal neurological examination findings, received baseline brain imaging and

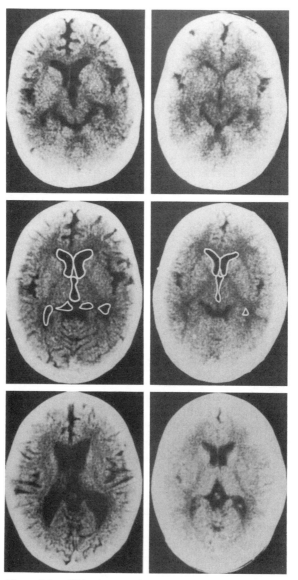

Figure 9.6.   CT brain images before and after continuous infusion AZT treatment that also show the trace technique that determined the ventricular area. (From DeCarli, C., Fugate, L., Falloon, J., Eddy, J., Katz, D.A., Friedland, R.P., Rapoport, S.I., Brouwers, P., & Pizzo, P.A. [1991]. Brain growth and cognitive improvement in children with human immune deficiency virus-induced encephalopathy after six months of continuous infusion zidovudine therapy. *Journal of Acquired Immune Deficiency Syndromes, 4,* p. 587; reprinted by permission.)

follow-up imaging 1 year later. An unspecified number of the children were receiving antiretroviral therapy. Of the 14 children, 10 survived the year. Of these 10, 4 children showed improvement on the basis of results of their neuroimaging studies. Again, there was no correlation between the neuroimaging changes and clinical improvement in this limited study.

In a larger study, the relationship among therapy-related changes in brain imaging, level of cognitive functioning, and immune response was analyzed in 77 children (Brouwers, DeCarli, et al., 1994). The antiretroviral therapies used were continuous infusion AZT, oral intermittent AZT, oral dideoxycytidine alone and in an alternating schedule with AZT, oral dideoxyinosine, and continuous infusion soluble recombinant CD4 alone and in combination with oral dideoxyinosine. These antiretroviral therapies all have differing degrees of CNS penetration, which may affect the impact of treatment on the CNS (Balis et al., 1989; Balis et al., 1992; Brouwers, DeCarli, et al., 1994). CT brain scan ratings were performed as reported previously (DeCarli et al., 1993) and showed no significant overall change in CT severity ratings. A significant positive correlation between CNS drug penetration and improved ventricular size suggested that better CNS penetration was associated with greater improvements on CT. A similar relationship was observed between changes in neurocognitive function and drug CNS penetration (Brouwers, DeCarli, et al., 1994).

In addition, when a subgroup analysis was used, a significant decline in CD4 percentage was associated with worsening of cortical atrophy and neurobehavioral decline. Significant increases in CD4 percentages were associated with neurobehavioral gains but not with improvements on CT scan (Brouwers, DeCarli, et al., 1994). These findings suggest that irreversible structural damage might have occurred during the course of the disease. These structural changes may not improve, despite functional improvements in neurocognitive function (DeCarli et al., 1991).

Cerebral calcifications worsened significantly independent of antiretroviral therapy, CNS drug penetration, or improvements in other imaging measures. This suggests that cerebral calcification, once present, does not reflect disease progression and, therefore, is not a good marker of therapeutic response. These findings also support the hypothesis that cerebral calcifications are independent of cerebral atrophy and may reflect a different neuropathological process (DeCarli et al., 1993).

In summary, longitudinal imaging studies have demonstrated significant neurological improvements with certain antiretroviral therapies, related to their CNS penetration. CNS penetration may, therefore, be important in choosing or developing future antiretroviral therapies, because neurological symptoms are one of the most common manifestations of pediatric HIV-1 infection.

The authors are aware of only one study that evaluated cerebral metabolic response to antiretroviral therapy (Brunetti et al., 1989). Three adults and one child underwent [¹⁸F]fluorodeoxyglucose (FDG) PET before and after AZT therapy. The adults received AZT orally, but the child received the drug as a continuous infusion (Pizzo et al., 1988). The first FDG PET scan revealed that the child had large areas of hypometabolism in the right frontal and parietal lobes, which normalized after 12 weeks of therapy (see Figure 9.5 on p. *xxxiii*). His IQ, which had dropped 28 points before he started antiviral therapy, returned to normal after 9 months of AZT therapy. The adults also showed signficant increases in cerebral metabolism in response to the oral AZT therapy; accompanying clinical improvement occurred in two of the three adults. Of note, a consistent increase in global cerebral metabolic rates suggested that the CNS effect of HIV-1 is diffuse, a finding that is consistent with the notion of circulating toxins.

FUTURE DIRECTIONS AND CONCLUSIONS

The use of brain imaging in children with HIV-1 has documented that abnormalities are common. Even when they are mild, lesions identified by CT are associated with neurobehavioral dysfunction and immune depletion, thereby suggesting that the CNS compromise associated with HIV-1 is a continuous process. HIV-1 infection of the brain, therefore, may occur early in the course of disease and can be clinically asymptomatic or presymptomatic. MRI and functional brain imaging may offer better detection of early signs of CNS damage from HIV-1 infection in children who are asymptomatic or mildly symptomatic. Quantitation of brain volumes and cerebral tissue types, such as gray and white matter, may serve to strengthen our understanding of structure–function relations in children with HIV-1, in whom direct effects of the virus are the primary mechanism for CNS manifestations. The potential therapeutic implications of identifying children with CNS HIV-1 infection who are presymptomatic remain to be determined.

In the later stages of the disease, reflected by severe immune dysfunction and elevated levels of viral burden, children are at increased risk for developing HIV-1–related CNS manifestations. Careful monitoring of neurological and psychological function in these patients, therefore, is warranted, as mentioned. In children with more advanced disease, MRI does not appear to offer much advantage over CT brain imaging with regard to the documentation of CNS involvement.

Neuroimaging also can be used as a noninvasive measure of cerebral response to treatment. Quantitative changes in brain structure and function before and after various antiretroviral therapies have been demonstrated. The degree of CNS penetration of an antiretroviral agent has been associated with the effectiveness of the treatment with respect to neurobehavioral function.

Some evidence suggests that the presence of cerebral calcifications in children with vertically acquired HIV-1 disease, when seen on CT brain scan, may indicate in utero infection and a poor prognosis. Such children warrant frequent evaluation and may require a more aggressive therapeutic approach.

Additional, larger longitudinal studies of the relations between neuroimaging variables and virological, immunological, neurological, and psychological measures may offer considerable information about the neuropathophysiology of HIV-1 and the possible cerebral response to therapy.

REFERENCES

Ajmani, A., Habte-Gabr, E., Zarr, M., Jayabalan, V., & Dandala, S. (1991). Cerebral blood flow SPECT with Tc-99m exametazine correlates in AIDS dementia complex stages: A preliminary report. *Clinical Nuclear Medicine, 16,* 656–659.

Andiman, W.A., Simpson, B.J., Olson, B., Dember, L., Silva, T.J., & Miller, G. (1990). Rate of transmission of human immunodeficiency virus type 1 infection from mother to child and short-term outcome of neonatal infection. *American Journal of Diseases of Children, 144,* 758–766.

Auger, I., Thomas, P., De Gruttola, V., Morse, D., Moore, D., Williams, R., Truman, B., & Lawrence, C.E. (1988). Incubation periods for paediatric AIDS patients. *Nature, 336,* 575–577.

Balis, F.M., Holcenberg, J.S., & Poplack, D.G. (1989). General principles of chemotherapy. In P.A. Pizzo & D.G. Poplack (Eds.), *Principles and practice of pediatric oncology* (pp. 165–205). Philadelphia: J.B. Lippincott.

Balis, F.M., Pizzo, P.A., Butler, K., Hawkins, M., Brouwers, P., Husson, R., Jacobsen, F., Blaney, S., Gress, J., Jarosinski, P., & Poplack, D. (1992). Clinical pharmacology of 2′,3′-dideoxyinosine in human immunodeficiency virus-infected children. *The Journal of Infectious Diseases, 165,* 99–104.

Belman, A.L. (1990). AIDS and pediatric neurology. *Neurology Clinics, 8*, 571–603.

Belman, A.L., Diamond, G., Dickson, D., Horoupian, D., Liena, J., Lantos, G., & Rubinstein, A. (1988). Pediatric acquired immunodeficiency syndrome: Neurologic syndromes. *American Journal of Diseases of Children, 142*, 29–35.

Belman, A.L., Lantos, G., Horoupian, D., Novick, B.E., Ultmann, M.H., Dickson, D.W., & Rubinstein, A. (1986). AIDS: Calcification of the basal ganglia in infants and children. *Neurology, 36*, 1192–1199.

Belman, A.L., Ultmann, M.H., Horoupian, D., Novick, B., Spiro, A.J., Rubinstein, A., Kurtzberg, D., & Cone-Wesson, B. (1985). Neurological complications in infants and children with acquired immune deficiency syndrome. *Annals of Neurology, 18*, 560–566.

Blanche, S., Rouzioux, C., Guihard, M.L., Veber, F., Mayaux, M.J., Jacomet, C., Tricoire, J., Deville, A., Vial, M., Firtion, G., De Crepy, A., Douard, D., Robin, M., Courpotin, C., Ciraru-Vigneron, N., Le Deist, F., & Griscelli, C. (1989). A prospective study of infants born to women seropositive for human immunodeficiency virus type 1. *New England Journal of Medicine, 320*, 1643–1648.

Blanche, S., Tardieu, M., Duliege, A., Rouzioux, C., Le Deist, F., Fukunaga, K., Caniglia, M., Jacomet, C., Messiah, A., & Griscelli, C. (1990). Longitudinal study of 94 symptomatic infants with perinatally acquired human immunodeficiency virus infection: Evidence for a bimodal expression of clinical and biological symptoms. *American Journal of Diseases of Children, 144*, 1210–1215.

Bose, S., Moss, H., Brouwers, P., Pizzo, P., & Lorion, R. (1994). Psychological adjustment of HIV-infected school age children. *Journal of Developmental and Behavioral Pediatrics, 15*, S26–S33.

Bottomley, P.A., Cousins, J.P., Pendrey, D.L., Wagle, W.A., Hardy, C.J., Eames, F.A., McCaffrey, R.J., & Thompson, D.A. (1992). Alzheimer dementia: Quantification of energy metabolism and mobile phosphoesters with P-31 NMR spectroscopy. *Radiology, 183*, 695–699.

Bottomley, P.A., Hardy, C.J., Cousins, J.P., Armstrong, M., & Wagle, W.A. (1990). AIDS dementia complex: Brain high-energy phosphate metabolite deficits. *Radiology, 176*, 407–411.

Brouwers, P., Belman, A.L., & Epstein, L. (1991). Central nervous system involvement: Manifestations and evaluation. In P.A. Pizzo & C.M. Wilfert (Eds.), *Pediatric AIDS: The challenge of HIV infection in infants, children, and adolescents* (1st ed., pp. 318–335). Baltimore: Williams & Wilkins.

Brouwers, P., Belman, A.L., & Epstein, L. (1994). Organ specific complications: Central nervous system involvement: Manifestations, evaluation, and pathogenesis. In P.A. Pizzo & C.M. Wilfert (Eds.), *Pediatric AIDS: The challenge of HIV infection in infants, children, and adolescents* (2nd ed., pp. 433–455). Baltimore: Williams & Wilkins.

Brouwers, P., DeCarli, C., Civitello, L., Moss, H., Wolters, P., & Pizzo, P. (1995). Correlation between computed tomographic brain scan abnormalities and neuropsychological function in children with symptomatic human immunodeficiency virus disease. *Archives of Neurology, 52*, 39–44.

Brouwers, P., DeCarli, C., Tudor-Williams, G., Civitello, L., Moss, H., & Pizzo, P. (1994). Interrelations among patterns of change in neurocognitive, CT brain imaging, and CD4 measures associated with anti-retroviral therapy in children with symptomatic HIV infection. *Advances in Neuroimmunology, 4*, 223–231.

Brouwers, P., Moss, H., & Poplack, D. (1992). Retrospective and prospective studies of the effect of preventive central nervous system therapy on neuropsychological functioning in long-term survivors of childhood cancer. In B.F. Last & A.M. van Veldhuizen (Eds.), *Developments in pediatric psychosocial oncology* (pp. 79–89). Lisse, The Netherlands: Swets & Zeitlinger.

Brouwers, P., Moss, H., Wolters, P., Eddy, J., & Pizzo, P. (1989). Neuropsychological profile of children with symptomatic HIV infection prior to antiretroviral therapy [Abstract]. *Proceedings of the V International Conference on AIDS*, 316.

Brouwers, P., Moss, H., Wolters, P., El-Amin, D., Tassone, E., & Pizzo, P. (1992). Neurobehavioral typology of school-age children with symptomatic HIV disease [Abstract]. *Journal of Clinical and Experimental Neuropsychology, 14*, 113.

Brouwers, P., Tudor-Williams, G., DeCarli, C., Moss, H., Wolters, P., Civitello, L., & Pizzo, P. (1995). Relation between stage of disease and neurobehavioral measures in children with symptomatic HIV disease. *AIDS, 9*, 713–720.

Brouwers, P., van der Vlugt, H., Moss, H., Wolters, P., & Pizzo, P. (1995). White matter changes on CT brain scan are associated with neurobehavioral dysfunction in children with symptomatic HIV disease. *Child Neuropsychology, 1*(2), 93–105.

Brunetti, A., Berg, G., DiChiro, G., Cohen, R.M., Yarchoan, R., Pizzo, P.A., Broder, S., Eddy, J., Fulham, M.J., Finn, R.D., & Larson, S.M. (1989). Reversal of brain metabolic abnormalities following treatment of AIDS dementia complex with 3'-azido-2',3'-dideoxythymidine (AZT, zidovudine): A PET-FDG study. *Journal of Nuclear Medicine, 30,* 581–590.

Burns, D.K. (1992). The neuropathology of pediatric acquired immunodeficiency syndrome. *Journal of Child Neurology, 7,* 332–346.

Butler, K.M., Husson, R.N., Balis, F.M., Brouwers, P., Eddy, J., El-Amin, D., Gress, J., Hawkins, M., Jarosinski, P., Moss, H., Poplack, D., Santacroce, S., Venzon, D., Wiener, L., Wolters, P., & Pizzo, P.A. (1991). Dideoxyinosine in children with symptomatic human immunodeficiency virus infection. *New England Journal of Medicine, 324,* 137–144.

Butler, K.M., Husson, R.N., Lewis, L.L., Mueller, B.U., Venzon, D., & Pizzo, P.A. (1992). CD4 status and P24 antigenemia: Are they useful predictors of survival in HIV-infected children receiving antiretroviral therapy? *American Journal of Diseases of Children, 146,* 932–936.

Centers for Disease Control and Prevention. (1994). *HIV/AIDS Surveillance Report, 5*(4), 1–33.

Chamberlain, M.C. (1993). Pediatric AIDS: A longitudinal comparative MRI and CT brain imaging study. *Journal of Child Neurology, 8,* 175–181.

Chamberlain, M.C., Nichols, S.L., & Chase, C.H. (1991). Pediatric AIDS: Comparative cranial MRI and CT scans. *Pediatric Neurology, 7,* 357–362.

Chatkupt, S., Mintz, M., Epstein, L.G., Bhansali, D., & Koenigsberger, M.R. (1989). Neuroimaging studies in children with human immunodeficiency virus type 1 infection [Abstract]. *Annals of Neurology, 26,* 453.

Chrysikopoulos, H.S., Press, G.A., Grafe, M.R., Hesselink, J.R., & Wiley, C.A. (1990). Encephalitis caused by human immunodeficiency virus: CT and MR imaging manifestations with clinical and pathologic correlation. *Radiology, 175,* 185–191.

Civitello, L., Brouwers, P., DeCarli, C., & Pizzo, P. (1994). Calcification of the basal ganglia in children with HIV infection [Abstract]. *Annals of Neurology, 36,* 506.

Civitello, L.A., Brouwers, P., & Pizzo, P. (1993). Neurological and neuropsychological manifestations in 120 children with symptomatic human immunodeficiency virus infection [Abstract]. *Annals of Neurology, 34,* 481.

Cogo, P., Laverda, A.M., & Ades, A.E. (1990). European Collaborative Study: Neurologic signs in young children with human immunodeficiency virus infection. *Pediatric Infectious Disease Journal, 9,* 402–406.

Cohen, S.E., Mundy, T., Karassik, B., Lieb, L., Ludwig, D.D., & Ward, J. (1991). Neuropsychological functioning in human immunodeficiency virus type 1 seropositive children infected through neonatal blood transfusion. *Pediatrics, 88,* 58–68.

Connor, E.M., Sperling, R.S., Gelber, R., Kiselev, P., Scott, G., O'Sullivan, M.J., VanDyke, R., Bey, M., Shearer, W., & Jacobson, R.L. (1994). Reduction of maternal–infant transmission of human immunodeficiency virus type 1 with zidovudine treatment. *New England Journal of Medicine, 331,* 1173–1180.

Curran, J.W., Jaffe, H.W., Hardy, A.M., Morgan, W.M., Selik, R.M., & Dondero, T.J. (1988). Epidemiology of HIV infection and AIDS in the United States. *Science, 239,* 610–616.

Davis, L., Hjelle, B.L., Miller, V.E., Palmer, C.L., Llewellyn, A.L., Merlin, T.L., Young, S.A., Mills, R.G., Wachsman, W., & Wiley, C.A. (1992). Early viral brain invasion in iatrogenic human immunodeficiency virus infection. *Neurology, 42,* 1736–1739.

DeCarli, C., Civitello, L.A., Brouwers, P., & Pizzo, P.A. (1993). The prevalence of computed tomographic abnormalities of the cerebrum in 100 consecutive children symptomatic with the human immunodeficiency virus. *Annals of Neurology, 34,* 198–205.

DeCarli, C., Fugate, L., Falloon, J., Eddy, J., Katz, D.A., Friedland, R.P., Rapoport, S.I., Brouwers, P., & Pizzo, P.A. (1991). Brain growth and cognitive improvement in children with human immune deficiency virus-induced encephalopathy after six months of continuous infusion zidovudine therapy. *Journal of Acquired Immune Deficiency Syndromes, 4,* 585–592.

DePaula, M.D.N., Queiroz, W., Llan, Y.C., Rodreguez Taveras, C.J., Janini, M., & Soraggi, N.C. (1991). Pediatric AIDS: Differentials in survival [Abstract]. *Proceedings of the VII International Conference on AIDS,* 190.

Diamond, G.W., Kaufman, J., Belman, A.L., Cohen, L., Cohen, H.J., & Rubinstein, A. (1987). Characterization of cognitive functioning in a subgroup of children with congenital HIV infection. *Archives of Clinical Neuropsychology, 2,* 1–16.

Dickson, D.W., Belman, A.L., Park, Y.D., Wiley, C., Haroupian, D.S., Llena, J., Kure, K., & Lyman, W.D. (1989). Central nervous system pathology in pediatric AIDS: An autopsy study. *Acta Pathological Microbiological Immunological Scandinavica, 97*(Suppl. 8), 40–57.

Dickson, D.W., Lee, S.C., Hatch, W., Mattiace, L.A., Brosnan, C.F., & Lyman, W.D. (1994). Macrophages and microglia in HIV-related CNS neuropathology. *Research Publications of the Association for Research on Nervous and Mental Disorders, 72*, 99–118.

Dickson, D.W., Llena, J.F., & Weidenheim, K.M. (1990). Central nervous system pathology in children with AIDS and focal neurologic signs—stroke and lymphoma. In P.B. Kozlowski, D.A. Snider, P.M. Vietze, & H.M. Wisniewski (Eds.), *Brain in pediatric AIDS* (pp. 147–157). Basel, Switzerland: Karger.

Epstein, L.G., Berman, C.Z., Sharer, L.R., Khademi, M., & Desposito, F. (1987). Unilateral calcification and contrast enhancement of the basal ganglia in a child with AIDS encephalopathy. *American Journal of Neuroradiology, 8*, 163–165.

Epstein, L.G., DiCarlo, F.J., Jr., Joshi, V.V., Connor, E.M., Oleske, J.M., Kay, D., Koenigsberger, M.R., & Sharer, L.R. (1988). Primary lymphoma of the central nervous system in children with acquired immunodeficiency syndrome. *Pediatrics, 82*, 355–363.

Epstein, L.G., & Gendelman, H.E. (1993). Human immunodeficiency virus type 1 infection of the nervous system: Pathogenic mechanisms. *Annals of Neurology, 33*, 429–436.

Epstein, L.G., Sharer, L.R., & Goudsmit, J. (1988). Neurological and neuropathological features of human immunodeficiency virus infection in children. *Annals of Neurology, 23*(Suppl.), 19–23.

Epstein, L.G., Sharer, L.R., Joshi, V.V., Fojas, M.M., Koenigsberger, M.R., & Oleske, J.M. (1985). Progressive encephalopathy in children with accquired immune deficiency syndrome. *Annals of Neurology, 17*, 488–496.

Epstein, L.G., Sharer, L.R., Oleske, J.M., Connor, E.M., Goudsmit, J., Bagdon, L., Robert-Guroff, M., & Koenigsberger, M.R. (1986). Neurologic manifestations of human immunodeficiency virus infection in children. *Pediatrics, 78*, 678–687.

European Collaborative Study. (1992). Age-related standards for T lymphocyte subsets based on uninfected children born to human immunodeficiency virus infected women. *Pediatric Infectious Diseases Journal, 11*, 1018–1026.

Frank, Y., Lim, W., Kahn, E., Farmer, P., Gorey, M., & Pahwa, S. (1989). Multiple ischemic infarcts in a child with AIDS, varicella zoster infection, and cerebral vasculitis. *Pediatric Neurology, 5*, 64–67.

Gayle, H.D., & D'Angelo, L.J. (1991). Epidemiology of accquired immunodeficiency syndrome and human immunodeficiency virus infection in adolescents. *Pediatric Infectious Disease Journal, 10*, 322–328.

Goedert, J., Mendez, H., Drummond, J., Robert-Guroff, M., Minkoff, H., Holman, S., Stevens, R., & Rubinstein, A. (1989). Mother to infant transmission of human immunodeficiency virus type 1: Association with prematurity or low anti-gp 120. *Lancet, 2*, 1351–1354.

Hittelman, J. (1990). Neurodevelopmental aspects of HIV infection. In P.B. Kozlowski, D.A. Snider, P.M. Vietze, & H.M. Wisniewski (Eds.), *Brain in pediatric AIDS* (pp. 64–71). Basel, Switzerland: Karger.

Hittelman, J., Willoughby, A., Mendez, H., Nelson, N., Gong, J., Mendez, H., Holman, S., Muez, L., Goedert, J., & Landesman, S. (1991). Neurodevelopmental outcome of perinatally-acquired HIV infection on the first 24 months of life [Abstract]. *Proceedings of the VII International Conference on AIDS*, 65.

Husson, R.N., Saini, R., Lewis, L.L., Butler, K.M., Patronas, N., & Pizzo, P.A. (1992). Cerebral artery aneurysms in children infected with human immunodeficiency virus. *Journal of Pediatrics, 121*, 927–930.

Jarvik, J.G., Lenkinski, R.E., Grossman, R.I., Gomori, J.M., Schnall, M.D., & Frank, I. (1993). Proton spectroscopy of HIV-infected patients: Characterization of abnormalities with imaging and clinical correlation. *Radiology, 186*, 739–744.

Kauffman, W.M., Sivit, C.J., Fitz, C.R., Rakusan, T.A., Herzog, K., & Chandra, R.S. (1992). CT and MR evaluation of intracranial involvement in pediatric HIV infection: A clinical–imaging correlation. *American Journal of Neuroradiology, 13*, 949–957.

Kozlowski, P.B., Sher, J.H., Dickson, D.W., Llena, J.F., Sharer, L.R., Cho, E., & Kanzer, M.D. (1990). Central nervous system in pediatric HIV infection: A multicenter study. In P.B. Kozlowski, D.A. Snider, P.M. Vietze, & H.M. Wisniewski (Eds.), *Brain in pediatric AIDS* (pp. 132–146). Basel, Switzerland: Karger.

Krupp, L.B., Lipton, R.B., Swerdlow, M.L., Leeds, N.E., & Llena, J. (1985). Progressive multifocal leukoencephalopathy clinical and radiographic features. *Annals of Neurology, 17*, 344–349.

Kure, K., Llena, J.F., Lyman, W.D., Soeiro, R., Weidenheim, K.M., Hirano, A., & Dickson, D. (1991). Human immunodeficiency virus-1 infection of the nervous system. *Human Pathology, 22*, 700–710.

Levy, R.M., Bredesen, D.E., & Rosenblum, M.L. (1985). Neurological manifestations of AIDS: Experience of UCSF and review of the literature. *Journal of Neurosurgery, 62,* 475–495.

Martin, A. (1994). HIV, cognition, and the basal ganglia. In I. Grant & A. Martin (Eds.), *Neuropsychology of HIV infection* (pp. 234–259). New York: Oxford University Press.

Masliah, E., Achim, C.L., Ge, N., De Teresa, R., & Wiley, C.A. (1994). Cellular neuropathology in HIV encephalitis. *Research Publications of the Association for Research in Nervous and Mental Disorders, 72,* 119–131.

McCardle, P., Nannis, E., Smith, R., & Fischer, G. (1991). Patterns of perinatal HIV-related language deficit [Abstract]. *Proceedings of the VII International Conference on AIDS, 187.*

Medley, A., Anderson, R., Cox, D., & Billard, L. (1987). Incubation period of AIDS in patients infected via blood transfusion. *Nature, 328,* 719–721.

Menon, D.K., Ainsworth, J.G., Cox, I.J., Coker, R.C., Sargentoni, J., Coutts, G.A., Baudouin, C.J., Kocsis, A.E., & Harris, J.R.W. (1992). Proton MR spectroscopy of the brain in AIDS dementia complex. *Journal of Computer Assisted Tomography, 16,* 538–542.

Miller, M.J., & Remington, J.S. (1991). Toxoplasmosis in infants and children with HIV infection or AIDS. In P.A. Pizzo & C.M. Wilfert (Eds.), *Pediatric AIDS: The challenge of HIV infection in infants, children, and adolescents* (pp. 234–259). Baltimore: Williams & Wilkins.

Mitchell, W.G., Nelson, M.D., Contant, C.F., Bale, J.F., Jr., Wilson, D.A., Bohan, T.P., & Fernstermacher, M.J. (1993). Effects of human immunodeficiency virus and immune status on magnetic resonance imaging of the brain in hemophilic subjects: Results from hemophilic growth and development study. *Pediatrics, 91,* 742–746.

Moss, H.A., Brouwers, P., Wolters, P.L., Wiener, L., Hersh, S.P., & Pizzo, P.A. (1994). The development of a Q sort behavior rating procedure for pediatric HIV patients. *Journal of Pediatric Psychology, 19,* 27–46.

Moss, H.A., Wolters, P., Brouwers, P., Hendricks, M., & Pizzo, P. (in press). Impairment of expressive behavior in pediatric HIV-positive patients. *Journal of Pediatric Psychology.*

Murphy, D.G., Bottomley, P.A., Salerno, J.A., DeCarli, C., Mentis, M.J., Grady, C.L., Teichberg, D., Giacometti, K.R., Rosenberg, J.M., Hardy, C.J., Schapiro, M.B., Rapoport, S.I., Alger, J.R., & Horwitz, B. (1993). An in vivo study of phosphorus and glucose metabolism in Alzheimer's disease using magnetic resonance spectroscopy and PET. *Archives of General Psychiatry, 50,* 341–350.

Oleske, J., Minnefor, A., Cooper, R., Jr., Thomas, K., dela Oruz, A., Ahdieh, H., & Guerrero, I. (1983). Immune deficiency syndrome in children. *Journal of the American Medical Association, 249,* 2345–2349.

Oxtoby, M. (1990). Epidemiology of pediatric AIDS in the United States. In P.B. Kozlowski, D.A. Snider, P.M. Vietze, & H.M. Wisniewski (Eds.), *Brain in pediatric AIDS* (pp. 1–8). Basel, Switzerland: Karger.

Park, Y.D., Belman, A.L., Kim, T.S., Kure, K., Llena, J.F., Lantos, G., Bernstein, L., & Dickson, D.W. (1990). Stroke in pediatric acquired immunodeficiency syndrome. *Annals of Neurology, 28,* 303–311.

Pascal, S., Resnick, L., Barker, W.W., Loewenstein, D., Yashii, F., Chang, J.Y., Boothe, T., & Sheldon, J. (1991). Metabolic asymmetries in asymptomatic HIV-1 seropositive subjects: Relationship to disease onset and MRI findings. *Journal of Nuclear Medicine, 32,* 1725–1729.

Pelton, S.I., & Klein, J.O. (1991). Bacterial diseases in infants and children with infections due to HIV. In P.A. Pizzo & C.M. Wilfert (Eds.), *Pediatric AIDS: The challenge of HIV infection in infants, children, and adolescents* (pp. 199–208). Baltimore: Williams & Wilkins.

Persaud, D., Chandwani, S., Rigaud, M., Leibovitz, E., Kaul, A., Lawrence, R., Pollack, H., DiJohn, D., Krasinski, K., & Borkowsky, W. (1992). Delayed recognition of human immunodeficiency virus infection in preadolescent children. *Pediatrics, 90,* 688–691.

Pizzo, P.A., Eddy, J., Falloon, J., Balis, F., Murphy, R., Moss, H., Wolters, P., Brouwers, P., Jarosinski, P., Rubin, M., Broder, S., Yarchoan, R., Brunetti, A., Maha, M., Nusinoff-Lehrman, S., & Poplack, D. (1988). Effect of continuous intravenous infusion of zidovudine (AZT) in children with symptomatic HIV infection. *New England Journal of Medicine, 319,* 889–896.

Pohl, P., Riccabona, G., Hilty, E., Deisenhammer, F., Rossler, H., Zangerle, R., & Gerstenbrand, F. (1992). Double tracer SPECT in patients with AIDS encephalopathy: A comparison of 123I-IMP with 99Tcm-HMPAO. *Nuclear Medicine Communications, 13,* 586–592.

Pohl, P., Vogl, G., Fill, H., Rossler, H., Zangerle, R., & Gerstenbrand, F. (1988). Simple photon emission computed tomography in AIDS dementia complex. *Journal of Nuclear Medicine, 29,* 1382–1386.

Portegies, P., de Gans, J., Lange, J.M., Derix, M.M., Speelman, H., Bakker, M., Danner, S.A., & Goudsmit, J. (1989). Declining incidence of AIDS dementia complex after introduction of zidovudine treatment. *British Medical Journal, 229,* 819–821.

Porter, S.B., & Sande, M.A. (1992). Toxoplasmosis of the central nervous system in the acquired immunodeficiency syndrome. *New England Journal of Medicine, 327,* 1643–1648.

Price, D.B., Inglese, C.M., Jacobs, H., Haller, J.O., Kramer, J., Hotson, G.C., Loh, J.P., Schlusselberg, D., Menez-Bautista, R., Rose, A.L., & Fikrig, S. (1988). Pediatric AIDS: Neuroradiologic and neurodevelopmental findings. *Pediatric Radiology, 18,* 445–448.

Rogers, M., Thomas, P., Starcher, E., Noa, M., Bush, T., & Jaffe, H. (1987). Acquired immunodeficiency syndrome in children: Report of the Centers for Disease Control National Surveillance, 1982 to 1985. *Pediatrics, 79,* 1008–1014.

Rosci, M.A., Pigorini, F., Bernabei, A., Pau, F.M., Volpini, V., Merigliano, D.E., & Meligrana, M.F. (1992). Methods for detecting early signs of AIDS dementia complex in asymptomatic HIV-1 infected subjects. *AIDS, 6,* 1309–1316.

Rottenberg, D.A., Moeller, J.R., Strother, S.C., Sidtis, J.J., Navia, B.A., Dhawan, V., Ginos, J., & Price, R.W. (1987). The metabolic pathology of AIDS dementia complex. *Annals of Neurology, 22,* 700–706.

Roy, S., Geoffrey, G., Lapointe, N., & Michaud, J. (1992). Neurological findings in HIV-infected children: A review of 49 cases. *Canadian Journal of Neurological Sciences, 19,* 453–457.

Scott, G.B., Hutto, C., Makuch, R.W., Mastrucci, M.T., O'Connor, T., Mitchell, C.D., Trapido, E.J., & Parks, W.P. (1989). Survival in children with perinatally acquired human immunodeficiency virus type 1 infection. *New England Journal of Medicine, 321,* 1791–1796.

Sharer, L.R., Epstein, L.G., Cho, E., Joshi, V.V., Meyenhofer, M.F., Rankin, L.F., & Petito, C.K. (1986). Pathologic features of AIDS encephalopathy in children: Evidence for LAV/HTLV-III infection of brain. *Human Pathology, 17,* 271–284.

Tatsch, K., Schielke, E., Bauer, W.M., Markl, A., Einhaupl, K.M., & Kirsch, C.M. (1990). Functional and morphological findings in early and advanced stages of HIV infection: A comparison of 99mTc-HMPAO SPECT with CT and MRI studies. *Nuklearmedizin, 29,* 252–258.

Tovo, P.A., de Martino, M., Gabiano, C., Cappello, N., D'Elia, R., Loy, A., Plebani, A., Zuccotti, G.V., Dallacasa, P., Ferraris, G., Caselli, D., Fundaro, C., D'argenio, P., Galli, L., Principi, N., Stegagno, M., Ruga, E., & Palomba, E. (1992). Prognostic factors and survival in children with perinatal HIV-1 infection. *Lancet, 339,* 1249–1253.

Tsoukas, C.M., & Bernard, N.F. (1994). Markers predicting progression of human immunodeficiency virus-related disease. *Clinical Microbiology Reviews, 7,* 14–28.

Ultmann, M.H., Belman, A.L., Ruff, H.A., Novick, B.E., Cone-Wesson, B., Cohen, H.J., & Rubinstein, A. (1985). Developmental abnormalities in infants and children with acquired immune deficiency syndrome (AIDS) and AIDS-related complex. *Developmental Medicine & Child Neurology, 27,* 563–571.

Ultmann, M.H., Diamond, G.W., Ruff, H.A., Belman, A.L., Novick, B.E., Rubinstein, A., & Cohen, H.J. (1987). Developmental abnormalities in children with acquired immunodeficiency syndrome (AIDS): A follow up study: *International Journal of Neuroscience, 32,* 661–667.

Wechsler, D. (1974). *Manual for the Wechsler Intelligence Scale for Children–Revised.* New York: Psychological Corporation.

Whitt, J.K., Hooper, S.R., Tennison, M.B., Robertson, W.T., Golds, S.H., Burchinal, M., Wells, R., McMillian, C., Whaley, R.A., Combest, J., & Hall, C.D. (1993). Neuropsychologic functioning of human immunodeficiency virus-infected children with hemophilia. *Journal of Pediatrics, 122,* 52–59.

Wiley, C.A., Belman, A.L., Dickson, D.W., Rubinstein, A., & Nelson, J.A. (1990). Human immunodeficiency virus within the brains of children with AIDS. *Clinical Neuropathology, 9,* 1–6.

Wolters, P., Brouwers, P., Moss, H., El-Amin, D., Gress, J., Butler, K., & Pizzo, P. (1991). The effect of dideoxyinosine on the cognitive functioning of children with HIV infection after 6 and 12 months of treatment [Abstract]. *Proceedings of the VII International Conference on AIDS,* 194.

Wolters, P., Brouwers, P., Moss, H., & Pizzo, P. (1994). Adaptive behavior of children with symptomatic HIV infection before and after zidovudine therapy. *Journal of Pediatric Psychology, 19,* 47–61.

Wolters, P., Brouwers, P., Moss, H., & Pizzo, P. (1995). Differential receptive and expressive language functioning of children with symptomatic HIV disease and relation to CT scan brain abnormalities. *Pediatrics, 95,* 112–119.

Wolters, P., Moss, H., Eddy, J., Pizzo, P., & Brouwers, P. (1989). The adaptive behavior of children with symptomatic HIV infection and the effects of AZT therapy [Abstract]. *Proceedings of the V International Conference on AIDS*, 194.

Working Group of the American Academy of Neurology AIDS Task Force. (1991). Nomenclature and research case definitions for neurological manifestations of human immunodeficiency virus-type 1 infection. *Neurology, 41*, 778–785.

10

Predicting Outcomes for Infants and Young Children by Using Neuroimaging Technology

_____ *Rachelle Tyler and Judy Howard* _____

It is estimated that 10%–17% of children in the United States exhibit a developmental disability before reaching 17 years of age. Included in this category are children with speech and language difficulties, learning disabilities, visual and/or auditory impairment, seizures, cerebral palsy, and mental retardation—all conditions that have a significant impact on the health and educational functioning of children (Boyle et al., 1994; First & Palfrey, 1994). Therefore, because early intervention is critical for promoting the best possible quality of life for children with disabilities, it is imperative that we devise strategies for early identification of risk factors that can provide a basis for health care, early education, and social support services (Aylward, 1992; Beckwith, 1989; Bennett & Guralnick, 1991; Sigman et al., 1989). When considered within the overall contexts of child development and early intervention, a wide variety of existing tools, including neuroimaging techniques, can be useful for identifying, at a very early date, certain risk factors that are predictive of later developmental problems.

In evaluating the predictive usefulness of risk factors, it is imperative that professionals consider the complexity of the developmental process and the multiple variables that can influence developmental outcomes. The following discussion of the models of development and evaluation tools used in the field of child development in the mid-1990s provides the necessary context in which to place the information that can be inferred from neuroimages of a young child's brain. What we learn from neuroimaging may provide other important clues for predicting which path the developmental process may take for a given child (Bodensteiner et al., 1994; Dietrich & Bradley, 1988; Hack et al., 1994; Holland et al., 1986; Holzman et al., 1995; Lee et al., 1986; Roth et al., 1993; Van de Bor et al., 1993; Weisglas-Kuperus et al., 1992).

THEORIES OF DEVELOPMENTAL PROGRESSION

Researchers have generated three primary theoretical models to describe the process of child development: One theory posits that development is shaped by biological factors; another views environmental factors as the primary influences within the developmental process; and the third considers the interaction between these two types of factors to be instrumental in determining overall development (Lewis & Fox, 1986; Sameroff & Chandler, 1975). The biological model is based on the assumption that, at the outset, each infant has capabilities that are inherent in his or her own biological makeup. This neurobiological configuration may be the result of a combination of elements that include genetics, prenatal influences, and perinatal factors. The belief is that these initial capabilities remain consistent over time and that they are predictive of later outcomes. The environmental model, in contrast, supports the position that the nature of the environment, be it negative or positive, is predictive of the later outcome. The postnatal environment in this model primarily consists of parents and their individual characteristics, such as level of education, socioeconomic status, and emotional availability to the child.

The interactive model takes into account both the infant's biological capabilities and the nature of his or her postnatal environment, viewing development as an ongoing, interactive process between the infant and the environment (i.e., usually the parents) (Lewis & Fox, 1986; Sameroff & Chandler, 1975). Much of the research that has been conducted on the follow-up of infants who are at risk suggests that the interactive model probably is the most useful of the three models (Karmiloff-Smith, 1991). The interactive model has been supported by findings that indicate that infants who are at risk biologically, in general, have better outcomes when they are raised in sensitive, responsive, and supportive caregiving environments; this finding upholds the notion of neuroplasticity—that is, infants have the capacity to respond to environmental influences and to alter behavioral responses on the basis of the nature of the environmental input (Beckwith, 1989; Beckwith & Parmelee, 1986; Bennett & Guralnick, 1991; Duffy & Als, 1988; Sigman, 1982; Sigman et al., 1989; Sigman et al., 1992).

MEASURES USED TO IDENTIFY INFANTS AT RISK

In the mid-1990s, historical, neurodevelopmental, and behavioral organization measures commonly are used during infancy and toddlerhood to identify behaviors that may denote an increased risk for cognitive, language, social, and/or motor difficulties in a child's future. Some investigators also have used electroencephalograms (EEGs) and evoked potentials that reflect brain wave activity in an attempt to identify risk status and predict developmental outcomes (Beckwith & Parmelee, 1986; Doberczak et al., 1988; Molfese & Holcomb, 1989; Molfese & Molfese, 1994; Prechtl, 1977, 1990, 1992; Weisglas-Kuperus et al., 1992).

Although neuroimaging techniques are well-established tools for diagnosing disorders in infants and young children (Holzman et al., 1995; Roth et al., 1993; Weisglas-Kuperus et al., 1992), their usefulness in predicting developmental outcomes began to be explored only in the 1980s (Bodensteiner et al., 1994; Dietrich & Bradley, 1988; Holland et al., 1986). Techniques such as cranial ultrasonography, computed tomography (CT), magnetic resonance imaging (MRI), and, more recently, positron emission tomography (PET) have been shown to have significant potential to serve as valuable tools for identifying infants who are at risk at a very early stage. They also, however, have been shown to have the potential to mislead professionals and parents alike in their attempts to predict developmental outcomes. When neuroimaging techniques are used with infants and young children, it is critical to remember that a very young child's brain is a developing brain (Duffy & Als, 1988; Sigman, 1982), and an image of that brain at an isolated point in time may not provide a road map for the developmental process overall (Chugani, 1994; Chugani & Phelps, 1991; Chugani et al., 1987; Kerrigan et al., 1990). This is the case because such an image can neither provide a picture of the environment in which a child is reared and its influence on child development nor anticipate the rehabilitative process or the collateral systems within the brain that may emerge to compensate when neuroanatomical circuits are dysfunctional (Kerrigan et al., 1990).

Historical Measures

Historically, infants and young children who are at risk for later developmental problems initially have been identified on the basis of their pre- or perinatal histories — specifically, on the basis of events, such as prematurity, birth asphyxia, or prenatal exposure to alcohol and/or other drugs (Cohen et al., 1982; Lewis & Fox, 1986). This approach has its foundation in retrospective analyses that indicate that children who have motor disabilities (e.g., cerebral palsy) or language impairments that produce learning problems often have histories of pre- or perinatal complications (Cohen et al., 1982; Lewis & Fox, 1986). As a result, when attempting to identify children who are at risk for these difficulties, investigators have used obstetric complications scales that incorporate factors, such as mother's age, health, illnesses during pregnancy, previous obstetrical history, and complications during delivery. In addition, postnatal complications scales have been used to record the infant's medical complications, such as the presence or absence of respiratory difficulty, infections, and seizures, and surgical history.

Neurodevelopmental Measures

Since the 1970s, investigators have used standardized neonatal assessment scales to evaluate neurobehavioral responses (Brazelton, 1973; Parmelee & Michaelis, 1971; Prechtl, 1977). These various scales have many similarities. In all cases, the newborn is presented with various auditory, visual, and tactile stimuli and is placed in a variety of positions (e.g., seated, lying on back or stomach), and then the infant's responses are noted and recorded on scales ranging from very deviant to optimal. To perform well on such evaluations, the infant's nervous system must be sufficiently mature to maintain some regularity in involuntary functions, such as heart rate and respiration. When these functions can proceed in an organized manner, the infant may be able to exert control over states of arousal, such as sleep and wakefulness, when he or she is presented with various stimuli. The ability to control states of arousal that are appropriate to presented stimuli indicates a higher organization of the infant's nervous system. Optimal performance is evidenced when an infant responds appropriately to stimuli, modifies responses under different circumstances, and, finally, actively seeks interaction with the examiner (Brazelton, 1973; Parmelee & Michaelis, 1971; Prechtl, 1977). Deviant performances, as rated by these scales, are not necessarily predictive of outcome, but they do identify infants who have greater difficulty with self-regulation, thereby indicating the need for greater caregiver input. Although the anatomical correlates of complex behaviors are not well understood in the mid-1990s, techniques such as cranial ultrasound, anatomical MRI, functional MRI, and PET hold promise for advancing our knowledge of brain–behavior relationships.

Another neurodevelopmental tool used during early infancy is the assessment of visual attention (Sigman et al., 1992). When this measure is used, the evaluator presents the infant with a visual stimulus and records how long the infant fixates on the stimulus before looking away (i.e., total fixation time). Evidence supports the notion that infants with longer total fixation times on a given area of the target are equipped with less mature nervous systems. This is thought to be the case because such infants have greater difficulty either making sense of the visual stimulus or making the transition of looking away (Sigman et al., 1992). In the future, findings obtained through assessments of visual attention may be confirmed by neuroimaging techniques, such as PET, which may support the notion of impaired visual processing by demonstrating that the visual cortex and/or associated areas are not functioning properly.

Behavioral Organization Measures

Another measure that increasingly has been used to evaluate toddlers' abilities to organize and sequence play activities is the spontaneous play test. This test has been used with the following groups of children: those who are developing typically (Fenson et al., 1976; Largo & Howard, 1979); those who were born prematurely (Ungerer & Sigman, 1983); those who have autism (Mundy et al., 1987; Stone et al., 1990); those who have mental retardation (Motti et al., 1983; Mundy et al., 1988); and those who were prenatally exposed to alcohol and/or other drugs (Beckwith et al., 1994). During early childhood, children learn by exploring the material world through spontaneous play. The developmental progression includes an increasing ability to make play more complex (i.e., containing more sequences), less self-focused, and more symbolic (i.e., using one object to represent another). Spontaneous play tests generally involve counting play events within a certain period of time, noting the types of play events that occur, and rating those events according to a child's developmental age. Among children who have mental retardation, scores on spontaneous play tests consistently have been found to reflect mental as opposed to chronological ages. No such consistency in spontaneous play scores has been found among children who were prenatally exposed to drugs and who score within the normal range on standardized intelligence tests. Many children who experienced prenatal drug exposure exhibit patterns of disorganized play that cannot be correlated with specific mental ages. In terms of predictive value, a play score that is inconsistent with a child's mental age has been associated with a later learning problem in some studies (Cicchetti, 1987, 1990).

Electrophysiological Measures

The above-described neurobehavioral assessments provide a global view of those behaviors in infants and young children that reflect central nervous system (CNS) functioning. In addition, from pioneering research conducted in the 1960s (Dreyfus-Brisac, 1962), we have knowledge of evolving patterns of electrophysiological activity in different parts of the brain during the maturation of both children who were born prematurely and those who were not. On the basis of this research, EEGs have been used to show that certain patterns are typical of specific gestational ages and that persistence of these patterns beyond the normal periods during which they would be expected to occur may be predictive of poorer cognitive outcomes (Beckwith & Parmelee, 1986).

More specific electrophysiological measures that have been used with infants include evoked potentials that evaluate brain wave activity, such as that reflecting auditory functioning (Molfese, 1989). In such assessments, the infant is presented with an auditory stimulus, the interval between the presentation of the stimulus and the appearance of appropriate brain wave activity is measured, and whether appropriate brain wave activity occurs is noted. With the use of a specialized test to evaluate auditory evoked responses (or auditory evoked potentials) that are recorded from the temporal lobe, the ability of an infant to discriminate between speech and nonspeech auditory stimuli has been correlated with his or her speech and language development at 3 years of age (Molfese, 1989; Molfese & Molfese, 1994).

In addition, quantitative EEG (q EEG) has allowed investigators to begin mapping areas of neuroanatomical functioning as it translates into cortical surface activity. Rather than examining potential brain activity by imaging the metabolism of injected radioisotopes, investigations use q EEG to analyze electrophysiological activity to determine relative differences in activity. Most investigators, however, describe findings as they relate to conditions such as psychiatric disorders and learning disabilities. Although no investigations into the ability of qEEG analyses to predict developmental or cognitive outcomes in children had been performed when this book went to press in 1996 (Duffy, 1994), this technique may prove useful as we move toward a better understanding of the relationships between these measures and outcomes.

Environmental Measures

Measures of the home environment range from evaluations of maternal education, marital status, and socioeconomic status (Hollingshead, 1975) to the Home Observation for Measurement of the Environment inventory, which is a yes/no checklist completed in the home setting (Caldwell & Bradley, 1984), and to scales for rating in-home observations of various caregiving behaviors (Ainsworth, 1976; Egeland & Sroufe, 1981). Evaluations of the home environment during early infancy have been shown to be critical in predicting later cognitive abilities and school performance among children who are at risk biologically (Cohen & Parmelee, 1983; Sigman et al., 1989; Sigman et al., 1992).

Another postnatal/environmental factor that must be considered in any attempt to predict outcomes—regardless of whether biological risk is involved—is the nature of the attachment between the primary caregiver (usually the mother) and the infant. The fundamental basis of an infant's future optimal development is a secure attachment to a caregiver (Bowlby, 1969), who must be accessible and responsive to the infant's needs. When this basis has been established, the infant is emotionally available for stimulation from and exploration of the environment (Ainsworth, 1979). Measures that have been used to evaluate attachment/caregiving include observations of mother–infant face-to-face behaviors in a laboratory setting to assess mothers' contingent responses or sensitivity to infants' cues (Tronick & Weinberg, 1990) and observations of children's attachment behaviors toward their mothers in a laboratory setting (Ainsworth et al., 1978). Studies of typically developing, full-term infants have shown that those infants who have secure attachments with their primary caregivers score better on developmental tests and measures of language ability at 2 years of age than do those who do not have secure attachments (Matas et al., 1978). Moreover, studies have shown that infants who were born prematurely (i.e., infants at risk biologically), and who subsequently experienced sensitive caregiving early in life, were more advanced developmentally at 12 years of age than were those who did not experience such nurturing environments (Cohen et al., 1992).

Neuroimaging Measures

Neuroimaging techniques, such as ultrasonography, CT, MRI, and PET, also have been widely used in infants and young children (Chugani & Phelps, 1991; Chugani et al., 1987; Fitzhardinge et al., 1981; Hack et al., 1994; Lee et al., 1986). Ultrasonography has been used more widely with newborns, whereas CT, MRI, and PET have been used more commonly with older infants and children (Barnes, 1992). Static conditions, including structural lesions, such as intracranial hemorrhages, strokes, and tumors, can be identified through ultrasonography, CT, and MRI. MRI, on the one hand, identifies such lesions with greater clarity than do the other two techniques (Gelfand, 1989). PET, on the other hand, has an advantage over CT and MRI in that it yields an image of brain metabolism. A brief overview of ultrasonography is presented in this chapter. For discussions of CT, MRI, and PET, see Chapter 2.

Ultrasonography

Ultrasonography involves the use of a transducer to convert electrical activity into ultrasonic energy and vice versa. The transducer, a device that uses a high-frequency energy wave, moves particles so that they vibrate in a uniform fashion. When the energy
is directed to an area in which no tissue is present, as in the case of fluid, no sound
waves are propagated. When tissue is present, the waves reflect toward the source,
and juxtaposed tissues that vibrate in a like fashion form a cohesive unit, producing
what appears as a structure or image on the monitor or screen (Noce, 1990). As a
screening tool, ultrasonography can be used to visualize infant CNS structures, such
as the cerebral hemispheres, ventricles, midline structures (e.g., the corpus callosum),
and cerebellum. After an infant reaches approximately 6 months of age, the growth of
his or her CNS renders ultrasonography a less effective measure because the anterior
fontanelle, which provides the "window" for the ultrasound examination, begins to
close (Barnes, 1992).

In fetuses and young infants, ultrasonography has been used extensively since
the 1970s to examine the CNS, which is composed of tissues with varying densities
that vibrate at varying rates (Dixon & Bejar, 1989; Hack et al., 1994; Roth et al., 1993;
Synnes et al., 1994; Weisglas-Kuperus et al., 1992). In fetal screening, ultrasound provides images of structures such as the spinal column and of head size (see Figure 10.1).
Furthermore, ultrasound remains the best method for gaining a view of intracranial
hemorrhages, cysts, and large malformations, such as missing structures and enlarged
ventricles, in newborns. In general, ultrasound examinations are performed on infants
who are at risk for CNS lesions as a result of premature birth, perinatal asphyxia (lack
of oxygen), and/or congenital anomalies (because an anomaly in one organ system
prompts clinicians to examine other systems). The procedure can be performed without administering sedatives or removing the infant from the newborn nursery.

PREDICTING OUTCOMES

Even before neuroimaging techniques became available for research and clinical use,
considerable information was available regarding the effectiveness of measures taken
during infancy in predicting outcomes for children who were considered to be at risk
on the basis of their medical histories (Cohen et al., 1982; Parmelee et al., 1994). Since
the mid-1970s, for example, investigators have approached outcome assessments in infants with perinatal histories of premature birth through various measures and have
described outcomes as they relate to medical and early neurobiological factors in combination with environmental factors (Beckwith, 1989; Duffy & Als, 1988; Lewis & Fox,
1986; Sigman, 1982; Sigman et al., 1992). A similar process has occurred in the study
of infants with histories of prenatal exposure to alcohol and/or other drugs (Azuma &
Chasnoff, 1993; Beckwith et al., 1994; Brooks-Gunn et al., 1994; Howard, 1994; Howard
et al., 1995; Rodning et al., 1989). With the advent of neuroimaging technology, researchers have begun to combine neuroimaging techniques with these other measures
to identify risk factors more clearly and, thereby, improve our ability to predict developmental outcomes.

Predicting Outcomes for
Children Who Were Born Prematurely

Advances in neonatal intensive care unit technology have enabled pediatricians to provide successful medical interventions for increasing numbers of premature babies, in-

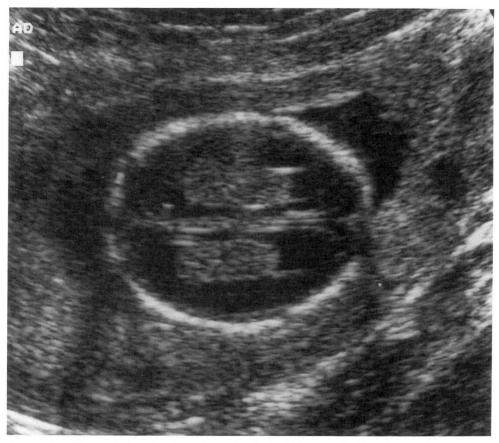

Figure 10.1.   Ultrasound of a typical fetus at gestational age of 16–17 weeks. The white oval is the skull, and the dark areas within the oval area are the cerebral hemispheres.

cluding infants with very low birth weights. We know that, compared with full-term birth, premature birth often is associated with a greater risk for complications such as hemorrhages to the infant's brain. Moreover, premature infants, as a group, have an increased incidence of neurological problems (e.g., cerebral palsy) and cognitive or learning difficulties as they progress through childhood (Hack et al., 1994).

In a study of 79 infants who were born prematurely, had a mean gestational age of 30 weeks (normal gestation is between 37 and 42 weeks) and a mean birth weight of 1,136 grams (approximately 2.5 pounds), and were free of major congenital anomalies, Weisglas-Kuperus et al. (1992) examined the association of cerebral ultrasonography findings, neonatal neurological evaluations, and perinatal conditions with outcomes at 3.6 years of age. Each newborn underwent a cranial ultrasound examination and a neo-natal neurological evaluation, and neurological and neurodevelopmental (cognitive) assessments were conducted at 3.6 years of age. The study found that those children who, as newborns, had abnormal neurological examinations, as well as enlarged ven-tricles and severe bleeding in the brain, which extended into the white matter, as shown by ultrasonographic evaluation, had a much higher incidence of neurological abnormalities at 3.6 years of age. Those children whose ultrasonographic evaluations did not show enlarged ventricles or bleeding into the white matter, whether additional ultrasonographic findings were normal or abnormal, were neurologically intact at 3.6 years. Although bleeding into the white matter and enlarged ventricles were associated with later neurological impairment, no significant relationship was found between neonatal cerebral ultrasound findings and intelligence at 3.6 years of age. Therefore, findings obtained from ultrasound were helpful in defining *groups* of children who were at low, intermediate, and high risk for later neurological deficits. Neither neurological nor cognitive outcomes, however, could be predicted accurately for *individual* children, and a great deal of variance in neurological and cognitive outcomes could not be explained on the basis of neonatal ultrasound examination. In conclusion, neonatal ultrasound examinations were most predictive when they were considered in combination with another measure—newborn neurological evaluation.

In another longitudinal study in which ultrasonography was used to examine infants who had been born prematurely from birth to 8 years of age, Roth et al. (1993) followed 206 children who were born at gestational ages of less than 33 weeks and who either had a birth weight of less than 1,250 grams (approximately 2.75 pounds) or required mechanical ventilation. In this study, ultrasonographic findings that indicated enlarged ventricles and bleeding into the white matter/cerebral atrophy, combined with a history of mechanical ventilation, were significant predictors of both neurological and cognitive disabilities. Moreover, independent of ultrasonographic findings, infants who required mechanical ventilation performed more poorly on language tasks at 8 years of age than did those who did not require mechanical ventilation. As in the previous study, ultrasonography was most predictive when it was considered in combination with other measures—in this case, medical history of mechanical ventilation.

Finally, in a longitudinal study in which neuroimaging techniques were used to predict outcomes in infants who were born prematurely with very low birth weights, Hack et al. (1994) assessed outcomes in school-age children as they related to maternal risk factors, neonatal complications, and cerebral ultrasonography results. These investigators studied 68 children with birth weights of less than 750 grams (approximately 1.65 pounds) and compared them with 65 children who had birth weights between 750 grams and 1,499 grams (approximately 3.30 pounds) and with 61 children who were born full-term at normal birth weights (weights between 2,700 grams [approximately 5.95 pounds] and 3,900 grams [approximately 8.59 pounds]). They found that infants who had major cerebral abnormalities (bleeding into the white matter or cerebral atrophy), as revealed by ultrasonography, as well as oxygen dependence for at least 36 weeks past corrected gestational age, were more likely to be identified as having mental retardation at school age, regardless of social risk factors. Major ultrasonographic abnormalities also were associated with cerebral palsy, and infants who were oxygen dependent for at least 36 weeks past corrected gestational age were more likely to have visual impairments at 6–7 years of age, compared with infants who were not oxygen dependent for this extended period. The authors concluded that, although outcomes in school-age children were related to both biological and social risk factors, major developmental outcomes (e.g., mental retardation, cerebral palsy) were associated more closely with neonatal complications than with social disadvantage among this population of very low birth weight children. Therefore, in this study, in those infants with the lowest birth weights, medical measures (i.e., ultrasonographic findings, oxygen dependency) were more predictive in determining outcomes than were social risk factors, such as maternal age, education, and socioeconomic status.

These three longitudinal studies begin to provide clarification about the use-fulness of neonatal ultrasonographic evaluations in predicting developmental out-come. It appears that a static picture that shows enlarged ventricles, as well as evi-dence of bleeding into the adjacent brain matter, is highly predictive of future neurological problems, such as cerebral palsy. Ultrasonographic findings are not, how-ever, as predictive of later intellectual functioning. One reason may be that these stud-ies contain no reports of environmental influences beyond the mother's level of educa-tion and socioeconomic status. They do not take into account early maternal caregiving or the early interaction between the primary caregiver and infant, which have been shown to have an effect on cognitive functioning (Beckwith & Parmelee, 1986; Sigman et al., 1989; Sigman et al., 1992).

Predicting Outcomes for Children Who Were Prenatally Exposed to Alcohol and/or Other Drugs

Prenatal exposure to alcohol and/or other drugs has been recognized as a medical prob-lem since the 1960s (Finnegan, 1981; Finnegan et al., 1975; Jones & Smith, 1973; Jones et al., 1973; Smith, 1979; Wilson et al., 1979). Only since the mid- to late 1980s, how-ever, have researchers and clinicians sought to take a closer look at outcomes for these children beyond infancy. As a result of the widespread cocaine abuse that emerged in the United States during the mid-1980s, women of childbearing age have come to rep-resent a growing population of drug abusers; this increase in the number of female substance abusers has resulted in the rise in the number of infants who are identified as having been prenatally exposed to alcohol and/or other drugs (Chasnoff, 1988; Vega et al., 1993). As these numbers have risen, concern has grown regarding medical, neu-rological, cognitive, and social outcomes for these children as they progress through childhood and into adulthood. Correspondingly, increasing numbers of investigators have turned their attention toward evaluation and follow-up of these infants and chil-dren from both medical and developmental standpoints (Azuma & Chasnoff, 1993; Beckwith et al., 1994; Billman et al., 1991; Bingol et al., 1987; Chasnoff et al., 1992; Chasnoff et al., 1989; Hadeed & Siegel, 1989; Handler et al., 1991; Howard, 1994; How-ard et al., 1995; Rodning et al., 1989; Young et al., 1992).

The predictive validity of neuroimaging for children who were prenatally exposed to alcohol and/or other drugs is less clear than is that for infants who were born prema-turely and without prenatal substance exposure. This discrepancy exists largely be-cause investigators only began to study this population on a longitudinal basis in the 1980s. When this book went to press in 1996, longitudinal studies had yet to be under-taken to examine findings obtained through neuroimaging as they relate to long-term neurological or intellectual outcomes. A few investigators, however, had begun to de-scribe early findings determined by neuroimaging techniques.

One of the first of these studies examined in utero 43 fetuses exposed to cocaine (Mitchell et al., 1988). When the investigators measured the biparietal diameters of the heads by using ultrasound in these fetuses, they found that approximately 46% of the fetuses exposed to substances had suboptimal head growth compared with the fetuses of mothers who did not abuse substances. Many studies have confirmed the finding of small head sizes in infants who were prenatally exposed to heroin and/or methadone (Lifschitz et al., 1985; Vargas et al., 1975), cocaine (Azuma & Chasnoff, 1993; Chasnoff et al., 1992; Coles et al., 1991; Handler et al., 1991; Howard et al., 1995; Zuckerman et al., 1989), and alcohol (Bingol et al., 1987; Day & Richardson, 1991). The finding is significant in that it is recognized that head circumference reflects brain growth, which can be a predictor of future intellectual development (Dorman, 1991).

In another study, Dixon and Bejar (1989) used ultrasonography to investigate 74 full-term newborns who were prenatally exposed to substances (cocaine, methamphetamine) and 87 infants who were not prenatally exposed to substances. They found cranial abnormalities in 31.5% of the infants who were prenatally exposed to drugs, compared with 5.3% of infants who were not exposed to drugs. These abnormalities consisted of intraventricular hemorrhages and signs of necrosis and cavitary lesions in the basal ganglia, frontal lobes, and posterior fossa—areas of the brain that subserve motor function and cognition.

Heier et al. (1991) used ultrasonography, CT, and MRI to evaluate 43 newborns who were prenatally exposed to cocaine and 62 newborns who were not prenatally exposed to alcohol and/or other drugs. Ultrasound was used as a screening method, followed by CT or MRI to obtain images with higher resolution of structural abnormalities identified through ultrasound. Heier et al. (1991) found that 17% of the infants who were prenatally exposed to alcohol and/or other drugs had cortical infarctions, compared with 2% of the infants who had not been prenatally exposed to drugs. Of the newborns who had been prenatally exposed to cocaine, 12% also had midline defects compared with 0% of infants who had not been prenatally exposed to alcohol and/or other drugs. Although the children who were enrolled in these neuroimaging studies as newborns were not followed over the long term with respect to cognitive development or school performance, the presence of such abnormal findings during the neonatal period may indicate an increased risk for neurological or developmental difficulties (including learning and/or attention problems) as the youngsters progress through childhood.

Qualitative PET also has been used to assess brain metabolism among children who were prenatally exposed to substances. One pilot study evaluated six preschool-age children who had been prenatally exposed to phencyclidine (PCP, a synthetic hallucinogenic drug originally developed for use as an anesthetic) and who had been followed since birth in connection with a larger study (Tyler et al., 1993). As in most cases of prenatal substance exposure, all of the children had been exposed to multiple substances, including cocaine, alcohol, and nicotine, in addition to the mothers' primary substance of abuse (PCP). At the time of this pilot, in 1993, PET was approved for research involving children with histories of speech and language difficulty or cognitive delay, and functional MRI had not yet become available at the institution at which the research was conducted. The six children chosen for the pilot study exhibited global developmental delay or speech and language delay based on standardized developmental evaluations performed at 2 years of age. All six children had been born full-term and experienced no perinatal complications other than the history of prenatal drug exposure.

Within the pilot study, when the children ranged in age from 4 to 6 years, the children were assessed with the use of a standardized developmental test, measurement of growth parameters, and PET. In addition, mothers/caregivers were interviewed regarding the children's behaviors both at home and in their school/preschool settings. Through qualitative analyses of the PET scans, three of the six children were found to have right frontal lobe hypometabolism (see Figure 10.2. on p. *xxxiii*). All three of these children had normal head circumferences and developmental quotients within the low to normal range. Two of the three youngsters had problems sustaining attention, as determined by their behavior during the developmental evaluations and by information obtained during interviews of the caregivers. The remaining three children in the pilot had no qualitative evidence of focal abnormalities, had microcephaly, and had developmental quotients within the retarded to very low normal range.

These preliminary data are of interest in light of findings reported by Zametkin et al. (1990), who found evidence of reductions in cerebral glucose metabolism in the frontal lobe among a cohort of adults with childhood histories of attention-deficit/hyperactivity disorder and no prenatal alcohol and/or other drug exposure. The etiological basis for the neurofunctional findings obtained in the pilot study remains unknown, and we do not know whether childhood findings of neurofunctional (hypometabolism of the right frontal lobe) and behavioral (problems in sustaining attention) effects will persist into adolescence and adulthood. It may be that environmental factors will mitigate the attention problems, compensatory systems within the CNS will improve the hypometabolism, and/or a combination of factors will influence outcomes in ways we have yet to determine.

In 1996, studies in which investigators have examined the interactions between environmental factors and neuroimaging findings had yet to be undertaken. As a result, we do not know the effects of environmental input on functions and structures identified through neuroimaging techniques. We do know, however, that a positive postnatal environment is associated with better cognitive outcomes overall.

CONCLUSIONS

As the 20th century draws to a close, we continue to investigate reliable measures for predicting long-term neurological, cognitive, and school-related outcomes for infants and young children who are at risk. Methods used since the 1960s have included assessment of pre- and postnatal events, evaluation of home environments, neurobehavioral and neurodevelopmental testing, and electrophysiological and neuroimaging measures. Results obtained through many of these techniques have been evaluated as predictors of outcomes as children who are at risk progress beyond infancy. It appears that developmental outcome for groups of children, much less individual children, cannot be predicted through the use of a single tool. Rather, to increase predictability, a combination of measures must be used.

When it is used in conjunction with clinical data, neuroimaging is a valuable tool for identifying infants who display neuroanatomical characteristics that place them at risk for adverse neuromotor outcomes, such as cerebral palsy. It has proved less useful, however, in attempts to predict cognitive outcomes. Provided that a child has not experienced a major CNS insult, the environment appears to be a major factor in predicting later cognitive functioning; significant environmental influences include not only the early caregiving environment, but also the medical care, educational services, and community social supports that guide the child as she or he learns and grows. In the future, neuroimaging findings may help us to predict outcomes even more accurately.

FUTURE DIRECTIONS

Functional neuroimaging represents an exciting field for future research. When this book went to press in 1996, no investigative studies had been undertaken to evaluate the effects of environmental influences on the central nervous system functioning as viewed through neuroimaging techniques. From a behavioral standpoint, however, the environment often has been shown to have a significant effect on cognitive and emotional outcomes in children. In the future, therefore, functional neuroimaging, such as PET and functional MRI, may serve as a useful adjunct to other forms of developmental evaluation in predicting outcomes for children. Two areas, in particular, seem appropriate for research in this field. Future investigations, for example, could compare, over the long term, neurobehaviors and changes in functional neuroimages of children who experienced early trauma (e.g., birth asphyxia, postnatal bleeds, shaken baby syndrome). In addition, in light of research that indicates that many young children who are diagnosed with mild mental retardation have been raised in environments that lack appropriate care and stimulation (Ramey, MacPhee, & Yeates, 1982), future studies could examine children who are at risk and who have not experienced CNS trauma to determine the influences of enriched versus deprived environments on child development and neuroimaging findings. Such studies could evaluate how environmental influences alter imaging findings and determine whether these findings are translated into developmental outcomes in behavior and cognition.

REFERENCES

Ainsworth, M.D.S. (1976). *System of rating maternal-care behavior.* Princeton, NJ: Educational Testing Service.

Ainsworth, M.D.S. (1979). Infant–mother attachment. *American Psychologist, 34*(10), 932–937.

Ainsworth, M.D.S., Blehar, M.C., Waters, E., & Wall, S. (1978). *Patterns of attachment: A psychological study of the strange situation.* Hillsdale, NJ: Lawrence Erlbaum Associates.

Aylward, G.P. (1992). The relationship between environmental risk and developmental outcome. *Developmental and Behavioral Pediatrics, 13*(3), 222–229.

Azuma, S.D., & Chasnoff, I.J. (1993). Outcome of children prenatally exposed to cocaine and other drugs: A path analysis of three-year data. *Pediatrics, 92*(3), 396–402.

Barnes, P.D. (1992). Imaging of the central nervous system in pediatrics and adolescence. *Pediatric Clinics of North America, 39*(4), 743–776.

Beckwith, L. (1989). Preventive interventions with parents of premature infants. In S.E. Goldston, C.M. Heinicke, R.S. Pynoos, & J. Yager (Eds.), *Preventing mental health disturbances in childhood* (pp. 41–54). Washington, DC: American Psychiatric Press.

Beckwith, L., & Parmelee, A.H. (1986). EEG patterns of preterm infants, home environment, and later IQ. *Child Development, 57*, 777–789.

Beckwith, L., Rodning, C., Norris, D., Phillipsen, L., Khandabi, P., & Howard, J. (1994). Spontaneous play in two-year-olds born to substance-abusing mothers [Special issue]. *Infant Mental Health Journal, 15*(2), 189–201.

Bennett, F.C., & Guralnick, M.J. (1991). Effectiveness of developmental intervention in the first five years of life. *Pediatric Clinics of North America, 38*(6), 1513–1528.

Billman, D., Nemeth, P., Heimler, R., & Sasidharan, P. (1991). Prenatal cocaine exposure (PCE): Advanced Bayley psychomotor scores [Abstract]. *Pediatric Research, 29*, 251A.

Bingol, N., Fuchs, M., Diaz, V., Stone, R.K., & Gromisch, D.S. (1987). Teratogenicity of cocaine in humans. *Journal of Pediatrics, 110*(1), 93–96.

Bodensteiner, J., Schaefer, G.B., Breeding, L., & Cowan, L. (1994). Hypoplasia of the corpus callosum: A study of 445 consecutive MRI scans. *Journal of Child Neurology, 9*(1), 47–49.

Bowlby, J. (1969). *Attachment and loss: Attachment* (Vol. 1). New York: Basic Books.

Boyle, C.A., Decoufle, P., & Yeargin-Allsopp, M. (1994). Prevalence and health impact of developmental disabilities in U.S. children. *Pediatrics, 93*(3), 399–403.

Brazelton, T.B. (1973). *Neonatal Behavior Assessment Scale.* Philadelphia: J.B. Lippincott.

Brooks-Gunn, J., McCarton, C., & Hawley, T. (1994). Effects of in utero drug exposure on children's development: Review and recommendations. *Archives of Pediatric and Adolescent Medicine, 148*, 33–39.

Caldwell, B., & Bradley, R. (1984). *Home Observation for Measurement of the Environment.* Little Rock: University of Arkansas.

Chasnoff, I.J. (1988). *A first: National hospital incidence study.* Chicago: National Association for Perinatal Addiction Research.

Chasnoff, I.J., Griffith, D.R., Freier, C., & Murray, J. (1992). Cocaine/polydrug use in pregnancy: Two-year follow-up. *Pediatrics, 89*(2), 284–289.

Chasnoff, I.J., Griffith, D.R., MacGregor, S., Dirkes, K., & Burns, K.A. (1989). Temporal patterns of cocaine use in pregnancy: Perinatal outcome. *Journal of the American Medical Association, 261*(12), 1741–1744.

Chugani, H.T. (1994). Development of regional brain glucose metabolism in relation to behavior and plasticity. In G. Dawson & K.W. Fischer (Eds.), *Human behavior and the developing brain* (pp. 153–175). New York: Guilford Press.

Chugani, H.T., & Phelps, M.E. (1991). Imaging human brain development with positron emission tomography. *Journal of Nuclear Medicine, 32*(1), 23–25.

Chugani, H.T., Phelps, M.E., & Mazziotta, J.C. (1987). Positron emission tomography of human brain development. *Annals of Neurology, 22*(4), 487–496.

Cicchetti, D. (1987). Developmental psychopathology in infancy: Illustration from the study of maltreated youngsters. *Journal of Consulting and Clinical Psychology, 55*, 837–845.

Cicchetti, D. (1990). The organization and coherence of socioemotional, cognitive, and representational development: Illustrations through a developmental psychopathology perspective on Down syndrome and child maltreatment. In R. Thompson (Ed.), *Nebraska Symposium on Motivation* (Vol. 36, pp. 275–382). Lincoln: University of Nebraska Press.

Cohen, S., Parmelee, A., Sigman, M., & Beckwith, L. (1982). Neonatal risk factors in preterm infants. *Applied Research in Mental Retardation, 3*, 265–278.

Cohen, S.E., & Parmelee, A.H. (1983). Prediction of five-year Stanford-Binet scores in preterm infants. *Child Development, 54*, 1242–1253.

Cohen, S.E., Parmelee A.H., Beckwith, L., & Sigman, M. (1992). Biological and social precursors of 12-year competence in children born preterm. In C.W. Greenbaum & J.G. Auerbach (Eds.), *Longitudinal studies of children at psychological risk: Cross-national perspectives* (pp. 65–78). Norwood, NJ: Ablex Publishing Corp.

Coles, C., Platzman, K., Smith, I., James, M., & Falek, A. (1991). Effects of cocaine, alcohol, and other drugs used in pregnancy on neonatal growth and neurobehavioral status. *Neurotoxicology and Teratology, 13*(4), 1–11.

Day, N.L., & Richardson, G.A. (1991). Prenatal alcohol exposure: A continuum of effects. *Seminar in Perinatology, 14*(4), 271–279.

Dietrich, R.B., & Bradley, W.G., Jr. (1988). Normal and abnormal white matter maturation. *Seminars in Ultrasound, CT, and MRI, 9*(3), 192–200.

Dixon, S.D., & Bejar, R. (1989). Echoencephalographic findings in neonates associated with maternal cocaine and methamphetamine use: Incidence and clinical correlates. *Journal of Pediatrics, 115*(5), 770–778.

Doberczak, T.M., Shanzer, S., Senie, R.T., & Kandall, S.R. (1988). Neonatal neurologic and electroencephalographic effects of intrauterine cocaine exposure. *Journal of Pediatrics, 113*(2), 354–358.

Dorman, C. (1991). Microencephaly and intelligence. *Developmental Medicine and Child Neurology, 33*, 267–272.

Dreyfus-Brisac, C. (1962). The electroencephalogram of the premature infant. *World Neurology, 3*, 5–12.

Duffy, F.H. (1994). The role of quantified electroencephalography in psychological research. In G. Dawson & K.W. Fischer (Eds.), *Human behavior and the developing brain* (pp. 93–133). New York: Guilford Press.

Duffy, F.H., & Als, H. (1988). Neural plasticity and the effect of a supportive hospital environment on premature newborns. In J.F. Kavanagh (Ed.), *Understanding mental retardation: Research accomplishments and new frontiers* (pp. 179–206). Baltimore: Paul H. Brookes Publishing Co.

Egeland, B., & Sroufe, L. (1981). Attachment and early maltreatment. *Child Development, 52*, 45–52.

Fenson, L., Kagan, J., Kearsley, R.B., & Zelazo, P.R. (1976). The developmental progression of manipulative play in the first two years. *Child Development, 47*, 232–236.

Finnegan, L.P. (1981). Maternal and neonatal effects of drug dependence in pregnancy. In J.H. Lowinson & P. Ruiz (Eds.), *Substance abuse: Clinical problems and perspectives* (pp. 545–581). Baltimore: Williams & Wilkins.

Finnegan, L.P., Kron, R.E., Connaughton, J.F., Jr., & Emich, J.P. (1975). Neonatal abstinence syndrome: Assessment and management. *Addictive Diseases: An International Journal, 2*(1), 141–158.

First, L.R., & Palfrey, J.S. (1994). The infant or young child with developmental delay. *New England Journal of Medicine, 330*(7), 478–483.

Fitzhardinge, P.M., Flodmark, O., Fitz, C.R., & Ashby, S. (1981). The prognostic value of computed tomography as an adjunct to assessment of the term infant with postasphyxial encephalopathy. *Journal of Pediatrics, 99*(5), 777–781.

Gelfand, M.J. (1989). Advances in nuclear imaging. *Annals of Emergency Medicine, 18*(2), 1310–1314.

Hack, M., Taylor, H., Klein, N., Eiben, R., Schatschneider, C., & Mercuri-Minich, N. (1994). School-age outcomes in children with birth weights under 750 g. *New England Journal of Medicine, 331*(12), 753–759.

Hadeed, A.J., & Siegel, S.R. (1989). Maternal cocaine use during pregnancy: Effect on the newborn infant. *Pediatrics, 84*, 205–210.

Handler, A., Kistin, N., Davis, F., & Ferré, C. (1991). Cocaine use during pregnancy: Perinatal outcomes. *American Journal of Epidemiology, 133*(8), 818–825.

Heier, L.A., Carpanzano, C.R., Mast, J., Brill, P.W., Winchester, P., & Deck, M.D.F. (1991). Maternal cocaine abuse: The spectrum of radiologic abnormalities in the neonatal CNS. *American Journal of Neuroradiology, 12*, 951–956.

Holland, B.A., Hass, D.K., Norman, D., Brant-Zawadzki, M., & Newton, T.H. (1986). MRI of normal brain maturation. *American Journal of Neuroradiology, 7*, 201–208.

Hollingshead, A.B. (1975). *Four factor index of social status.* Unpublished manuscript, Yale University, New Haven, CT.

Holzman, C., Paneth, N., Little, R., Pinto-Martin, J., & the Neonatal Brain Hemorrhage Study Team. (1995). Perinatal brain injury in premature infants born to mothers using alcohol in pregnancy. *Pediatrics, 95*(1), 66–73.

Howard, J. (1994). Barriers to successful intervention. In D. Besharov (Ed.), *When drug addicts have children: Reorienting child welfare's response* (pp. 91–100). Washington, DC: Child Welfare League of America/American-Enterprise Institute.

Howard, J., Beckwith, L., Espinosa, M., & Tyler, R. (1995). Development of infants born to cocaine-abusing women: Biologic/maternal influences. *Neurotoxicology and Teratology, 17*(4), 403–411.

Jones, K.L., & Smith, D.W. (1973). Recognition of the fetal alcohol syndrome in early infancy. *Lancet, 1*, 999–1001.

Jones, K.L., Smith, D.W., Ulleland, C.N., & Streissguth, A.P. (1973). Pattern of malformation in offspring of chronic alcoholic mothers. *Lancet, 1*, 1267–1271.

Karmiloff-Smith, A. (1991). Beyond modularity: Innate constraints and developmental change. In S. Carey & R. Gelman (Eds.), *The epigenesis of mind: Essays on biology and cognition* (pp. 173–197). Hillsdale, NJ: Lawrence Erlbaum Associates.

Kerrigan, J.F., Chugani, H.T., & Phelps, M.E. (1990). Regional cerebral glucose metabolism in clinical subtypes of cerebral palsy. *Pediatric Neurology, 7*(6), 415–425.

Largo, R.H., & Howard, J.H. (1979). Developmental progression in play behavior of children between nine and thirty months. I. Spontaneous play and imitation. *Developmental Medicine and Child Neurology, 21*, 299–310.

Lee, B.C.P., Lipper, E., Nass, R., Ehrlich, M.E., de Ciccio-Bloom, E., & Auld, P.A.M. (1986). MRI of the central nervous system in neonates and young children. *American Journal of Neuroradiology, 7*, 605–616.

Lewis, M., & Fox, N.A. (1986). Infant assessment: Challenges for the future. In M. Lewis (Ed.), *Learning disabilities and prenatal risk* (pp. 307–331). Chicago: University of Illinois Press.

Lifschitz, M.H., Wilson, G.S., O'Brian Smith, E., & Desmond, M.M. (1985). Factors affecting head growth and intellectual function in children of drug addicts. *Pediatrics, 75*(2), 269–274.

Matas, L., Arend, R.A., & Sroufe, L.A. (1978). Continuity of adaptation in the second year: The relationship between quality of attachment and later competence. *Child Development, 49*, 547–556.

Mitchell, M., Sabbagha, R.E., Keith, L., MacGregor, S., Mota, J.M., & Minoque, J. (1988). Ultrasonic growth parameters in fetuses of mothers with primary addiction to cocaine. *American Journal of Obstetrics and Gynecology, 159*(5), 1104–1109.

Molfese, D.L. (1989). The use of auditory evoked responses recorded from newborn infants to predict later language skills. *Birth Defects, 25*(6), 47–62.

Molfese, D.L., & Molfese, V.J. (1994). Short-term and long-term developmental outcomes: The use of behavioral and electrophysiological measures in early infancy as predictors. In G. Dawson & K.W. Fischer (Eds.), *Human behavior and the developing brain* (pp. 493–517). New York: Guilford Press.

Molfese, V.J., & Holcomb, L.C. (1989). Predicting learning and other developmental disabilities: Assessment of reproductive and caretaking variables. *Birth Defects, 25*(6), 1–23.

Motti, F., Cicchetti, D., & Sroufe, L.A. (1983). From infant affect expression to symbolic play: The coherence of development in Down syndrome children. *Child Development, 54*(5), 1168–1175.

Mundy, P., Sigman, M., Kasari, C., & Yirmiya, N. (1988). Nonverbal communication skills in Down syndrome children. *Child Development, 59*, 235–249.

Mundy, P., Sigman, M., Ungerer, J., & Sherman, T. (1987). Nonverbal communication and play correlates of language development in autistic children. *Journal of Autism and Developmental Disorders, 17*(3), 349–364.

Noce, J.P. (1990). Fundamentals of diagnostic ultrasonography. *Biomedical Instrumentation & Technology, 24*, 456–459.

Parmelee, A.H., & Michaelis, M.D. (1971). Neurological examination of the newborn. In J. Hellmuth (Ed.), *Exceptional infant* (Vol. 2, pp. 3–23). New York: Brunner/Mazel.

Parmelee, A.H., Sigman, M., Garbanati, J., Cohen, S., Beckwith, L., & Asarnow, R. (1994). Neonatal electroencephalographic organization and attention in early adolescence. In G. Dawson & K.W. Fischer (Eds.), *Human behavior and the developing brain* (pp. 537–554). New York: Guilford Press.

Prechtl, H. (1977). *The neurological examination of the full-term newborn infant: Clinics in developmental medicine* (Vol. 63, 2nd ed.). Philadelphia: J.B. Lippincott.

Prechtl, H.F.R. (1990). Qualitative changes of spontaneous movements in fetus and preterm infant are a marker of neurological dysfunction [Editorial]. *Early Human Development, 23*, 151–158.

Prechtl, H.F.R. (1992). The organization of behavioral states and their dysfunction. *Seminars in Perinatology, 16*(4), 258–263.

Ramey, C.T., MacPhee, D., & Yeates, K.O. (1982). Preventing developmental retardation: A general systems model. In L. Bond & J. Joffe (Eds.), *Facilitating infant and early childhood development*. Hanover, NH: University Press of New England.

Rodning, C., Beckwith, L., & Howard, J. (1989). Characteristics of attachment organization and play organization in prenatally drug-exposed toddlers. *Development and Psychopathology, 1*, 277–289.

Roth, S., Baudin, J., McCormick, D., Edwards, A., Townsend, J., Stewart, A., & Reynolds, E. (1993). Relation between ultrasound appearance of the brain of very preterm infants and neurodevelopmental impairment at eight years. *Developmental Medicine and Child Neurology, 35*, 755–768.

Sameroff, A.J., & Chandler, M.J. (1975). Reproductive risk and the continuum of caretaking casualty. In F.D. Jorowitz, M. Hetherington, S. Scarr-Salapatek, & G. Siegel (Eds.), *Review of child development research* (Vol. 4, pp. 187–244). Chicago: University of Chicago.

Sigman, M. (1982). Plasticity in development: Implications for intervention. In L.A. Bond & J.M. Joffee (Eds.), *Facilitating infant and early childhood development* (pp. 98–120). Hanover, NH: University Press of New England.

Sigman, M., Beckwith, L., Cohen, S.E., & Parmelee, A.H. (1989). Stability in the biosocial development of the child born preterm. In M.H. Bornstein & N.A. Krasnegor (Eds.), *Stability and continuity in mental development: Behavioral and biological perspectives* (pp. 29–42). Hillsdale, NJ: Lawrence Erlbaum Associates.

Sigman, M., Cohen, S.E., Beckwith, L., Asarnow, R., & Parmelee, A.H. (1992). The prediction of cognitive abilities at 8 and 12 years of age from neonatal assessments of preterm infants. In S.L. Friedman & M. Sigman (Eds.), *The psychological development of low birthweight children* (pp. 299–314). Norwood, NJ: Ablex Publishing Corp.

Smith, D.W. (1979). The fetal alcohol syndrome. *Hospital Practice, 14*, 121–128.

Stone, W.L., Lemanek, K.L., Fishel, P.T., Fernandez, M.C., & Altemeier, W.A. (1990). Play and imitation skills in the diagnosis of autism in young children. *Pediatrics, 86*(2), 267–272.

Synnes, A.R., Ling, E.W.Y., Whitfield, M.F., Mackinnon, M., Lopes, L., Wong, G., & Effer, S.B. (1994). Perinatal outcomes of a large cohort of extremely low gestational age infants (twenty-three to twenty-eight completed weeks gestation). *Journal of Pediatrics, 125*(6, Part 1), 952–960.

Tronick, E., & Weinberg, K. (1990). *Mother-infant interactive paradigms for evaluating the socioemotional development of infants.* Paper presented at the National Institute on Drug Abuse, Washington, DC.

Tyler, R., Chugani, H., & Howard, J. (1993). A pilot study of cerebral glucose utilization in children with prenatal drug exposure. *Annals of Neurology, 34*(3), 460.

Ungerer, J., & Sigman, M. (1983). Developmental lags in preterm infants from one to three years of age. *Child Development, 54*, 1217–1228.

Van de Bor, M., Ens-Dokkum, M., Schreuder, A.M., Veen, S., Brand, R., & Verloove-Vanhorick, S.P. (1993). Outcome of periventricular-intraventricular hemorrhage at five years of age. *Developmental Medicine and Child Neurology, 35*, 33–41.

Vargas, G.C., Pildes, R.S., Vidyasagar, D., & Keith, L.G. (1975). Effect of maternal heroin addiction on 67 liveborn neonates. *Clinical Pediatrics, 14*(8), 751–757.

Vega, W.A., Kolody, B., Hwang, J., & Noble, A. (1993). Prevalence and magnitude of perinatal substance exposures in California. *New England Journal of Medicine, 329*(12), 850–854.

Weisglas-Kuperus, N., Baerts, W., Fetter, W., & Sauer, P. (1992). Neonatal cerebral ultrasound, neonatal neurology and perinatal conditions as predictors of neurodevelopmental outcome in very low birthweight infants. *Early Human Development, 31*, 131–148.

Wilson, G.S., McCreary, R., Kean, J., & Baxter, J.C. (1979). The development of preschool children of heroin-addicted mothers: A controlled study. *Pediatrics, 63*(1), 135–141.

Young, N.K., Wallace, V.R., & Garcia, T., (1992). Developmental status of three to five year-old children who were prenatally exposed to alcohol and other drugs. *School Social Work Journal, 16*, 1–15.

Zametkin, A.J., Nordahl, T.E., Gross, M., King, C., Simple, W.E., Rumsey, J., Hamburger, S., & Cohen, R.M. (1990). Cerebral glucose metabolism in adults with hyperactivity of childhood onset. *New England Journal of Medicine, 323*(20), 1361–1366.

Zuckerman, B., Frank, D.A., Hingson, R., Amaro, H., Levenson, S.M., Kayne, H., Parker, S., Vinci, R., Aboagye, K., Fried, L.E., Cabral, H., Timperi, R., & Bauchner, H. (1989). Effects of maternal marijuana and cocaine use on fetal growth. *New England Journal of Medicine, 320*(12), 762–768.

III

Future Directions and Clinical Applications in the Use
— of Neuroimaging with Children —

This book reflects an effort to present cutting-edge information about advances in the use of neuroimaging procedures to better understand a range of childhood disorders. In this context, it is important to note that the quality and robustness of data derived from neuroimaging studies of children diagnosed with a particular developmental disorder depend, in large part, on a number of conceptual and methodological factors. These factors include the care with which the samples under study are defined and classified, the quality of the tests and procedures that are used in the diagnosis of children, the reliability and validity of the activation tasks that are used in those neuroimaging studies that assess brain function or processing, and the level of detail provided about the specific neuroimaging procedures used. In this section, Drs. G. Reid Lyon and Judith M. Rumsey summarize a series of conceptual and methodological issues that should be considered before conducting neuroimaging studies with children and when interpreting neuroimaging data obtained from studies of particular clinical groups.

11

Neuroimaging and Developmental Disorders
Comments and Future Directions
———— G. Reid Lyon and Judith M. Rumsey ————

The chapters in this volume, in addition to addressing specific topics in neuroimaging, appear to speak with one voice about the complexity of the brain and the role of neuroscience in unraveling the brain's mysteries. Likewise, each chapter demonstrates how neuroscience, in general, and neuroimaging, in particular, can contribute to the field's understanding of the developing brain and of the factors that can interfere with its healthy development. Each chapter presents evidence that researchers have learned a great deal about the developing brain and its workings since the mid-1980s and that a significant contributor to this emerging knowledge has been the field of neuroimaging.

Many of this book's contributors have expressed the prescient observation that along with the explosion of technology that now allows the imaging of both the structures and functions of the brain comes the realization that neuroimaging remains immature in its applications. As noted throughout this volume, many neuroimaging modalities now exist. These modalities range from those that provide detailed anatomical information (e.g., magnetic resonance imaging [MRI]) to those that provide information about, and images of, the functions of the brain. With respect to the latter modalities, three-dimensional functional imaging of task-related changes in blood flow and metabolism can be obtained with positron emission tomography (PET). Improved resolution has become available with functional magnetic resonance imaging (fMRI), which can potentially provide a radiation-free window to the functioning of the child's brain.

Although PET and fMRI will likely predominate functional neuroimaging in the immediate future, additional techniques that may offer more direct measures of neuronal activity and further improvements in resolution are emerging. The temporal resolution of both PET (when used to measure regional cerebral blood flow) and fMRI is limited by regional hemodynamic response times, typically on the order of seconds. Furthermore, when fMRI is used, venous drainage of activated regions may give rise to apparent activation at locations distant from the site of neural activity. Another technique, magnetoencephalography (MEG), records magnetic signals proportional to electroencephalographic waves emanating from brain electrical activity. As discussed by George et al. (1995), this technique may be used to better resolve both the time course of neuronal activity contributing to regions of activation and the source of activations that depend on slower hemodynamic changes. The convergence of evidence from both fMRI and MEG may increase confidence in observations obtained with either method alone. When used in conjunction with other imaging modalities, MEG may provide a means to define the sequence of neuronal events contributing to an fMRI or a PET image.

Each imaging technique, therefore, has unique advantages and limitations, and it is expected that questions in adult and developmental neuroscience will be addressed by convergent applications of multiple neuroimaging modalities. Research to identify which brain-mapping modality is most effectively suited to which investigative purpose continues. Given the intensity of this research, it is expected that technical developments in neuroimaging will continue to occur at rapid rates. In view of this speed, it will be important to apply refined and/or new neuroimaging techniques within a research and clinical context informed by theoretical, conceptual, and methodological rigor. In short, no matter how elegant, advanced, and exciting a particular technological neuroimaging advance may be, its usefulness in understanding brain–behavior relationships depends on its theoretical and conceptual context, for it is this background that provides the foundation for the scientific questions that are posed. Continued collaboration among scientists across disciplines is critical to provide this context. As Fox (1993) has stressed

> Experiments need to be built on theoretical frameworks already established by neuropsychology and cognitive psychology. Data analysis strategies need to be informed by our colleagues in mathematics, statistics, physics, and computer science. Computational modeling needs to advance from the level of the local network to that of the neural system and must be applied to the growing body of knowledge. Databases relating experimental conditions, observed activations, and proposed models need to be created and effectively shared. The field will mature only if laboratories privileged to have instruments capable of mapping the human brain perceive the need for human brain mapping to be a convergence of disciplines, rather than a discipline in isolation. (p. 2)

This chapter discusses a number of conceptual and methodological issues of importance to neuroimaging studies with children. The application of neuroimaging techniques to the study of the developing brain in children poses unique challenges in addition to any technical adjustments that may be required to help the child adapt to the neuroimaging environment (i.e., ensuring a child's comfort, cooperation, and ability to remain motionless for required lengths of time). These challenges include 1) the definition of patient samples, 2) the understanding of normal and abnormal structural brain development, and 3) the ability to achieve a good fit between theoretical constructs and task-related activations in functional studies.

DEFINING CLINICAL GROUPS AND UNDERSTANDING VARIABILITY

The chapters in this book reflect efforts to better understand the effects of medical conditions on the developing brain and the neurobiological substrates of developmental disorders. A comprehensive grasp of these issues requires both an understanding of common group characteristics and an understanding of the variability within a given group. This requirement applies equally to disorders with known etiologies, such as pediatric acquired immunodeficiency syndrome (AIDS) and genetic disorders, and to developmental disorders of unknown etiologies, such as reading disorders and autism. The ability to image individual differences in both the structure and the function of the brain can be used to elucidate differences in how children and adults with such disorders behave, learn, and progress.

It is important to note that, in each chapter, the value of the findings derived from neuroimaging depends on the methodological precision with which the classification, definition, identification, and measurement of children or adults studied have been conducted. Otherwise-compelling findings about a disorder are sometimes downgraded to interesting or spurious findings, because the results cannot be replicated or generalized. This devaluation of findings frequently occurs as a result of heterogeneity within a diagnostic group. Brain and behavioral impairments, even in disorders with known biological etiologies, may vary considerably, both quantitatively (i.e., in severity) and qualitatively (i.e., the brain and/or behavior may be differentially affected across individuals). This heterogeneity presents an even greater problem for developmental disorders with unknown or poorly understood etiologies than for those with identified etiologies.

One source of such variability is the high comorbidity, or clinical overlap, seen in many childhood disorders. A prime example is the frequent co-occurrence of attention deficit disorders in children with dyslexia. Research suggests that attention deficit disorders and dyslexia are associated with different cognitive and behavioral deficits (Wood & Felton, 1994), thereby supporting their status as independent disorders and stimulating the search for separate brain-based correlates, genetic markers, and treatments (see Chapter 5). Failure to distinguish among children with and without comorbid disorders increases heterogeneity and impedes the search for brain-based correlates. The longitudinal classification study of dyslexia discussed in Chapter 4 provides an example of how the explicit investigation of comorbidity adds conceptual and interpretive strength to the study of a heterogeneous disorder such as dyslexia.

Conversely, different disorders sometimes share cognitive and neurobehavioral features and respond to similar behavioral interventions and/or therapeutic medications, which suggests some commonality in their underlying neurobiology. For instance, children with limited general intelligence (reflected in low IQ scores) and specific reading disability display similar phonological deficits (Stanovich & Siegel, 1994); and children diagnosed with neurofibromatosis-1, Turner syndrome, and attention-deficit/hyperactivity disorder (ADHD) may all display deficits in "executive function" (see Chapters 5 and 7). The identification of the biological substrates of specific symptoms that span different disorders, therefore, may also enrich neuroscientists' understanding of a range of developmental disorders.

For developmental disorders with unknown etiologies, the search for biological correlates and markers may be facilitated by an improved understanding of underlying cognitive or neuropsychological deficits. The identification of essential, or "core," deficits (e.g., phonological deficits in dyslexia, discussed in Chapters 3 and 4) may provide a bridge for linking diagnostic categories reflecting behavioral syndromes with brain-based abnormalities—be they structural or functional. The identification of associated deficits, which account for the variability within a diagnostic category, will pave the way for correlating specific symptoms or features with variability in brain structure and function. Knowledge of such deficits may provide the basis for defining more homogeneous subgroups within diagnostic categories and thereby facilitate the identification of biological markers. Such knowledge moves the field closer to understanding the individual child and has implications for prognosis and intervention.

Although remarkable progress has been made in the empirically based diagnosis of behavioral disorders, the need remains for the continued refinement of classification systems. The classification of childhood disorders presents a more formidable challenge than does the classification of adult disorders. The clinical picture in childhood disorders frequently changes with development and is affected by both biological and environmental influences. Some symptoms may improve with intervention and compensation; and other, new symptoms may emerge as brain systems subserving other cognitive functions mature or environmental demands increase. Improved classification can facilitate the identification of brain-based abnormalities. In turn, neuroimaging findings may suggest revisions of existing clinical classifications.

ANATOMICAL NEUROIMAGING

The Need for Normal Developmental Data

The need remains for a truly normative database and a better understanding of normal development of brain structure. Patient groups should be compared with truly normal control groups; that is, children recruited from the community, evaluated, and determined to be healthy and free of neurodevelopmental and behavioral problems before scanning. This is important because medical or patient control subjects with scans that are clinically read as normal may nonetheless show subtle deviations in brain structure or function when more sensitive quantitative techniques are applied.

Knowledge of normal development will help clarify the need for strict versus relaxed controls for age in studies of developmental disorders. Such knowledge would be especially helpful for determining whether some disorders are associated with lags versus deviations in development. For rare disorders and small-sample studies, an understanding of normal development would be helpful in identifying which ages and/or genders of subjects can reasonably be included in a single group. For example, in neuroimaging studies of autistic children, researchers may have greater confidence in small-sample studies of patients who vary widely in age if age-related effects are known to be minimal. For studies of sexually dimorphic brain structures or those that show steep or prolonged developmental curves, small-sample studies must be more restrictive in patient age and gender. Knowledge of normal variability of brain structures across ages and genders permits investigators to determine the numbers of subjects needed to demonstrate differences of varying magnitudes among groups.

Image Analysis

The exquisite spatial resolution and flexibility of MRI (with respect to imaging planes and pulsing sequences [see Chapter 2]) are exploited by data analytic techniques that permit a more precise characterization of brain anatomy in subtle developmental disorders and in disease states in which subtle changes must be tracked over time. Such changes include disease-related processes, such as medial temporal sclerosis in partial complex seizures of temporal lobe origin (see Chapter 8), and therapeutic effects in pediatric AIDS (see Chapter 9). Advances in anatomical MRI data analysis include volumetric measures of the whole brain as well as individual brain structures; improved techniques for differentiating and measuring gray matter and white matter; and three-dimensional renderings that can be used to more accurately measure curved surfaces of interest, such as the planum temporale.

Techniques for differentiating gray and white matter may provide measures that are more sensitive than are volume measures for tracking stages of disease and therapeutic effects, as suggested in Chapter 9. The curved surface of the planum temporale has contributed to inaccurate definitions and measures in disorders such as dyslexia (see Chapters 3 and 4). Thanks to technological advances, measurement of the planum may be approached with three-dimensional surface-rendering algorithms that permit a much closer approximation of its true area (see Chapter 3). Also of great interest are methods of cortical parcellation to subdivide and measure functional brain anatomy as seen on MRI scans; these methods began to be developed in the 1990s (see Rademacher et al., 1992). Figure 11.1 on page *xxxiv* illustrates the application of one such cortical parcellation method to delineate the complex gyral topography of the brain on coronal MRI slices.

Defining Relationships Among Brain Structures

Correlations among deviations in diverse brain structures may help researchers understand the neural networks involved in developmental disorders and ascertain how development has gone awry. Few, if any, studies have defined the relationship of deviations in one structure with those in another. It is hoped that future studies will explore and establish such relationships. For example, deviations in the normal leftward asymmetry of the planum temporale and deviations in posterior portions of the corpus callosum, through which neuronal connections from the planum travel, have been found in some studies of dyslexia (see Chapter 3). As of 1996, however, no studies reported had examined the relationship between these two anomalous features of the dyslexic brain. The determination of meaningful relationships between anomalies should further the creation of theories of abnormal brain development. Anatomical deviations that are not linked might be related to dissociable symptom clusters, which would help explain the clinical heterogeneity seen in many disorders.

Brain–Behavior Correlations

Clarification of brain–behavior relationships also requires the establishment of links between deviations in brain anatomy associated with disorders and the behavioral features of those disorders (see Chapter 1). Behavioral syndromes and disease states are frequently variable in their clinical presentation. Studies that establish links between deviations in brain anatomy and specific features of disorders will further investigators' understanding of the biological bases of complex disorders. In adult schizophrenia, for example, reductions in the size of limbic structures (i.e., hippocampus, amygdala) have been related to positive psychotic symptoms, whereas negative symptoms (e.g., cognitive deficits) have not been correlated with the sizes of these structures (Bogerts et al., 1993). Cognitive deficits may be associated with changes elsewhere in the brain, such as the frontal lobes.

Studies to establish such links require behavioral measures with established construct validity, clarification of the nature of the behavioral deficits associated with various disorders, and state-of-the-art anatomical measures. Patterns of neuropsychological deficits associated with lateralized brain lesions in adults with acquired neuropathology either may fail to lateralize in the same way in children or may require more sensitive anatomical measures for lateralization to be demonstrated (see Chapter 1). An example rests with MRI findings in Turner syndrome, which is thought to be characterized by specific visuospatial deficits with relatively intact verbal skills—a behavior pattern that would suggest right-lateralized pathology in adults. Studies reviewed in Chapter 7 (e.g., Murphy et al., 1993) have reported bilateral, rather than lateralized, reductions of parieto-occipital brain regions. Nonetheless, more refined anatomical measures, such as ratios of gray matter to white matter in these regions, have revealed abnormalities that are lateralized to the right parietal region, consistent with neuropsychological hypotheses based on the adult lesion literature.

Other qualitative MRI findings may also serve as important biological correlates of behavior and development. Cortical anomalies such as those seen in autism (see Chapter 6) and hyperintensities in conditions such as neurofibromatosis-1 (see Chapter 7) may provide new markers for establishing brain–behavior relationships in the developing child. T2-weighted hyperintensities (i.e., unidentified bright objects or signals) associated with neurofibromatosis-1 show some correlation with reductions in IQ (see Chapter 7), findings that were revealed only when patients' IQs were compared with those of their siblings. Correlations between the number of locations of these hyperintensities and sibling-referenced reductions in IQ are seen in children with neurofibromatosis-1 with hyperintensities, whereas children with neurofibromatosis-1 without hyperintensities showed no such reductions in IQ. The fact that the number, rather than the volume, of these hyperintensities has been related to cognitive loss is consistent with a connectionist or network model.

Brain–behavior relationships may continue to be sought for other biological markers, such as genetic markers. Future studies should address the effects of various genetic factors on brain structure and function and discuss how different genetic etiologies diverge or converge in their effects on neuropsychological abilities and behavioral pathology. For example, when varied etiologies result in impaired reading or attention, one might ask whether they do so by affecting common systems in the brain (e.g., through their effects on a final common pathway) or whether they take multiple neural routes to impairing abilities within these domains (Pennington, 1995).

Once appropriate measures and markers have been identified in cross-sectional studies, longitudinal studies might clarify the clinical course of developmental brain disorders. Anatomical correlates of declining abilities (e.g., the suspected decline in IQ in males with fragile X syndrome, which is discussed in Chapter 7) might be associated with a lack of normal change or development in certain structures. Maturational improvements in function observed in disorders such as ADHD (see Chapter 5) might be accompanied by convergence with normal brain development. Therapeutic improvements, such as those observed in pediatric AIDS (see Chapter 9), might be associated with some normalization of affected neural tissue or compensatory development.

FUNCTIONAL NEUROIMAGING

In the functional domain, fMRI is likely to assume a leading role in future studies of relatively healthy children, whereas improved PET techniques may continue to play a role in studies of children with neurological disorders and those of adults with refractory developmental disorders. As noted in Chapter 2, both techniques are capable of yielding information that is interpretable for each individual studied.

Activation Tasks

Functional neuroimaging provides information about the localization of neural activity associated with cognitive or other tasks. It may, therefore, be used to elucidate the brain regions and neural networks involved in various forms of cognitive processing. It may be used in studies of individuals with medical illness or developmental disorders to determine which brain regions are affected and to provide clues about functional brain reorganization and compensation. Tasks shown to elicit activation in certain brain regions or circuits in normal individuals may be used to probe the integrity of those regions and systems in individuals with disordered development.

Such studies may involve asking the child (or adult) to respond to a task that requires perceiving sounds, performing motor movements, reading, decision making, or discriminating among visual stimuli. The interpretation of functional neuroimaging data typically assumes that the task used to elicit a brain response is a valid measure of the construct under study. Tasks may be selected and developed on the basis of 1) a thorough understanding of the behavioral literature relevant to the task; 2) their relevance to the disorder under study; and 3) the existing neuropsychological, neuroanatomical, and neurophysiological literature concerning localization of function. When one is designing tasks for studies of disordered development, one hopes to achieve confluence of these factors.

Tasks taken from the behavioral literature most typically require modification to fit the constraints imposed by the neuroimaging situation. Complex tasks must frequently be broken down into simpler tasks involving elemental operations. In general, the subject completes many items of one type to achieve a steady state of cognitive activity, which is to be captured in the time window permitted by the imaging technique. This repetition provides a sufficient number of trials to achieve reasonable statistical power and a good signal-to-noise ratio. Such requirements may limit both the ability of such tasks to fully capture the phenomena they seek to represent and the ability of researchers to study highly integrative brain functions.

As discussed in Chapter 2, activations seen with functional neuroimaging methods (e.g., PET, fMRI) reflect two scanning conditions: 1) the experimental task of primary theoretical interest and 2) the task or condition that serves as a baseline contrast. The baseline task is, therefore, as much a determinant of activation as is the experimental task. The neurophysiological signature that is associated or time locked to the experimental task may be derived by subtracting from it the pattern of blood flow or signal intensity obtained during a baseline condition. Baseline tasks are, therefore, subject to scrutiny as measures of the constructs they are purported to represent.

Many study designs to date have employed hierarchical subtraction techniques to segregate specific cognitive operations. In such designs, series of tasks that reflect a number of sequential, elemental operations thought to be involved in cognitive processing are devised. Scans obtained during the first task in such a chain are subtracted from those obtained during the second task; scans obtained during the second task are subtracted from those obtained during the third task; and so on, to capture sequential stages of information processing and to identify the localized brain regions associated with each operation. Such designs assume serial models of processing; that is, they assume that researchers can segregate individual components of the brain-based processes they seek to capture and that these component processes occur sequentially, with each stage being completed before information is sent to the next stage or level. Such designs are probably most appropriate for studying sensory and motor functions, but they may be inappropriate for studying more central, elaborative processes, such as levels of language processing (Demonet et al., 1993).

Increasingly, serial models of brain function are being replaced by models that acknowledge reciprocal neural connections and distributed neural networks. In the domain of language, information processing is hypothesized to occur in cell ensembles or networks that are linked and that operate simultaneously and in parallel (Mesulam, 1990). Consistent with this hypothesis, physiological recordings obtained during linguistic tasks have shown that Broca's area and Wernicke's area are activated simultaneously, not consecutively (Fried et al., 1981). Such results are not well captured by hierarchical subtraction designs (Demonet et al., 1993; Sergent et al., 1992). Rather, such results are more consistent with study designs that compare tasks that differ in emphasis or that direct attention to a particular aspect of processing. For example, a syntax task may be contrasted with a semantic task, given that semantic processing cannot be entirely eliminated or segregated during the study of syntax.

The physical constraints imposed by scanners can also lead to task designs that imperfectly reflect the processes they seek to represent. For instance, in fMRI, even subtle movements (e.g., those generated when speaking) create artifacts and degrade the images obtained. Tasks involving silent reading or other mental operations and simple button-press responses are preferable from a technical standpoint. Task formats involving decision making (multiple choice or yes/no formats) and button presses to indicate decisions, therefore, are more compatible with the constraints of the fMRI situation than are activities such as speaking or reading aloud. Such formats may, however, result in the activation of brain regions other than those of primary theoretical interest, thereby decreasing the relevance of the task to the phenomenon of interest.

Lexical decision-making tasks in which subjects view words silently, make decisions about them, and respond by pressing a button have been shown to predominantly activate frontal brain regions rather than posterior language regions, which are activated when subjects read aloud (Price et al., 1994; Chapter 4). Activations associated with reading silently and those associated with reading aloud also differ in their localization (Bookheimer et al., 1995). Technological improvements that enhance the adaptability of fMRI to allow a variety of stimuli (e.g., auditory, visual, tactile) and a variety of behavioral responses (including speech) will, therefore, be beneficial. This flexibility already is available with PET.

There is also a need to better understand task-related factors that are secondary to the hypotheses or purposes of functional imaging studies, such as the rate at which task items are presented and the effects of practice (Price et al., 1994), which may influence brain activations. Variations in these factors across studies may lead to apparently inconsistent results. Models for understanding the direct influences of such variables are needed to determine the specification of such parameters, which frequently are chosen arbitrarily with unknown effects.

The application of functional neuroimaging to clinical populations also requires consideration of task-performance levels. When patients with neuropsychological deficits are studied using tasks hypothesized to assess those deficits, they may be expected to perform worse than the control subjects. Given this difference, interpretation of physiological differences may be problematic. Tasks designed to eliminate performance deficits may sidestep the phenomenon of primary interest. Solutions to this dilemma may include the use of brain–behavior correlations to better link the quality of performance to brain activity. Another solution may be the use of parametric designs, discussed in Chapter 2, to characterize differences in brain activity at varying levels of difficulty or rates of performance.

Although the tasks that have been used with PET and fMRI techniques through 1996 are experimental in nature, it is possible that they eventually will assume a clinically useful role. Currently, Wada testing, in conjunction with language and memory tasks, is used to localize brain regions essential to language and memory functions before surgery for intractable seizures. It is conceivable that, in the future, fMRI and PET scanning may play a role in presurgical evaluations as well as in a variety of diagnostic evaluations. Tasks might, for example, be developed for the early identification of children at greatest risk for reading and attention disorders or for the evaluation of medication effects. Such techniques might also evaluate behavioral and educational interventions with respect to their effects on brain function and organization or reorganization. Studies of this nature with children with reading disability, sponsored by the National Institute of Child Health and Human Development, National Institutes of Health, Bethesda, Maryland, have been undertaken at several research sites.

Neural Networks

Functional imaging techniques should be applied both to identify specific regions involved in well-defined behavioral functions and to understand neural networks and their organizational qualities in children with normal development and in those with childhood disorders, including those without imageable anatomical lesions. This use may be especially important for disorders such as autism, which has resisted researchers' attempts to define a clear neurological basis (see Chapter 6). Network analyses, such as those described by Horwitz et al. (1995), may be used to characterize the interactions among brain regions during specific cognitive tasks and to determine how these interactions change in normal development, developmental disorders, and disease. For example, network approaches have begun to be applied to problems as diverse as mapping functional interactions within normal brains during cognitive challenges and tracking changes in brain organization after surgery for adult brain disorders, such as Parkinson's disease (Grafton et al., 1994).

Figure 11.2 on page *xxxiv* illustrates the application of a network approach to understanding cognitive processes involved in the abilities to match faces (i.e., object discrimination) and to locate dots in a spatial task. As is shown in Figure 11.2, the functional networks that were active for the two tasks differed. When subjects matched faces, occipitotemporal pathways were activated. When subjects performed a dot-location task in which they mentally rotated designs (i.e., a spatial operation), occipitoparietal pathways were activated (McIntosh et al., 1994). These visual tasks activated two different pathways that closely corresponded to the "what" and "where" pathways that have been described in nonhuman primates. The ventral, occipitotemporal pathway (the so-called what pathway) subserves object recognition, and the dorsal, occipitoparietal pathway (the so-called where pathway) subserves spatial operations. The ability to demonstrate these sorts of neural networks in healthy humans may provide a sound basis for testing their integrity in developmental disorders.

The initial applications of functional neuroimaging techniques to an understanding of developmental disorders have begun to produce exciting findings. It is clear that the practical problems associated with working with children in scanners are being solved. More challenging, perhaps, is the need for continued progress in determining how best to capture the neural correlates of the core underlying deficits in developmental disorders.

CONCLUSION

In this chapter, the authors attempt to identify a number of conceptual and methodological issues of importance in designing and interpreting neuroimaging studies. The need to ensure that the children under study are classified and defined in a manner that permits clear communication among scientists and clinicians and that fosters replicability in future studies is emphasized. In studies designed to elucidate structural brain correlates, it is imperative that anatomical imaging use accurate, sensitive measures of brain anatomy. Tasks used in functional neuroimaging studies should possess good construct validity; be specifically relevant to the disorder of interest; and activate, in healthy individuals, the intended brain regions or networks based on a priori hypotheses derived from a sound knowledge of functional neuroanatomy, neurophysiology, and neuropsychology. Much remains to be learned about how best to adapt tasks found in the behavioral literature to the neuroimaging situation and about how secondary variables affect patterns of activation demonstrated with functional imaging. Future adaptations of imaging techniques to permit tasks to more adequately represent the cognitive variables of interest may also help ensure that patterns of activation demonstrated with imaging reflect the sought-after neural correlates. Finally, the authors discuss a number of needs and acknowledge exciting advances in both the anatomical and functional realms. It is hoped that this discussion stimulates continued gains in neuroscientists' knowledge of developmental disorders.

REFERENCES

Bogerts, B., Lieberman, J.A., Ashtari, M., Bilder, R.M., Degreef, G., Lerner, G., Johns, C., & Masiar, S. (1993). Hippocampus-amygdala volumes and psychopathology in chronic schizophrenia. *Biological Psychiatry, 33,* 236–246.

Bookheimer, S.Y., Zeffiro, T.A., Blaxton, T., Gaillard, W., & Theodore, W. (1995). Regional cerebral blood flow during object naming and word reading. *Human Brain Mapping, 3,* 93–106.

Demonet, J.F., Wise, R., & Frackowiak, R.S.J. (1993). Language functions explored in normal subjects by positron emission tomography: A critical review. *Human Brain Mapping, 1,* 39–47.

Fox, P.T. (1993). Editorial. *Human Brain Mapping, 1,* 1–2.

Fried, J., Ojemann, G.A., & Fetz, E.E. (1981). Language related potentials specific to human language cortex. *Science, 212,* 353–356.

George, J.S., Aine, C.J., Mosher, J.C., Schmidt, D.M., Ranken, D.M., Schlitt, H.A., Wood, C.C., Lewine, J.D., Sanders, A., & Belliveau, J.W. (1995). Mapping function in the human brain with magnetoencephalography, anatomical magnetic resonance imaging, and functional magnetic resonance imaging. *Journal of Clinical Neurophysiology, 12,* 406–431.

Grafton, S.T., Sutton, J., Couldwell, W., Lew, M., & Waters, C. (1994). Network analysis of motor system connectivity in Parkinson's disease: Modulation of thalamocortical interactions after pallidotomy. *Human Brain Mapping, 2,* 45–55.

Horwitz, B., McIntosh, A.R., Haxby, J.V., & Grady, C.L. (1995). Network analysis of brain cognitive function using metabolic and blood flow data. *Behavioral Brain Research, 66,* 187–193.

McIntosh, A.R., Grady, C.L., Ungerleider, L.G., Haxby, J.V., Rapoport, S.I., & Horwitz, B. (1994). Network analysis of cortical visual pathways mapped with PET. *Journal of Neuroscience, 14,* 655–666.

Mesulam, M.M. (1990). Large-scale neurocognitive networks and distributed processing for attention, language, and memory. *Annals of Neurology, 28,* 597–613.

Murphy, D., DeCarli, C., Daly, E., Haxby, J., Allen, G., White, B., McIntosh, A., Powell, C., Horwitz, B., Rapoport, S., & Schapiro, M. (1993). X-chromosome effects on female brain: A magnetic resonance imaging study of Turner's syndrome. *Lancet, 342,* 1197–1200.

Pennington, B.F. (1995). Genetics of learning disabilities. *Journal of Child Neurology, 10,* 69–77.

Price, C.J., Wise, R.J.S., Watson, J.D.G., Patterson, K., Howard, D., & Frackowiak, R.S.J. (1994). Brain activity during reading: The effects of exposure duration and task. *Brain, 117,* 1255–1269.

Rademacher, J., Galaburda, A.M., Kennedy, D.N., Filipek, P.A., & Caviness, V.S. (1992). Human cerebral cortex: Localization, parcellation, and morphometry with magnetic resonance imaging. *Journal of Cognitive Neuroscience, 4,* 352–374.

Sergent, J., Zuck, E., Levesque, M., & Macdonald, B. (1992). Positron emission tomography study of letter and object processing: Empirical findings and methodological considerations. *Cerebral Cortex, 2,* 68–80.

Stanovich, K.E., & Siegel, L.S. (1994). Phenotypic performance profile of children with reading disabilities: A regression-based test of the phonological-core variable-difference model. *Journal of Educational Psychology, 86,* 24–53.

Wood, F.B., & Felton, R.H. (1994). Separate linguistic and attentional factors in the development of reading. *Topics in Language Disorders, 4,* 42–57.

Index

Page references followed by *f*, *t*, and *n* indicate figures, tables, and notes, respectively.